O 300062214

The Facts of Life

The Facts of Life

The Creation of Sexual Knowledge in Britain, 1650–1950

Roy Porter

and

Lesley Hall

YALE UNIVERSITY PRESS   NEW HAVEN AND LONDON   1995

Set in Baskerville by Best-set Typesetter Ltd., Hong Kong
Printed and bound in Great Britain by The Bath Press, Avon

Library of Congress Cataloging-in-Publication Data

Porter, Roy
    The facts of life: the creation of sexual knowledge in
Britain, 1650–1950/Roy Porter and Lesley Hall
        p.   cm.
    Includes bibliographical references and index.
    ISBN 0–300–06221–4
    1. Sexology—Great Britain—History.   2. Sex
instruction literature—Great Britain—History.
I. Porter, Roy, 1946–   . II. Title.
HQ18.G7H35   1995
306.7′0941—dc20   94–21091
                                                                      CIP

A catalogue record for this book is available from the
British Library.

I wish either my father or my mother, or indeed both of them, as they were in duty both equally bound to it, had minded what they were about when they begot me.

Laurence Sterne, *Tristram Shandy*, Book I, ch. i

Contents

List of Illustrations

All illustrations © Wellcome Institute Library

Preface and Acknowledgements

This book is scarcely an instance of *ejaculatio praecox*, and the authors are grateful to Robert Baldock of Yale University Press for his patience in tolerating its slow coming. Roy Porter was the principal author of Chapters 1 to 5, and Lesley Hall of Chapters 6 to 11.

We record here our gratitude to the Harry Ransom Humanities Research Center at the University of Texas at Austin for awarding Lesley Hall a research fellowship to visit the Center to consult their rich collections, and to the Wellcome Trust for the additional travel funding that enabled her to take up this fellowship. Others acknowledged are the staff at the British Library Department of Manuscripts, with particular thanks to Dr Anne Summers; David Doughan and all at the Fawcett Library at London Guildhall University; Gervase Hood, former archivist at the Royal College of Obstetricians and Gynaecologists; Kim Collis and other staff of the Sheffield City Archives; Dr James McGrath of the University of Strathclyde Library; Dorothy Sheridan and her colleagues in the Tom Harrisson-Mass Observation Archives at the University of Sussex (Material copyright the Trustees of the Mass Observation Archives at the University of Sussex reproduced by permission of the Curtis Brown Group Ltd, London); the archivists at the Royal Society; the curators of the John Johnson Ephemera Collection in the Bodleian Library; and Margaret Chekri of the Family Planning Association.

Above all the authors thank their colleagues in the Wellcome Institute Library, in particular the Reader Services team for locating books, processing inter-library loans and photocopying, and the rest of the Contemporary Medical Archives Centre staff, with particular gratitude to Isobel Hunter for drawing attention to the unpublished autobiography of V. H. Mottram.

Lesley Hall thanks friends and colleagues who have long supported and encouraged her in this field: Dorothy Porter, Heather Creaton, Greta Jones, Barbara Brookes, Lara Marks, Dick Soloway, Angus

McLaren and Naomi Pfeffer, and also Dr Liz Stanley, with the wish that she had known earlier of her work on the Mass Observation 'Little Kinsey' survey. As always, Ray McNamee deserves the George Henry Lewes Memorial Award for supportive male companionship.

Roy Porter would like to thank Caroline Overy, nonpareil as a research assistant, and Sally Bragg, Kathleen Game, Frieda Houser and Jan Pinkerton for typing revision after revision.

Part I

FROM THE RESTORATION TO VICTORIA

Introduction: Histories of Sex

Dismissing it as 'an hoary old debauchee acknowledged by no-one', the prominent twentieth-century surgeon, D'Arcy Power, concluded that the first popular sex manual in the English language, a work that had appeared as long ago as 1690, 'at its best is a mere catchpenny production written for the prurient-minded and the less said about it the better'.[1] Power would be gratified to find that his counsel has been widely heeded. Scholars have judged study of sexual manuals rather *infra dig.*, and very little indeed has been said about them – and not just the early ones, but their Victorian and early twentieth-century progeny too.

Power's advice obviously has a quaint ring: the 'less said about sex manuals the better' mimics our hackneyed idea of the 'Victorian'[2] conviction that sex itself, indeed the body as a whole, verges on the unmentionable. In the course of the following three hundred pages, by contrast, a great deal will be said about sexual knowledge and sexual advice. This book is the first scholarly survey of the rise of English-language treatises of sexual knowledge and guidance, and it closely scrutinizes teachings about sexual functions and disorders, physical and moral tenets about sexual activity, prescribed and proscribed coital positions, and views about sexual pleasures and proprieties.

Advice books were often prefaced with warnings of the 'Do Not Read On Unless . . .' type. We want all our readers to read on, but we wish, nevertheless, to issue a caution right at the outset, though one of a different kind. We wish to make it clear that there are many topics connected with sex and sexual inquiries which do not fall within the scope of the book as we have conceived it, and about which, consequently, little will be written. Above all, this is not a history of British sex or sexuality, or of sexual activities and attitudes at large. It has virtually nothing to say about many of the subjects integral to what is today understood as sexuality in its full sense: there will be almost no discussion about child sexuality (or today's favourite topic, child sexual abuse), about male and female homosexuality, about the perversions, about cross-dressing and trans-sexualism, about the politics of prostitution and pornography, about erotic paintings, prints and poetry, about the oral tradition and sexual folklore, about the construction and reconstruction of gender difference and shifting stipulations of male and female roles in culture and society.[3] This list of omissions could be dramatically extended. All are significant topics that deserve consideration within the history of sexuality at large. To some degree, they have already been written about by others;[4] to a large degree they remain to be investigated and interpreted. But they are not central to this book. To prevent misunderstandings, it must be emphasized here that our primary aim is not to discuss how often, when, where, with whom and with what enjoyment (if any) Britons actually had sex. It is not even to explore broad cultures of sexuality and the interplay of sexuality with morals, religion, philosophy, aesthetics, gender and politics, its connections with love[5] or personal identity or the social order. This book does not research representations of sex in poetry, plays, novels, essays, paintings, cartoons and jokes.[6] It does not investigate the dialectics between sex, the family, society and the state, or concentrate on the associations between sex, sexuality and the creation and recreation of gender.[7] Neither is its main focus the changing scientific comprehension of sexual biology or the mechanics of conception, fertilization and other aspects of what became embryology, gynaecology and venereology.[8] There are, doubtless, dozens of other aspects of the histories of sex and sexuality whose absence from this book will surprise or disappoint certain readers.

The aim of this book is to survey attempts in Britain,[9] over a three-hundred-year span, to create a literature and a discipline of sexual information and advice: our work is an examination of the codification of sexuality. And through surveying the relevant authors and publications, *The Facts of Life* aims to examine the underlying politics of sexual knowledge: the structures of authority and subjection, permission and prohibition within which sexual knowledges were articulated, and the key debates that raged on such matters. The core of this enterprise lies in writings dedicated to imparting to the public teachings about sex – together with discussion of their authors, contexts and impacts.

Sexual advice works are typically both descriptive and prescriptive. The emergent genre is far from monolithic; from ponderous tomes penned by physicians or authors who saw themselves as scientists, natural and social (including those now termed the founding fathers of sexology), it ranges to writings primarily intended to catch the public eye with a cocktail of the sensational and the titillating or to promote quackish sexual medicines and appliances. This book does not pretend that there is a single, progressive, heroic tale to be told, commencing with initial, erroneous or mealy-mouthed works and leading up to the (putatively) superior sex writings available today, be they *More Joy of Sex*, the latest *Kinsey Report*, or the 1994 survey of *Sexual Behaviour in Britain*.[10] Like everything else, sexual advice literature is to be understood as of its time, not measured against some transcendental scale of merit. We have attempted to avoid judgmentalism and anachronism, while recognizing that it is the responsibility of the historian to act as an interpreter.

Even within this defined field, limitations of knowledge and space have led us to be rather selective. For one thing, we have not undertaken a comprehensive survey of *all* or even most of the writings through which sexual knowledge and advice were being conveyed. At any moment, scores of books and pamphlets were available, offering direct or indirect sexual instruction, from encyclopaedic reference works to erotic prints and magazines, bawdy verse, self-improvement literature, broadsheets and other advertising material – to say nothing of tomes like the Bible. Study of the place of sex instruction within popular culture at large is an important topic. Ephemeral books – like the anonymous *Marriage Promoted. In a Discourse of its Ancient and Modern Practice, Both under Heathen and Christian Common-Wealths* (1690) or the equally anonymous *The Ladies Dispensary, or, Every Woman her own Physician* (1770), or, in a later era, the tastefully bound and gilt-lettered *The Marriage Ring: A Gift-Book for the Newly Married, and Those Contemplating Marriage* (undated, late nineteenth century) by W. Landels, D.D., or the woman doctor, Gladys Cox's *The Woman's Book of Health: A Complete Guide to Physical Wellbeing* (mid-1930s), issued under the auspices of the *Lady's Companion* – have never seriously been examined, but this will have to await another time and place.[11] Rather we have focused on a succession of the most prominent books, writers and institutions from *Aristotle's Master-Piece*, near the close of the seventeenth century, to Marie Stopes, Eustace Chesser and others in the twentieth century. That there are drawbacks in concentrating on big names and a hallowed succession is obvious, but there is also, it should be insisted, much historical value in this approach. For the fact of the matter is that, throughout the period covered by this volume, a handful of texts were quite inordinately influential. Rather as readers went to the Bible for religion, Mrs Beeton for cookery recipes, Old Moore for the full moon or Burke for the peerage, so they read Venette's *Conjugal Love* or Marie Stopes's *Married Love* when they wanted to sort out their sex lives or know if they were pregnant. Such canonical texts created authority and respectability in a field where many effusions were deeply suspect. It was decent, for example, to give young folks a copy of *Aristotle's Master-Piece* as an engagement present, or for respectable wives to own a copy of Marie Stopes. We are not necessarily claiming that the works addressed in the chapters below were, in form and content, uniquely important; but they were, perhaps for fortuitous reasons, highly influential, and for that reason command prime attention.

We have been selective in our choice of texts, individuals and controversies, and also in our focus of attention. We have principally concerned ourselves with what is said about sexual activity, its conduct and regulation. Many of the works discussed range far more widely. Some of the early books, for instance, follow the consequences of coitus through to childbirth and beyond. We have not, however, analysed the obstetrical teachings of such texts.[12] Many books embed discussion of sexual intercourse in wider surveys of the afflictions of males and females, notably venereal diseases – various authors were touting their skills as VD surgeons or had remedial pills and potions to offer.[13] The present book deals with the pathologization of sex – for much sexual advice came in the form of dreadful warnings of the wages of sin – but it touches only marginally upon venereal disease as such. There is much else prominent in the literature covered below – discussion of the humours, of sexual anatomy, of foetal growth, and, above all else, of married relations – that will be under-represented in the following chapters.

This book also says less than ideally we would have wished about the impact of the texts and traditions examined. Great books do not automatically change the world, and historians have grown highly suspicious of mechanical notions of 'influence'. We cannot blithely assume that readers took the advice the manuals gave – that is, went and did what they were told: the 'command' model is inappropriate. Reading is not passive; people read actively and selectively, rejecting unwelcome advice and absorbing mainly what they believe already. Reading may confirm habits rather than change them. In any case, people do not always read the books they buy or are given: possession of a book (for status reasons, as an authority or a totem) may count for more than the reading of it. Or the reading of it may serve quite other purposes and afford other pleasures than its ostensible mission. Cook books, slimming books and gardening manuals are often read, not as aids to cooking, slimming or gardening but as pleasures in their own right, even as substitutes for cooking, slimming or gardening. The relationship between sex advice literature and the uses made of it is not self-evident but requires to be historically reconstructed.[14]

And here the problem is that, until well into the Victorian era and even beyond, we are largely lacking the evidence that would permit us to resolve these questions. We can be fairly confident what readers did with certain sorts of advice and improving literature. We know some at least, having bought arithmetic primers, did sums, because they did them in the margins and on the flyleaves of surviving copies of arithmetic books.[15] And we certainly have desultory scraps of evidence about the uses to which sex manuals were put. The writings of John Cannon, a Taunton apprentice of the early eighteenth century, graphically prove that *Aristotle's Master-Piece* could be used as an aid to mutual masturbation amongst a group of youngsters.[16] Similar slivers of information suggest that possession and circulation of such texts may have been the stimulus for sexual play, for individuals, couples or groups. But the number of people leaving detailed records of their sexual activities is pitiably small, and many of those – characters such as James Boswell – cannot be assumed to have been representative; just the opposite, in fact. We are in almost total ignorance of the personal sexual beliefs and behaviour of all but the tiniest minority in the world we have lost. Certainly, as Peter Gay has emphasized,[17] intimate secrets survive in the archives more than is sometimes assumed: the Victorians did not wholly deem matters sexual unfit for pen and paper. Yet it is safe to predict that we shall forever remain in the dark even about the bedroom athletics or pillow-talk of otherwise well-known public figures, about the Miltons as well as the mute inglorious Miltons.[18] Our evidence remains patchy in the extreme before we are aided by twentieth-century sources like the Stopes collection, and the archives of Mass Observation and recent oral histories afford historians more reliable windows on to the role played by the printed word in shaping sexual attitudes and practices.[19]

This work attempts to sketch a body of writings that have individually been neglected by historians and whose cumulative story has never adequately been told. Traditional histories of sex – for example the encyclopaedic compilations of Iwan Bloch[20] – naturally include some discussion, but there has hitherto been only one attempt to write a history of sex manuals in English, and that work is facetious and in any case perpetuates symptomatic misreadings by commencing only around 1880.[21] Whatever reading we may develop of British sex and sexuality, sexual practice and sexual culture, it must take cognizance of the fact that sex advice certainly did not start about 1880; it was not entirely the brainchild of Freud or the work of Marie Stopes, and it did not stem from a revolt against so-called Victorian prudery, Bowdlerism and Grundyism.

Historical analysis of the body of writings addressed in this book poses profound conceptual and interpretative issues. There has been deep and animated debate of late regarding the constitution of the sexual and its history.[22] It would be otiose to rehearse here all the theoretical positions currently being espoused, designed to demonstrate that sex and sexuality are not timeless, universal biological givens but historical and cultural constructs. But it is worth briefly trying to show how our text engages with such theorizings and has benefited from them.

We entirely accept, following the arguments of Foucault and others, that sex is not a natural datum awaiting discovery by doctors, scientists and others; we equally allow that the truth of sex has not (despite some conspiracy theories) been 'concealed' down the centuries by priests and moral vigilantes until finally 'revealed' by radicals and reformers.[23] Rather, sexuality was produced by the production of knowledge about it.[24] We intend that statement in various senses. In a banal way, sexuality could not exist in the culture without words, images, metaphors and symbols to represent it. Put more strongly, the sexual is such a complex and contested domain, mightily charged with associations and emotions, norms and values, that the terms in which it is posited determine the entity itself.

This further raises questions of knowledge and power: who commands the idiom through which the sexual is defined and prescribed? Is the language of sex the idiom of common speech, the jargon of medicine or of moral philosophy, the prerogative of experts? Is talking sex expressing oneself, regulating others or engaging in shared exchanges? Not least (and here the insights of Roland Barthes are important)[25] the discourse of sex conveys erotic pleasures that may be independent of the pleasures of coitus itself.

The valuable point made by Foucault is that sex must be understood as discursively produced. The equivocal nature of the relations between writing about sex and what might be going on in brains and bedrooms has radical implications for a history of sexual advice. The constitution of sexual knowledge clearly cannot be taken as a flight of steps towards truth or as some sudden epiphany. It may be reasonable to argue that a history of investigations into the solar system tells of a move from ignorance and error to information. But 'sexual knowledge' is not like astronomical inquiry (heavenly bodies are just objects; human bodies are subjects and objects simultaneously). The story of sexual knowledge is far more like the history of dancing. Dancing is an activity regulated by oral and written criteria of performance; there are definite notions of correctness; but its truth (the right steps and so forth) is itself governed by norms of performance that vary with groups, culture and time. Sex is similar. Sex advice books are thus continually creating and reinventing the object they are purporting to discover, depict, and even legislate for.[26]

It is partly on these grounds that Foucault sought to demystify histories of sex that claimed to chart a transition from repressed silence to

liberation and fulfilment in the modern era.[27] Foucault's argument has
a point. The notion of some grand sea-change from a traditional Christian society, in which sex was censored or muzzled, to a modern post-
Freudian world in which it is free and salvational has much mythic
mileage but will not stand historical scrutiny. Foucault was moreover
right to insist that the ages which supposedly repressed or suppressed
sexual discourse were, in reality, talking endlessly about it: as can be
seen from the latter half of this book, sexual writings flourished as never
before in the supposedly buttoned-up Victorian era.[28]

It is less clear, however, that Foucault's wholesale dismissal of the
'repressive hypothesis' is historically justified. To refute the repressive
hypothesis, Foucault seemed to think it sufficient to adduce the mere
fact of the multiplication of sexual discourse and its genres. What he
failed to do in respect of sexual discourse was to pay sufficient attention
to its tone and implications, those whom it included, those it excluded,
those it empowered, those it disqualified. At times Foucault seemed to
be implying that the presence and proliferation of discourse *ipso facto*
refuted the repressive hypothesis. That cannot be so. The following
chapters will concern themselves with the normative universe envisaged
by sex advice manuals, and the questions of who, within those universes,
was regarded as having powers, places and privileges. Far from
expecting to find Whiggish or anti-Whiggish patterns (progress –
deterioration) we believe that we hear a talking-shop of discourses and
an ebb and flow of opinion.

This leads naturally to the question of the contribution made by
feminist theorizings during the last generation to our understanding
of sex as a historical subject. Liberal histories of sex have assumed
that 'repression' was a truth and an evil reality, and that a historical
transition could be traced leading to emancipation. The writing of
histories would aid this process. Such traditional histories implicitly
assumed the male voice, and supposed that sexual emancipation was a
game in which there were only winners and no losers: men like Freud
would pioneer emancipation and women would thereby become eman-
cipated too. Feminists have exposed the male fantasy embedded in such
views.[29] They have shown that within patriarchy, sexuality has always
been posited upon gendered divisions, and that because males have
commanded political, military, economic and cultural power, it has
been men who have specified sexual roles and the sexual division of
labour. This has resulted in all manner of male-constructed fantasies
about the nature of the 'opposite sex' – virgin, vamp, maiden, whore,
the 'frigide', the *femme fragile* and *femme fatale*, and so forth: many
blatantly contradictory, and mostly victim-blaming.[30] Sex, many feminists have contended, has, on the contrary, been more like a zero-sum

game, involving gendered contests. One man's emancipation may be another woman's repression, exploitation or subordination. There is no *a priori* reason to suppose that the outlooks and interests of males and females in sexual relations are or have been identical, or even harmoniously complementary.

Such considerations are obviously crucial when approaching sex advice literature because, before the twentieth century, it was almost wholly written by males, even when anonymous or purporting to be penned by women. It necessarily viewed sex through male eyes. There was the private and subjective male viewpoint: a phallocentric dream of voluptuous pleasure. And there was the public male viewpoint: the hierarchical division of erotic and moral labour between man and woman, posited within the larger male-constructed domains of society and politics (the public and the private, 'separate spheres', and so forth).[31] For these reasons, it is essential to be alert to gender specification in the erotic worlds conjured up by sex advice, because that was a world entirely created by male writers, presupposing female complicity in male-centred visions of normative sexuality. To say this is not, of course, to imply that all sex advice literature flagrantly embodied gross male domination; but it is to point to the operation of arts of persuasion and also to the implicit assumption of the manifest rightness of male heterosexual maleness.[32]

This raises two other major issues. First, the matter of the interpretation of twentieth-century sex advice manuals written by women. It is possible – plausible, even – to see authors like Marie Stopes, Helena Wright and Stella Browne in the present century constituting a real breakthrough. At long last, women became authorities on these matters; women's views of sexual happiness and fulfilment became articulated, as women wrote for women's needs. Women's sexual *wants* at last became central. Certain feminist historians have celebrated this as making headway.[33] Others, notably Sheila Jeffreys in Britain and Andrea Dworkin in the USA, have demurred, viewing much of this genre of writing as 'patriarchal complicity', in other words, a form of collusion or betrayal.[34] In particular, such critics have drawn attention to the assumption in these writings that it is the wife's or woman's responsibility to provide sexual gratification to the male (to be whore as well as wife, mistress as well as mother) – and to the fact that implicitly they blame the female party for broken sex. Within a male culture the voice and purposes of the female advice-author are themselves problematic. It cannot simply be assumed that the female author contributes the woman's voice as a dissenting or autonomous point of view. Such advice – which might be seen as a particularly insidious charter for the male – provides matters for further analysis.[35]

Radical feminists have complained that such advice literature tacitly promotes 'compulsory heterosexuality'. That phrase is, of course, in itself tendentious, but it usefully points to aspects of the advice manuals that require analysis. First, it makes it clear that the 'facts of life' literature is concerned to establish sexual identity. A sense of self – as 'male', 'female', 'heterosexual', 'bisexual' or whatever – is not timeless and fixed. Recent historians have been at great pains to demonstrate how radically notions and norms of sexual identity have changed from Greek times to the present; today's categories like 'homosexual' and 'pervert' can be traced back barely a hundred years.[36] One of the functions of sexual advice literature has been to invent, create and criticize sexual identity.[37]

More specifically, sexual discourse has aimed to *limit* and create closures in sexual identity. Sex has been presented as natural, desirable and proper, but only within certain personae. In blunt and slightly anachronistic terms, until very recently the manuals have sanctified sex between heterosexual males and heterosexual females, who should preferably be married and monogamous. All other modes of sexual identity and sexual practice have been more or less unacceptable and often subject to censure and interdiction. For that reason, it is important to examine in the literature not just sexual facilitation but sexual stigmatization; encouragement of certain acts and identities implies curtailment or condemnation of others.

Last, the problem arises of situating this subject within wider histories. Narrowly, there is a history of texts. Rigorous postmodernists, influenced by Derrida and his devotees, may wish to argue that texts are all there is: hence sexuality is textuality.[38] We have a certain off-the-cuff sympathy for this sex/text position, since a few texts – *Aristotle's Master-Piece, Married Love* – have exercised quite extraordinary domination over our subject. But we have also sought to venture further. Texts have authors, and readers, and critics, and commentators. Texts can also affect attitudes, and attitudes may determine behaviour. According to our way of reading, those texts did not exist in splendid isolation. Themselves products of their times, they played their part in changing sexuality and sexual activities – albeit in ways which, at the personal level, are exceedingly tricky to document, at least before the present century.

Wider historical questions confront us: how are we to perceive the sexual history of the last few hundred years? Is it meaningful to go on using the large categories traditionally employed with such insouciance? People used to speak of 'Victorianism' in sex, implying puritanism and prudery.[39] Then Steven Marcus discovered the 'other Victorians': Victorians who were surprisingly involved in cultures of pornography.[40] Peter Gay then suggested that the real Victorians were more like the 'other Victorians' than ever suspected – that respectable Victorian paterfamiliases and their spouses often enjoyed a passionate and experimental eroticism.[41] The standard categories thus seem to be falling apart. Moreover, as emphasized by studies of the double standard[42] and of the class and gendered aspects of Victorian sex, it is deeply misleading to speak as if a single erotic universe governed all. The respectable family man who at home in his parlour was a paragon of sexual propriety might also keep his lower-class mistress or frequent the flagellants' brothel. The masses were not necessarily expected to subscribe to the same sexual morality as the proper bourgeoisie, or the raffish aristocracy for that matter;[43] and the deserving poor, though 'immoral' by middle-class standards, aimed to be seen to be pursuing a more respectable morality than the riff-raff.

Hence fine-textured research makes it difficult any longer to bandy around terms like 'the age of liberty', 'the Regency', or 'Victorianism'; at the very least it is necessary to specify more precisely which groups and genders are being referred to, and in what decades. And practice was often radically different from professions.

Nevertheless, awareness of complexity should not lead to interpretative nihilism and the denial of pattern and change. The sexual accent of the Restoration truly was different from that of the Commonwealth;[44] Evangelicalism ushered in distinct sexual goals from those common in the era of Wilkes[45] – indeed they were different precisely because they were revolts against the moralities of their elders and fathers. We must not deny the shifts in sexual mores, registered in and to some degree effected by the sexual advice literature studied in this book, but make it our business to understand the implications of such shifts; understand how a mind-set of sexual denial and suppression may simultaneously be a language of expression (of open secrets); understand how 'permissiveness' may become *compulsory* permissiveness and so a new oppression. We must comprehend what the sexual advice literature said, and equally tune in to the messages between the lines.

This book covers a period of nearly three centuries. We have divided it in two parts around the early Victorian years. This is not because we believe that the accession of Victoria *per se* wrought a radical transformation in public morals and sexual attitudes. But we do see changes occurring around that time. Before then, the field was dominated by a fairly small number of texts. In the Victorian era, these proliferated. Texts multiplied, conflicts grew, and issues hitherto present but subdued – questions of professional policing of lay knowledge, the authority of the medical profession, the involvement of the courts – were energetically discussed in the public domain. An age that deeply feared the social corrosion likely to follow from public knowledge of contraception or perusal of Krafft-Ebing endlessly aired its fears in public, ironic though that may seem to us. The first half of this volume lays the foundations with detailed discussion of a relatively small number of issues; the latter part of the book examines the later proliferation.

CHAPTER ONE

Contexts: from the Restoration to the Accession of Queen Victoria

The sexual history of Britain between the Restoration and Queen Victoria's accession has been popularly portrayed in bodice-ripping terms, starting with Charles II in bed with Nell Gwyn and culminating in the philandering of the disgustingly obese Prince Regent, and on the way taking in Boswell, Wilkes and the Regency rakes; Kitty Fisher, Harriette Wilson and a bevy of other *demi-mondaines,* and such male fantasy elements as John Cleland's *Memoirs of a Woman of Pleasure* (*Fanny Hill*) and Rowlandson's bawdy prints. Today academics tend to focus on the darker side of sexual history, on scapegoating and exploitation, and the attempts of the anxious and angry to police sexual behaviour through the Societies for the Reformation of Manners and the later Vice Societies, through prosecutions of prostitutes and attacks on the profanities on the stage, and through the Bowdlerizing crusade,[1] thanks to which Victorianism was in the saddle long before Victoria came to the throne, indeed before she was ever born.[2]

This attention to the deeds of libertines and the struggles of moral crusaders results in the Hollywood headline history of pre-Victorian sex; and, research has shown, this has about as much relation to the real sexual precepts and practices of the 'long eighteenth century' as the Hollywood sexual life depicted on celluloid or performed at the poolsides of Bel Air and Beverly Hills has to the sex life of ordinary Americans. For this reason, we are fortunate that major new studies over the last couple of decades have begun to cast light on the fine textures of post-Restoration sexuality. Historical demographers have traced changing patterns of marriage, legitimate births and bastards. We now know with some certainty that the great population rise after 1750 was largely due, not to a declining death rate, but to an increase in births, which in turn was due to earlier marriage combined with the higher incidence of bastardy. Certain barriers to the formation of unions and to sexual coupling were evidently crumbling, though explanations of such changes continue to be disputed.[3]

The place of sexual activity within village and market-town communities is now being explored. Sex occurred within frameworks of customs and expectations, themselves shaped by property, wealth and exchange, gender and rank. Nowadays we tend to label sexual actors by psychosexual type (heterosexual, gay, lesbian, and so forth); three or four centuries ago, the equivalent was probably the idea of 'reputation' – being godly and upright, or lewd, a whore or a whoremonger. Sexual reputation did not in any straightforward way hinge upon what one did: to be stigmatized as a whore did not mean that one earned a living by full-time prostitution – it was, rather, a flexible, negotiable community condemnation.

Amongst the 'respectable' sort – soldiers, sailors, whores and so forth would form striking exceptions – sexual intercourse was permissible within marriage and where expectations of marriage had been created and signalled amongst courting couples. Upon pregnancy, marriage would then normally and ideally take place,[4] and community sanctions were levelled against those who took or gave sex beyond the customary norms. In a tight-knit, face-to-face community, the loose woman would lose her reputation and perhaps her chance of finding a marriage partner; and the man who brought bastards into the world would be forced to marry, or flee. The value of sex was inscribed within rules and norms, and it was subject to an exchange economy in which the ultimate regulator was the balance between production and reproduction in an age which did not possess reliable means of contraception and which did not systematically attempt its practice. Like other commodities, sex held its value because demand outstripped supply.

Reputation for virtue was valuable, particularly in a woman, and public pressures were applied to limit sexual activity.[5] But it was also the business of the public to ensure that sufficient children were born for economic prosperity, or at least survival. Too many mouths to feed was an obvious disaster; too few, and shortages of labour, ratepayers and soldiers would follow. And while a wailing chorus of moralists in the later years of the seventeenth century and the early years of the eighteenth condemned England as a nation of fornicators and harlots, there was equal concern amongst political arithmeticians about the decay of population, a lack of hands to the plough or sailors and soldiers for Her Majesty's forces. As we shall see, there was no contradiction in complaining in a single breath about sexual licence and about population decline, for sinful sex was widely assumed to be procreatively unproductive. Overall, the sexual life of the pre-Victorian lower orders still awaits proper research. Suffice to say that the early advice literature shows that individual sexual expression was routinely subordinated to the procreative strategies presupposed by wider moral and national agendas.[6]

Traditional marriage was not 'romantic'. Convictions about the institution of marriage emphasized dynastic policies amongst the ruling class (including the classic arranged marriage) and utilitarian considerations amongst the middling sort (a woman would seek a man capable of supporting her; a man would choose a capable housewife).[7] Recent studies have maintained that there was a new preference in the eighteenth century for what has been called 'affective individualism'. There was a growing idea of marrying for love, or at least with a view to emotional and erotic fulfilment; close feelings and sympathies between the partners were increasingly regarded as lying at the heart of a proper and happy marriage – ideas like these were circulated in didactic literature, in fiction, and in letters and diaries. Such 'affective individualism' paved the way for new sexual inflections: warmer and tenderer images of erotic attraction than in entrenched Christian teachings.[8] Within the sophisticated culture of Addisonian politeness, gentlemen were expected to act genteelly; but there was a new accent on femininity as a source and object of pleasure. Changing social roles, the growth of wealth and leisure (what critics denounced as 'luxury'), and, not least, new fashions, resulted in the ideal of the tender, soft, loving female and in the glamorization of women.[9]

Of course these were images, and they are not easy to relate to reality (it might be argued that ideals bear inverse relation to actualities). Well-documented accounts of the lives of the upper classes, particularly after 1750, suggest that leisured people, with time on their hands for the cultivation of intense personal lives, were investing huge psychic energies in the pursuit of personal passions and pleasures, in a manner begging to be called 'romantic'.[10] The erotic was becoming a central aspect of individual identity within a culture that nevertheless distinguished clearly between male and female roles – one moving, it has been argued, in the direction of 'separate spheres', heightening sexual difference.[11]

Ideals and institutions rarely function smoothly. Lawrence Stone's magnificent tetralogy of studies of marriage and divorce, drawing upon hitherto unused legal testimony, has demonstrated how radically sexual practice might depart from norms and precepts. Gentlemen were frequently coarse in their sexual behaviour – promiscuous and violent towards partners, especially when drunk – and wives not infrequently held as captives and sexual slaves. That may come as no surprise.

Less expected are the frequent displays of sexual forwardness from women provided by Stone's evidence. Despite stereotypes of women as passive, ladylike and ornamental, the evidence of divorce cases (not, of course, a representative sample), shows considerable sexual assertive-ness from women too – in using erotic bait to seduce males into marriage, in obtaining sexual pleasure through diverse erotic games. Moreover, whereas hand-me-down sexual stereotypes have assumed that premarital female virtue, that is, virginity, was essential to middle- and upper-class mores, Stone's evidence suggests that the respectable classes were prepared to indulge in erotic play before and outside marriage. It was not unknown for mothers to permit or even encourage daughters to sleep with suitors as a matrimonial bait. In short, when evaluating the sexual advice literature examined in the rest of this book, it is important not to be misled by an imagined repertoire of behaviour that bears little relation to reality.[12]

Sexual advice gave expression to certain contemporary intellectual movements. Broadly speaking, the tide of thought called the Enlighten-ment was influential in shaping notions of human nature, individuality, the self and the passions, intimate and social behaviour and the wider sense of destiny.[13] This is not to imply that sexual advice manuals were directly influenced by Locke, Hume or Kant. But we should not be surprised to find affinities between key Enlightenment ideas and sexual recommendations, in view of the fact that the Enlightenment was not just a theoretical philosophical system but directed to changing behaviour; and England was by common consent amongst the most Enlightened nations in Europe. Enlightenment outlooks filtered down through many channels: essays, fiction, coffee-house conversation, or the doctor's consultation. Not all sectors of society were equally affected. The Enlightenment began as an elitist movement within polite, male society. Because literacy was high and culture was becoming commercialized, England also had a growing general public eager to read about, see and share in the tastes of their betters.[14]

How far Enlightenment ideas (on sexuality as on anything else) percolated down through society remains debatable, and we should not presume that Enlightenment views on sexuality necessarily anticipated those of latter-day liberals. Attitudes towards eroticism are complex; sex is not something movements are simply 'for' or 'against'. Not least, we need to be cautious before attributing changing sexual behaviour to intellectual causes or influences. Demographic rise and the growing incidence of bastardy after 1750 attest to increased sexual activity amongst large sections of the population, but it might be premature to attribute this to a revolution in *sexual attitudes*, as supposed by some historians.[15] More probably population rise was a response to times in which social impediments to copulation and marriage were diminishing, and economic incentives to larger families were strong.

In their quest for lifestyles which were rational, liberal, polite and happy, advocates of the Enlightenment contrasted themselves to the common people, whom they regarded as leading lives dominated by custom and superstition, and the courtly aristocracy, whose mores were artificial, dissipated and useless. Rustic and courtly sexual habits were equally unacceptable to Enlightenment opinion. The sexual lives of the masses were seen as impoverished, limited by suspicious and guilt-ridden attitudes towards the body. Within popular faith, sensuality was associated with the Fall. Folk wisdom and proverbs predicted that those who wallowed in the lusts of the flesh paid for their pleasures: venereal diseases and bastards were the wages of sin. The violence of popular bawdy embodied subconscious male fears of cuckoldry, castration, impotence and female insatiability.[16]

Lower-class sex was also circumscribed by a domestic and village economy in which prudence dictated the regulation of family size and the production of offspring only under desirable circumstances. Pre-marital sexuality was controlled, and, especially in the seventeenth century, marriage was commonly postponed till the late twenties. Within marriage, abstinence and coitus interruptus helped to trim family size, affect being tailored to income. Family disgrace, community shame and the Church courts punished deviants.[17]

At the other social pole was the Restoration court, whose libertinism was notorious.[18] But much Restoration eroticism was obscenity, the desire to arouse being matched by a desire to shock. Rejection of Calvinist values was spearheaded by rakes like Rochester who were still Puritans at heart. Restoration pornography was misogynistic and aggressive, and its comedies cynical about love and marriage, encouraging defensive laughter at old goats, cuckolds and the impotent. 'Plainly many late seventeenth-century Englishmen shared an obsessive yet apprehensive view of sexuality,' Roger Thompson has written:

> For all their libertine philosophising and summonses to merriment, they seem profoundly inhibited and uncomfortable about the subject. They cannot treat it in a matter-of-fact, balanced way; they cannot laugh about it without sniggering, or describe it straightforwardly, joyously, even innocently. Their reaction is disproportionate, discordant, distorted and disassociated. Pepys cannot appreciate the pleasure and the fun in *L'Escholle des Filles*; he is tantalised, drunkenly horrified; he ejaculates, he destroys. Shame is the spur.[19]

Enlightened opinion rejected traditional plebeian behaviour and traditional courtly display alike. Critics attempted to set conduct upon a sounder footing, developing a sexual psychology grounded in a proper science of human nature. Rejecting original sin and the Calvinist corruption of the flesh, the enlightened argued that Nature was good, and that proper behaviour should seek to realize human nature, rather than to deny, fight and conquer it. Man's nature lay in his senses; its essence was a capacity to be happy. It was not only self-styled Utilitarians who believed that happiness and virtue were heads and tails of a single coin.

For the Third Earl of Shaftesbury and his followers, man had been programmed with faculties or senses like benevolence which produced pleasure. For others, like Locke, human nature was a *tabula rasa*, yet man had basic drives to pursue pleasure and avoid pain, all subsequent action being learnt by experience and fixed by association. In either case, pursuit of pleasure towards the goal of happiness became seen amongst Enlightenment writers as the behaviour dictated to man by Nature. 'Pleasure is now, and ought to be, your business,' Chesterfield told his son.[20] The tendency to produce happiness was the only ultimate yardstick of right and wrong, good and evil.

If Nature was good, then erotic desire, far from being sinful, itself became desirable. And the sexual instincts were undoubtedly natural. Being pleasure-giving, such passions were thus to be approved. 'The Venereal Act . . . when it is performed in obedience to nature,' argued the Scot, Robert Wallace, is 'highly delightful'.[21] There is, maintained Boswell, no 'higher felicity on Earth enjoyed by man than the parti-cipation of genuine reciprocal amorous affection with an amiable woman'.[22] 'Animal attraction' was, for Erasmus Darwin, 'the purest source of human felicity; the cordial drop in the otherwise vapid cup of life'.[23] Sex was also functional. David Hume argued that erotic attraction was the 'first and original principle of human society'.[24] Habitually associated with beauty and benevolence, it was a constructive rather than an anarchic passion.

These naturalistic and hedonistic assumptions – that Nature had made men to follow pleasure, that sex was pleasurable, and that it was natural to follow one's amorous urges – informed Enlightenment attitudes towards sexuality.[25] Thus Jeremy Bentham argued that the ascetic Pauline condemnation of fornication except within marriage was counter-utilitarian: 'when viewed in an unprejudiced point of view, and by the standard of utility, sexual gratification in those modes, against which popular antipathy is apt to rage with greatest fury, will be seen not to belong to the department of morality'.[26]

Such assumptions constitute the psychological morality shaping John Cleland's cunningly titled fiction of Fanny Hill: *Memoirs of a Woman of Pleasure* (1749). Throughout that work, the 'principle of pleasure' was presumed to be the *primum mobile* of human action.[27] The bawd, Mrs Cole, 'considered pleasure of one sort or another as the universal port of destination, and every wind that blew thither was a good one, provided that it blew nobody any harm'.[28] Of the pleasures, sex was reckoned to be supreme and fundamental. Fanny was 'guided by nature only'.[29] 'I began to enter into the true unalloy'd relish of that pleasure of pleasures,' Fanny recorded, 'when the warm gush darts through all the ravish'd inwards; what floods of bliss . . . too mighty for nature to sustain';[30] her sexual encounters with her beau were 'the most delicious hours of my life'.[31]

Furthermore, sexual urges were often portrayed as instinctual to the mechanical constitution of mankind: 'I had it now,' wrote Fanny Hill, 'I felt it now, and beginning to drive, he soon gave nature such a powerful summons down to her favourite quarters, that she could no longer refuse repairing thither; all my animal spirits then rush'd mechanically to that centre of attraction.'[32] And spreading sexual bliss was equated with the maximizing of public happiness. When Fanny ceased to be a kept woman and became a public prostitute, she saw herself 'passing thus from a private devotee to pleasure into a public one, to become a more general good, with all the advantages to put my person out to use either for interest or pleasure or both'.[33] In Enlightenment thought fabrics, the accent was on gratification. When Boswell wanted to ask Louisa when she would allow him to have sex with her, his question was 'How then can I be happy? What time?'[34]

Libidinal hedonism was all the more acceptable because it squared with broader Enlightenment outlooks. Enlightenment naturalism encouraged a certain materialism of outlook. The body became the seat of sensation and so the source of consciousness; for Condillac, touch was the prime sense.[35] In the mechanistic associationism of Hartley, Priestley and others, reductionism collapsed the distinctions between the psychological and the physiological. For Dr Erasmus Darwin, the very idea of beauty arose as a result of infantile association of the 'female bosom' with generosity and fertility.[36] The penis could be seen as 'a wonderful machine'.[37] Sexual aesthetics and action became intrinsic to the cause and effect inevitability of the mechanical universe.

Not least, Enlightenment hydraulic physiology could see regular genital discharges as cleansing, requisite for health. 'I was afraid I was going to have an attack of gout the other day,' wrote Lord Carlisle. 'I believe I live too chaste. 'Tis not a common fault with me.' Sire of fourteen children himself, Erasmus Darwin recommended marriage (that is, sexual outlet) as a cure for psychosomatic disorders.[38]

The Enlightenment was interested in the 'natural philosophy' of sex, its 'art and science', which, as Fanny Hill said, 'resided in the favourite centre of sense'.[39] It even toyed with a kind of sexual religion. The therapist James Graham set up a Temple of Health, which housed his celestial bed in a chamber called 'the holy of holies'. Erasmus Darwin's

Temple of Nature was a paean to the 'Deities of Sexual Love', for it was they who propelled evolutionary progress through the superfecundity of the generative powers. Life rose from asexual to sexual reproduction, which was 'the chef d'œuvre, the master piece of nature',[40] not only improving and diversifying the stock, but being more fun as well. Darwin's heroic poem celebrated the marriage of Cupid and Psyche: 'All forms of Life shall this fond pair, delight/And sex to sex the willing world unite.'[41]

So in Enlightenment thought sexuality saturated the universe. Cosmic poetry celebrated the recent confirmation of plant sexuality. Erasmus Darwin in *The Loves of the Plants* (which deployed a sexual taxonomy) depicted in mock-heroic manner the sexual liaisons of the plant world.[42] Darwin's evolutionary vision of life's development saw sexuality as the animating cause. Sexual desires were always threatening to overstock the environment; the survival of the best weeded out the rest.[43]

Viewed less as a sin or vice than as part of the economy of Nature, sexuality figured largely in eighteenth-century intellectual discussion, an object for inquiry. Travellers' reports and anthropological musings familiarized the English with the polygamous societies of the South Seas. For many this Polynesian image of a society without sexual possessiveness, guilt or jealousy was attractive; as also, doubtless, for males the prospect of legitimately enjoying several wives (Boswell called it being 'patriarchal'). 'Free love' was much discussed: Boswell maintained that even as a married man he should be free to follow his sexual instincts: predictably, he would not allow the same freedom to women.[44] Jeremy Bentham advocated divorce, partly to free women from sexual slavery: 'to be constrained to receive [an husband's unwanted] embraces, is a misery too great to be tolerated even in slavery itself'.[45]

Debate arose about sexuality as a facet of personal relations. The desirability of open sexual discussion was often stressed. 'It would be proper,' suggested Mary Wollstonecraft,

> to familiarise the sexes to an unreserved discussion of those topics which are generally avoided in conversation from a principle of false delicacy; and that it would be right to speak of the organs of generation as freely as we mention our eyes or our hands.[46]

Manuals appeared discussing sexual techniques, compatibility, venereal diseases, fertility, birth limitation and reproduction.[47]

Enlightenment England conceptualized sexuality as natural. As integral to human nature, it was an important component of happiness. As part of the universe, it was to be studied. But did such beliefs have any impact on sexual practice?

Amongst the most marked features of Georgian sexuality was its public stamp, its openness and visibility.[48] Pornography, both elite and popular, was prominent in the written and printed culture.[49] Pornographic journals began appearing from the 1770s, starting with the *Covent Garden Magazine* or *Amorous Repository*, which contained sexy stories and advertisements for prostitutes and brothels, including prices. Erotic and scatological prints were commonplace, engraved by such leading artists as Gillray, Rowlandson and Morland. Obscene references to royalty and politicians were the staple of cartoons (Pitt the Younger appeared as 'The Bottomless Pitt', 'stiff to everyone but a lady'). Newspapers advertised sexual services from gigolos to aphrodisiacs, VD cures and such abortifacients as Farrer's 'Catholic Pills' and Velno's 'Vegetable Syrup'. Adultery and 'innocence destroyed' were the staple of titillating novels like *The Innocent Adulteress* (1777) and *Fatal Follies* (1788), all too often read, critics deplored, by young ladies.

The Gothic novel offered sado-masochistic thrills. Helpless women were humiliated in *The Monk* (1796); the tyrannical father in *The Castle of Otranto* (1765) plotted to marry his son's bride. There was an extensive literature about prostitutes from *Moll Flanders* (1722) to *Fanny Hill* (1749), its tone warmer and less disgusted than that of its Restoration predecessors. The novels of Laurence Sterne drew on ingrained sexual *doubles entendres* in words, suggestion and situation.[50] Erotic literature sold well: *Memoirs of a Woman of Pleasure* reputedly made its publisher Ralph Griffiths £10,000.

Sexuality was high profile. In London, prostitutes numbered probably over 10,000, of all sorts from the kept woman to amateur and professional street-walkers, the whore who would perform for a glass of wine to the high-class and well-bred courtesan who, Casanova recorded, might cost 6 guineas for a night at a bagnio. Prostitutes plied their trade on the streets with little concerted interference and advertised in such directories as Jack Harris's *The Whoremonger's Guide to London*.[51]

Various sexual entertainments were catered for. Bagnios and seraglios met specialized tastes like flagellation. Men of pleasure had their own private clubs. There were shows which featured naked dancing and copulation, as for example the one run by Mrs Hayes where, she advertised, 'at 7 o'clock precisely 12 beautiful nymphs, spotless virgins, will carry out the famous Feast of Venus, as it is celebrated in Tahiti, under the instruction and leadership of Queen Oberea (which role will be taken by Mrs Hayes herself)'. Whores and their clients copulated in St James's Park – while James Boswell christened the recently opened Westminster Bridge one May evening in 1763:

At the bottom of the Haymarket I picked up a strong, jolly young damsel, and taking her under the arm I conducted her to Westminster Bridge, and then in armour complete did I engage her upon this noble edifice. The whim of doing it there with the Thames rolling below us amused me very much.[52]

There was a good deal of promiscuity, which few questioned. Maid-servants were fair game for male advances: rakes were not the worse thought of so long as they made arrangements for any resulting bastards. Although women were often victims of unwanted attentions, many seem to have been perfectly compliant. Young William Hickey was first seduced at the age of ten by a maid, Nanny Harris. An early memory was of awaking one morning to find himself between Nanny's legs: 'with one of my hands upon the seat of Love where I have no doubt she had placed it'.[53]

Men found no difficulty in getting sexual partners. Actresses and dancers were assumed to be sexually easygoing, and many females obviously felt better off as kept women than as servants or as wives. Some high-class *demi-mondaines* and courtesans, like Kitty Fisher and Fanny Murray, won fame and became much-prized artists' models and objects of public fascination. Women of easy virtue were not automatically turned into outcasts. In the 1780s Francis Place had as his master Mr France, a London leather-breeches maker who had three daughters.

His eldest daughter was and had been for several years a common prostitute. His youngest daughter, who was about seventeen years of age, had genteel lodgings where she was visited by gentlemen; and the second daughter . . . was kept by a captain of an East India ship, in whose absence she used to amuse herself as such women generally do.[54]

Evidently neither Place, nor France, nor the women were embarrassed by this situation. It was commonplace for respectable men to keep mistresses and to walk out in public with them, as for instance did the Duke of Grafton with Nancy Parsons.[55] Wives were often complaisant about their husbands' keeping mistresses (they might be glad of the chance of avoiding pregnancy). Well-to-do young men in London were expected to be gallants. 'Where,' demanded John Wesley,

is male chastity to be found? Among the nobility, among the gentry, among the tradesmen, or among the common people of England? How few can lay any claim to it at all? How few desire so much as the reputation of it! How numerous are they now even among such as are accounted men of honour and probity who are as fed horses, every one neighing after his neighbour's wife.[56]

At least in high society, adultery, *ménages à trois* and fluid sexual liaisons seem to have been handled in a civilized manner; they were certainly matters of intense gossip and amusement, but not necessarily causes of matrimonial breakdown, occasions for duels or psychic disaster. Wives were accustomed to putting up with their husbands' affairs. The Honourable Mrs Stuart, wife of James Archibald Stuart, informed Boswell

> That from what she had seen of life in this great town she would not be uneasy at an occasional infidelity in her husband, as she did not think it at all connected with affection. That if he kept a particular woman, it would be a sure sign that he had no affection for his wife; or if his infidelities were very frequent, it would also be a sign. But that a transient fancy for a girl, or being led by one's companions after drinking to an improper place, was not to be considered as inconsistent with true affection.[57]

Few men were ashamed of owning their bastards. Erasmus Darwin had two illegitimate daughters, whom he brought up openly on intimate terms with his second wife and their children. He founded a school in which they became the governesses. Bastards might even marry well: the illegitimate daughter of Sir Edward Walpole married Lord Waldegrave and, on his death, George III's brother, the Duke of Gloucester.

This public visibility and tolerance of sexuality encompassed a large slice of society, beyond the libertine elite of the Restoration court. Admittedly, other aspects of society were strait-laced, not least the Dissenting community. And, of course, the flaunting of sexuality was much more evident in large towns, above all London. Yet the openness of sexuality cannot be gainsaid. *A View of London and Westminster, Or the Town Spy* reckoned in 1725 that there were 107 brothels around Drury Lane alone, and in mid-century John Shebbeare noted that 'every print-shop has its windows stuck full with indecent prints to inflame desire through the eye, and singers in the streets charm your ears with lascivious songs to waken you to the same employment'. Francis Place confirmed that in the 1780s quite respectable shops sold pornography. The owner of one, Mrs Roach, 'used to open a portfolio to any boy or to any maidservant . . . the portfolio contained a multitude of obscene prints . . . she encouraged them to look at them . . . . This was common to other shops.'[58] The omnipresence of prostitutes, bawdy prints and

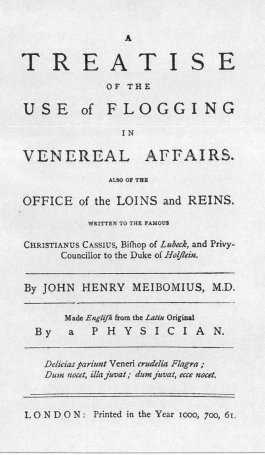

A

TREATISE

OF THE

USE of FLOGGING

IN

VENEREAL AFFAIRS.

ALSO OF THE

OFFICE of the LOINS and REINS.

WRITTEN TO THE FAMOUS

CHRISTIANUS CASSIUS, Bifhop of *Lubeck*, and Privy-Councillor to the Duke of *Holftein*.

By JOHN HENRY MEIBOMIUS, M.D.

Made *Englifh* from the *Latin* Original
By a PHYSICIAN.

Delicias pariunt Veneri *crudelia Flagra ;*
Dum nocet, illa juvat ; dum juvat, ecce nocet.

LONDON: Printed in the Year 1000, 700, 61.

1 By the eighteenth century the English had become notorious as a nation that derived sexual pleasure from beating.

titillating novels indicates that sexual indulgence and tolerance were not confined to a libertine fringe.

Sexual indulgence was publicly acceptable. Adventures were described by diarists like William Hickey without guilt or furtiveness. Seeking to enjoy himself on a sunny afternoon, Hickey would call in at a brothel, pick up some girls and escort them into the country or up the Thames. In a letter to David Hume, Lord Denbigh casually mentioned how he, in company with Lord Sandwich, Lord Mulgrave and Mr Banks, had taken 'two or three ladies of pleasure' up to Newbury for the better part of a week, noting that they intended 'to pass all this week and the next'.[59]

Sexual indulgence did not necessarily ruin a reputation, even that of a lady. 'No one is shocked,' complained Lady Mary Wortley Montagu, 'to hear that Miss So-and-So Maid of Honour, has got nicely over her confinement.'[60] Looking back from the more strait-laced nineteenth century, Francis Place observed how

> want of chastity in girls [of the tradesmen's class] was common, but it was not by any means considered so disreputable in master trades-men's families as it is now in journeymen mechanics' families. A tradesman's daughter who should now misconduct herself in the way mentioned would be abandoned by her companions, and probably by her parents.[61]

There was even greater freedom of expression. The *Monthly Review* believed that *Memoirs of a Woman of Pleasure* was a book not 'offensive to decency'. Robert Bage's novel *Mount Henneth* (1781) includes an episode in which the female characters discuss sexual intercourse after seeing a stallion copulating with a mare.[62]

In fact libertinism was often boasted about. Philandering was free and manly. Politicians such as John Wilkes and Charles James Fox gained as much in public acclaim from their sexual exploits as Pitt the Younger lost for lack of them. When Fox was charged in 1784 on a case of assault, he gave as his alibi that he had been in bed at the time with Mrs Armistead, who was willing to swear to it. He was much admired for his frankness. Sometimes sexual activity was represented as part of the Englishman's birthright. At the mock election at Garrett in Surrey, a man qualified for the franchise by having 'enjoyed a woman in the open air in the vicinity'. Cleland has Fanny Hill conceiving of herself as some sort of national utility: of her employment at the brothel she says there was an 'open public enjoyment' of her[63] – and yet there was freedom too: she was 'at [her] liberty to refuse the party'.[64]

Celebration of sexual freedom was often contrasted – in character-istic Enlightenment ways – to its opposites: the sick scourging of the flesh and the abomination of institutional chastity in Catholic monaster-ies and nunneries, and the denial of the passions by canting killjoy Puritans who, in the Enlightenment stereotypes, typically turn out to be Tartuffian hypocrites. Charles Surface and Tom Jones might be promiscuous, but they had good hearts, unlike such humbugs as Joseph Surface, who, while parading their virtue, turned out to be con-cupiscent, repressed lechers. In life and art, the Georgians did not demand that the sexually exuberant came to a sticky ending, and not all harlots' progresses were downhill all the way. Mrs Hayes, the society brothel keeper, retired reputedly worth £20,000, while the fictional Fanny Hill made £800 clear profit out of two years as a whore. Both *Fanny Hill* and *Moll Flanders* had happy endings; Fanny's career was described in typical Enlightenment terms as 'a rare alliance of pleasure with interest'.[65]

Elite public opinion and the authorities made little attempt to curb this sexual free-and-easy. There was no overriding public fear for most of the century that God's wrath was about to descend – though there were occasional and temporary panics, as after the London earthquakes of 1750. Though many fretted that sexual indulgence was leading to national corruption and anarchy, little was done about it. The general preference for liberty and decentralization over ministerial police action applied to sexual matters. The Church courts, hitherto the chief enforcers of sexual morals, were allowed to wither, though not quite disappear.[66] Parliament took no national, concerted action against prostitution, pornography or obscenity, though *ad hominem* charges were occasionally brought, especially when libel was involved or when there were personal axes to grind, as in the prosecution of John Wilkes's *Essay on Woman*.[67]

Enlightened culture tended to exonerate sexual misdeeds. Analysing crime, Henry Fielding exempted girl prostitutes from blame for their offences: they were 'whores through necessity'.[68] Similarly the Magdalen Hospital for Penitent Prostitutes was founded not to punish the whores, but out of 'pity' as a 'retreat', for the purpose of reform.[69] The age saw the setting up of the Foundling Hospital, and the Lock Hospital for treating venereal diseases, despite the views of some hard-liners that sexual crimes were thereby being condoned.

Some groups in Georgian England were doubtless horrified that rampant sexuality was undermining the moral fibre of God's chosen people. Early in the century, Societies for the Reformation of Manners were set up to bring prosecutions against prostitutes and pornographers, sabbath-breakers and swearers.[70] In 1787 the Proclamation Society was founded for the same purpose, developing into Wilberforce's Vice Society (1802). But these societies won only limited support, popular and official. The Societies for the Reformation of Manners were resented and ridiculed and their vigilante smut-hounds sometimes beaten up. They had declined by the 1740s.

The moving forces behind these anti-sex movements were deeply hostile to all facets of the Enlightenment. The early Reformation Societies were reincarnations of Stuart Puritanism. Attacks on the immorality of the stage came above all from the High Churchman Jeremy Collier. John Wesley, a passionate anti-Latitudinarian, attacked sexual indulgence: his *Arminian Magazine* talked of 'the deluge of depravity which has been pouring upon us'.[71] He was a Bowdlerizer *avant la lettre*. And not least the late eighteenth-century Evangelicals, who formed the core of the Vice Society, were entrenched against liberal politics (especially the French Revolution), rationalism and natural religion. In other words, there was a close alignment between sexual liberalism and endorsement of Enlightenment views.

Enlightenment opinion did not deem sex 'a good thing' *tout court.* Things were much more complicated. In sexuality, as in matters of child-rearing, personal freedom and politics, Enlightenment belief in liberty and indulgence had limits and ambiguities and intolerances of its own. The much-touted freedoms applied principally to males, while Enlightenment attitudes to women were highly ambiguous.[72] Ingrained misogynistic clichés saw women as men's playthings, or attributed a grotesque man-eating sexuality to women. 'I have my own private notions as to modesty,' stated Boswell, 'of which I would only value the appearance; for unless a woman has amorous heat, she is a dull companion.'[73]

Eighteenth-century English women were allowed a measure of freedom that shocked some foreign visitors. Englishwomen have 'no false modesty', noted Le Blanc. 'If a girl fancies a man and can't get to know him, she will send him a message with her proposal, or advertise.'[74] Enlightenment thought insisted that women were rational creatures, and there is much evidence from middle- and upper-class households of women being treated in a more egalitarian way, for example having greater choice of marriage partner.

Yet one strategy certain ladies followed to enhance their status as rational and refined creatures was to deflect attention from, or deny, their sexuality. Bluestockings like Hannah More highlighted female intellectual and moral abilities by repudiating the traditional emphasis on beauty and charm.[75] The radical intellectual Mary Wollstonecraft never resolved the tussle between two images of woman: the intellectual and the sensuous. In any case, liberal and Enlightened men no less than crusty reactionaries were unwilling to accord to women the full freedoms they sought for themselves. The fidelity of wives seemed essential to prevent bastards, who would bring confusion to family property and inheritance. The more Enlightenment sentimentality enhanced woman's special role as mother, the less was her scope for sexual independence.

Enlightenment mentalities were also frightened of plebeian sexuality. One didn't talk eroticism in front of the servants. The title of one of the more widely circulating pornographic magazines makes this point very clearly: *The Covent Garden Magazine, or Amorous Repository, Calculated Solely for the Entertainment of the Polite World* (1774). The fear was that sexual licence would slide into general disorder and anarchy. Moreover, as fast breeders the masses would outrun their ability to look after their own offspring, and the nation's capacity to absorb them. Economists and political arithmeticians were all too well aware of the swelling ranks of paupers and the vast increase in the poor rates. That late Enlightenment figure, Thomas Malthus, decreed that population growth had a tendency to outrun food supply. Failing voluntary moral checks amongst the poor (abstinence from sex by, for example, late marriage), positive checks, like famine or war, would supervene. Bentham and others devoted great effort to persuading the poor that it was in their interest to curb their sexuality so as to minimize poverty. Lower down the social scale, such rationalist radicals as Francis Place could see the wisdom of family limitation.

Enlightenment toleration of sexuality drew the line at certain groups, including the young. From early in the century there was a torrent of medical and moral opposition to masturbation, directed primarily against young people.[76] Such opposition came largely from those generally hostile to sexual liberalism, but it also arose from medical men and educators otherwise enlightened in their outlook, who were fearful that masturbation would jeopardize other cherished Enlightenment ideals. Warm and mutual relationships within the affectionate, companionate family were increasingly valued. The denial of original sin made childhood seem a time of innocence.[77] In these circumstances, teenage sexuality became problematized. Masturbation was a convenient explanation of why some people remained feeble in mind and body, plagued by lassitude and melancholy.

Enlightenment sexual tolerance extended only to heterosexuals.[78] The German traveller Von Archenholz noted that 'unnatural pleasures are held in great abhorrence with the men. In no country are such infamous pleasures spoken of with greater detestation.'[79] In London at least there were of course 'molly-clubs' for upper-class homosexuals, whose practices, if discreet, were tolerated. But buggery remained a capital felony, and the law was sometimes executed with full savagery against members of the lower classes. Some of the more notorious homosexual men of Georgian England, including William Beckford, found it prudent to live abroad or in seclusion. Enlightenment writers showed no sympathy towards homosexuality, endorsing the depiction of sodomy as 'a crime against nature' – the strongest term of condemnation they knew.[80]

Practically all Enlightenment figures recommended the pleasures of the flesh; but this is not of course to say they neglected or despised the pleasures of the mind. The two, Cleland has Fanny Hill insist, are mutually enhancing. It was only slightly eccentric thinkers like William Godwin who, from a radical stance, downgraded the body. Godwin believed that as men grew more rational, superior intellectual joys would increase and the vulgar taste for inferior bodily pleasures would atrophy. This would not threaten the regeneration of the species, since life would be ever more prolonged.[81]

Yet Enlightenment values opposed the blind and merely animal indulgence of sexual cravings. For sexuality to be enjoyable, it had to be refined, decent, polite. The Enlightenment legitimized sexuality on condition that it was made decorous. This civilized pursuit of pleasure took several forms. For many the emphasis was on the *rational* quest for sexual joy. Fanny Hill described one of her clients as a 'rational pleasurist':[82] 'he loved me with dignity in a manner equally remov'd from the sourness, the forwardness by which age is unpleasantly characteriz'd', while being 'much too wise to be asham'd of the pleasures of humanity'.[83] Sometimes the emphasis fell chiefly upon polished gentility. Fanny Hill recounted how she and others had found the secret of enjoying the most 'libertine pleasures' yet of reconciling 'even all the refinements of taste and delicacy with the most gross and determinate gratifications of sensuality'.[84] Sex should be neither savage nor sinful, but civilized: there was, she wrote, 'no stiffness, no reserve, no airs of pique, or little, but all was unaffectedly gay, cheerful, and easy'.[85]

An erotic etiquette needed to be negotiated which would guarantee pleasure without embarrassment. Polite society sought to have its liberties without offending. For example, at Devonshire House in the 1790s the Duke and Duchess shared a *ménage* with the Duchess's closest friend, Lady Elizabeth Foster. The Duke's legitimate children were brought up alongside his children by Lady Elizabeth. Yet propriety was strictly observed. Lady Elizabeth's illegitimate children were all born in secrecy abroad, as was a bastard of the Duchess by Lord Grey. The paternity of Lady Elizabeth's children was concealed from the children themselves. Similarly, for his part, James Graham the sex therapist emphasized the decorum of his lectures on generation: 'Ladies of rank and character are assured, that nothing will be said or seen, which can give even the smallest offence to the chastest and most delicate female eye or ear, and that every thing will be conducted with the most perfect decency and decorum.'[86] Above all, perhaps, the late Enlightenment cult of sensibility informed notions of decent sexuality.[87] Enlightenment thought regarded emotional refinement as enhancing sexuality. Francis Hutcheson claimed that

> The inclination to procreate is excited, or at least generally regulated in its choice of partner, by many delicate sentiments, and finer passions of the heart of the sweetest kind. . . . The esteem of virtue

and wisdom, the desire and love of innocence of manners, compla-
cence, confidence, and the tenderest good-will, are the most natural
incitements and concomitants of the amorous desire, and almost
obscure the brutal impulse towards the sensual gratification, which
might be had with persons of any character.[88]

Sexual attraction found expression in an aesthetic, elevated language,
brimful of feeling. Tenderness was underlined by the growing delicacy
of the language employed. *The Memoirs of a Woman of Pleasure* notably
contains no four-letter words. Sexual feelings were increasingly filtered
through sensibilities of ardour and Romantic passion. It was sentimental sex that gave *Tristram Shandy* and *A Sentimental Journey* their power.
Fanny Hill wrote of her own 'sensitive soul':[89] 'Love, that made me
timid, taught me to be tender too.'[90] For her the male member was a
'sensitive plant'.[91] In Mrs Cole's brothel, 'good manners and politeness
were inviolably observ'd; here was no gross ribaldry, no offensive or
rude behaviour or ungenerous reproaches to the girls for their
compliance with the humours and desires of the men'.[92] Within this
sentimental framework, Fanny fell in love with the man to whom she
gave her virginity, and eventually settled down with him.

Refined sexuality had its advantages. It was more erotic and also less
dangerous to health. Lord Chesterfield urged his son to get his sexual
experience with a refined Parisian lady rather than with a streetwalker
because it was more educative and the chances of catching pox were
slimmer:

> *Un arrangement*, which is, in plain English, a gallantry, is at Paris as
> necessary a part of a woman of fashion's establishment as her
> house. . . . A young fellow must therefore be a very awkward one to be
> reduced to, or of a very singular taste to prefer, drabs and danger to
> a commerce (in the course of the world not disgraceful) with a
> woman of health, education and rank.[93]

Above all, sex with sensibility seemed to solve that constant problem
of the English Enlightenment: how individuals could indulge selfish
passions without danger to the social order.

Within limits, English Enlightenment attitudes permitted free play of
individual sexuality, as they encouraged freedom of thought and
expression, religious toleration, and the free disposal of capital and
property. These attitudes carried over into action. Seventeenth-century
religious anxieties about the flesh were being dissolved. Doubtless, what
is often thought of as the 'Victorian' obsessional repression of sexuality

– seen as fatal both to individual psychic equilibrium and to family and social order – was long pre-Victorian in origins; but it sprang more from the repudiation of Enlightenment beliefs than from their fulfilment.

Rejection of Enlightenment sexuality crystallized in two movements. Romanticism dismissed Enlightenment sensuality as gross and materialistic. The idealization of love, and particularly of woman, was central to the Romantic quest. Blake wanted to liberate the body from prohibitions and inhibitions. But he also wanted to liberate it from Enlightenment politeness conventions and from merely natural desires. 'When Blake calls for the improvement of sensual enjoyment,' it has been said, 'it is as a means of freeing the individual from the merely vegetative and natural. The intensity of consummation becomes an annihilation of selfhood and an entry into the realm that transcends the temporal, the Eternal.'[94] Blake was an advocate of 'the lineaments of gratified desire', but he thought desire would be gratified only within the spiritual ideal of prelapsarian Adam reborn. Shelley longed in *Epipsychidion* (1821) for a unique, passionate and all-consuming ideal love, while also remaining an adherent of a Godwinian/Wollstonecraftian 'free love'. The mundane sexuality of the Enlightenment *homme moyen sensuel* was rejected by such Romantics in their quest for a more transcendental kind of love.

Contemporaneous with Romanticism was the movement, led by the Evangelicals, to banish hedonism in general, and sexuality in particular, from the respectable consciousness and from public life.[95] Pursuit of pleasure fell under deep suspicion. 'Let us give ourselves a little respite [on Sundays] from the fatigue of pleasure,' recommended Bishop Porteus.[96] One needed to be on guard against pleasure's darts: 'Novels generally speaking are instruments of abomination and ruin. A fond attachment to them is an irrefragable evidence of a mind contaminated, and totally unfitted for the serious pursuits of study, or the delightful exercises and enjoyments of religion.'[97] In his *Essay on the Stage*, the Methodist John Styles argued that 'in the choice of a wife, a gentleman should peremptorily reject every female who has been five times at a Theatre in the course of the last two years of her life'.[98] Of the many manifestations of pleasure, sexuality was the most sinister and sinful. Bowdlerism, Grundyism, prudery, anxiety and shame were called upon to put sexuality back in its rightful place. Sensuality came to be practically the antonym of respectability.

CHAPTER TWO

Medical Folklore in High and Low Culture: Aristotle's Master-Piece

From the late seventeenth century in the more advanced regions of Europe – England, France, the Netherlands, the German-speaking territories – and somewhat later in North America, sex advice literature started rolling off the presses. In time a trickle became a stream and then a flood. There were many such works, and they came in various forms, including books for women, books of 'secrets', midwifery manuals, and assorted erotica.[1] Works of popular medicine, astrological prediction, physiognomical lore, almanacs, and the new 'your questions answered' genre pioneered by the bookseller John Dunton, and much other writing aimed at ordinary readers contained snippets of information and advice pertaining to sexual etiquette and practice, pregnancy, fertility, childbirth and related topics.[2] Such books might recommend charms and potions to ensure success in love or guarantee potency or fecundity. They might disclose how to predict a baby's gender. They might explain birth defects and monstrosities. Sometimes they evoked the feats of great lovers, or thundered dire moral warnings against unbridled lust and unnatural practices.

The hotchpotch of ideas and information contained in books like Nicholas Culpeper's *Directory for Midwives* (1656 and many subsequent editions) derived from various sources.[3] There was an encyclopaedic tradition of wonders, marvels and monsters, whose long pedigree started with Pliny and continued via Isidore of Seville, Albertus Magnus, Bartholomaeus Anglicus and other medieval compilers.[4] Such sources were easily raided. So were various earlier writers on medicine, surgery and the body, for example Helkiah Crooke, author of *Microcosmographia* (1615)[5] and John Bulwer who wrote extensively on the body and its physiognomy, on gestures and on religious portents.[6] Also circulating were works containing tales of love, romantic heroes and memorable courtesans, pre-eminent amongst them being Jacques Ferrand's *De la Maladie d'amour, ou Mélancholie érotique* (1623),[7] though comparable

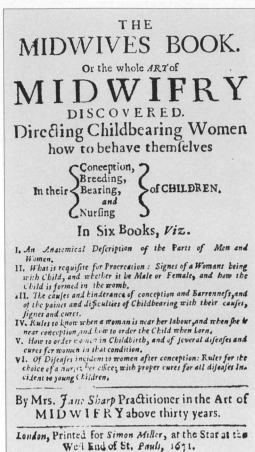

THE
MIDWIVES BOOK.
Or the whole *ART* of
MIDWIFRY
DISCOVERED.
Directing Childbearing Women
how to behave themselves

In their {Conception, Breeding, Bearing, and Nursing} of CHILDREN.

In Six Books, *Viz.*

I. *An Anatomical Description of the Parts of Men and Women.*

II. *What is requisite for Procreation : Signes of a Womans being with Child, and whether it be Male or Female, and how the Child is formed in the womb.*

III. *The causes and hinderance of conception and Barrennefs, and of the paines and difficulties of Childbearing with their causes, fignes and cures.*

IV. *Rules to know when a woman is near her labour, and when fhe is near conception, and how to order the Child when born.*

V. *How to order women in Childbirth, and of feveral difeafes and cures for women in that condition.*

VI. *Of Difeafes incident to women after conception: Rules for the choice of a nurfe, her office; with proper cures for all difeafes Incident to young Children.*

By Mrs. *Jane Sharp* Practitioner in the Art of
MIDWIFRY above thirty years.

London, Printed for *Simon Miller*, at the Star at the Weft End of St. *Pauls*, 1671.

2   Jane Sharp was one of the small number of midwives who wrote about her craft. Her book (1671) contained anatomical descriptions and accounts of procreation.

material could also be garnered from Robert Burton's colossal *Anatomy of Melancholy* (1621), which had gone through five editions by the time of Burton's death in 1640: the last third of Burton's *opus* was entirely devoted to the enigmatic and often calamitous power of love.[8]

A vast learned literature dealt with the body and its functions, conception and generation, 'women's problems' and the anatomical, physiological and psychological meanings of anatomical difference. At least from the twelfth century, such inquiries had been organized and reorganized in medico-surgical texts and in academic discourses expressed within the categories of scholasticism.[9] Some of this learning had specialized in the analysis of love, passion and lovesickness viewed as spiritual and (as we would say) psychological manifestations.[10] For their part, sixteenth- and seventeenth-century medical writers had built upon the new anatomy pioneered by Vesalius, Fabrizio and Falloppio, at Padua and other centres where dissection flourished, and pursued new studies of the anatomy of the penis and of women's reproductive organs.[11]

Against this background of energetic discussions of sexual anatomy and sexual activity, precisely what was novel in the second half of the seventeenth century? The issuing of books about matters sexual was not in itself new. Nor were the specific teachings contained in such books especially unusual. The era of the 'new science' trumpeted by Francis Bacon and eagerly taken up by those associated with the founding of the Royal Society might have been expected to produce radically new teachings about sexual anatomy and sexual activity; but that was not so. There is little in the advice literature of 1680 or 1720 that is not rooted in medieval and Renaissance texts. What is new is that such teachings were for the first time being condensed into handy, entertaining advice books targeted at the public at large.

We should not be surprised at such a development: the growth of literacy and the spread of consumer culture were creating highly favourable conditions. By the late seventeenth century, literacy was more or less universal amongst English males of the middling sort and above. Amongst the lower orders it was steadily rising: around 75 per cent of males in large towns like London were literate; figures for women, though lower, were also improving. Literacy is a problematic concept, but the non-stop output of chapbooks, broadsides, handbills and other forms of popular reading matter makes it clear that writers and stationers of the late seventeenth century believed there was a sizeable popular audience worth targeting.[12]

Interacting with rising literacy was the surge in commercial culture, the extension of regional and national markets in commodities and consumer items, thanks to better communications and to publicity engines such as newspapers: some historians write of a 'birth of a consumer society' or a 'consumer revolution' at this time. This is not the place to evaluate these claims;[13] suffice to say that more people were buying more goods, not least amongst which were reading matter including educational handbooks and works of self-culture, self-improvement and advice.[14]

Books and other printed materials thus formed a growth area: there was a print explosion associated with the rise of newspapers, magazines and periodicals.[15] And the rise of publications helped satisfy a hunger for self-improvement amongst countless small people – artisans, the petty bourgeoisie, provincial traders and so forth – stimulated by a galaxy of guides, handbooks and conduct manuals.[16] Buyers of newspapers, grammar books, arithmetic primers, almanacs, and the 'your questions answered' style of work pioneered by John Dunton's *Athenian*

Mercury[17] formed an eager market for the new, cheap, simple, helpful, entertaining books about love, sex and marriage.

A few books targeted at the common reader became highly successful, running into tens of editions and being energetically pirated, vulgarized and recycled. In France the bestseller by far was Nicolas Venette's *Tableau de l'amour conjugal*, which first appeared in 1686, went through over thirty editions in the eighteenth century (when its readership was chiefly bourgeois), before becoming in later generations the 'Bible of the French peasantry'. Venette's work was translated into English, German, Dutch and, eventually, Spanish, and it enjoyed a notable sale in Enlightenment England, though perhaps the title-page of a late eighteenth-century edition which claimed to be the 'twentieth edition' is yet another sexual boast. That international bestseller will be discussed in the following chapter. The most successful primer in English was *Aristotle's Master-Piece*. Surviving copies show that this work, typically printed sandwiched together with other pseudo-Aristotelian writings, went through over a score of editions in the eighteenth century, and far more in the nineteenth, in Britain and America as well. This chapter will address *Aristotle's Master-Piece* as an example of the teachings about sex and generation being offered to popular audiences in the pre-Victorian era.

Aristotle's Master-Piece presents problems of provenance scholars have hardly begun to tackle and which cannot be explored here. Segments of the sexual doctrines of Greek and Roman physicians and philosophers had been preserved, codified and rendered authoritative in encyclopaedic texts in the Middle Ages, and Renaissance humanism brought the publication of substantial scholarly discourses on sexual topics, culminating in Giovanni Sinibaldus's *Geneanthropeiae* (1642).[18] *Aristotle's Master-Piece* first appeared as an English text in 1684, relying heavily upon those works and a wide range of parallel sources. It is not, of course, by Aristotle;[19] its compiler or compilers, and the circumstances of its composition, remain unknown, though the medical popularizer William Salmon is believed to have had some hand in it.[20] Considering its vast circulation and staying power right into the present century, it has received oddly little scholarly attention – largely because it has been facilely dismissed for containing a 'great deal of nonsense'.[21] Condemning the work as 'an hoary old debauchee acknowledged by no-one',[22] the eminent physician, D'Arcy Power, concluded that it was 'a mere catchpenny production'.[23] Examining its fortunes in America, Otho Beall disparaged it as a scrapbook of 'pre-objective' and 'occult' sexual 'folklore', a 'medical anachronism' – a judgement that typecasts it all too neatly within clichés about popular and pre-scientific culture.[24] In a study focusing on nineteenth-century editions, Janet Blackman dubbed it an 'anachronism': 'it is almost,' she wrote, 'too exact in the imprecision or ineffectiveness of much of its advice, and this stems from lack of thought and explanation.'[25] If the work was so incompetent, one is left wondering why it sold so well.

The form and fortunes of *Aristotle's Master-Piece* pose problems that go to the heart of the issues raised in this book. Was it primarily a compilation of vernacular sexual and gynaecological know-how, or did it chiefly codify professional medical wisdom? What did readers want out of it? What did they get out of it? Did it gratifyingly confirm their prejudices, or did it open their eyes or solve their difficulties? Did it teach or titillate? Who actually read it – the married or the single, men or women? The sexually active or the sexually frustrated? And what pressures were placed upon publishers, and the hack writers and editors involved in modifying successive editions, to meet changing public expectations and accommodate new medical and scientific teachings?

Aristotle's Master-piece has been treated as a slapdash concoction of myths and old wives' tales. But properly examined, it will be seen to be a far more coherent work. It was constructed on a logical, sequential plan, and unfolded its teachings within a consistent intellectual paradigm. These aspects will be explored below and the connections examined between the teachings of *Aristotle's Master-Piece* and other sexual popularizations appearing in the succeeding decades.[26] It is not surprising, in view of the fact that it was an anonymous compilation reissued for over two hundred years, that there is no single, definitive text of *Aristotle's Master-Piece* reprinted verbatim down the ages. From the early eighteenth century, substantially distinct versions of the publication were circulating simultaneously. *Aristotle's Master-Piece* should not be seen as one single stem text adapted over time; the title was used to cover somewhat distinct variants. Even by the early eighteenth century, three fairly distinctive versions had appeared under that title. Two of these remained in print sporadically through the eighteenth century and beyond, and a radically distinct mutation appeared in the Victorian period. The publishing story is set out in the Appendices at the end of this chapter (pp. 54–64).

In outlook and content, what will for convenience be called Versions 1, 2 and 3 are broadly commensurable. As is evident from the chapter headings reproduced in the Appendix, they cover much the same ground, even though certain topics are treated in some versions but not in others. For example Versions 1 and 2 both contain chapters explaining how foetuses become endowed with a soul, whereas Version 3 has no such chapter. All three versions contain comparable sexual and medical information, explained in similar expressions and often in identical words. There is, however, one major and intriguing distinction between the first two versions and the third. The first two are essentially neutral in tone, conveying their information in a direct, didactic prose. By contrast, Version 3 (which, perhaps significantly, seems to have gone through the greatest number of reissues) is altogether more animated and jaunty, with an ear for the innuendo of popular bawdy.[27] In this version alone, seduction and conquest are treated with racy wit and sly irony. Version 3 praises chastity – 'virginity untouch'd and taintless, is the boast and pride of the fair sex' – but reserves a sting for the tail: 'but they generally commend it to put it off, as good as it is they care not how soon they are honesty rid of it'.[28] Similarly, the newly-wed husband is urged to embrace his bride, inflamed to feats of love by her charms; but if she is ugly, the advice is: do it in the dark![29] Moreover in Version 3 alone, each chapter has a tailpiece of light and mildly risqué doggerel. Rounding off the chapter on marriage, the husband announces his plan of campaign:[30]

> Now, my fair bride, new will I storm the mint
> Of love and joy, and rifle all that's in't;
> Now shall my infranchis'd hand, on ev'ry side,
> Shall o'er thy naked polish'd ivory slide.
> Freely shall now my longing eyes behold
> Thy bared snow, and thy undrained gold;
> No curtain now tho' of transparent lawn,
> Shall be before thy virgin treasure drawn,
> I will enjoy thee now, my fairest, come,
> And fly with me to love's elysium;
> My rudder with thy bold hand, like a try'd
> And skilful pilot, thou shalt steer and guide,
> My bark in love's dark channel, where it shall
> Dance, as the bounding waves to rise and fall.
> Whilst my tall pinnace in the Cyprian streight
> Rides safe at anchor and unlades the freight . . .
> Perform those rites nature and love requires
> Till you have quench'd each others amorous fires.

It may be a sign of the greater sexual frankness of this version that it opens, as does Venette's *Tableau*, with a long, nuts-and-bolts anatomical exposition 'of the parts of instruments of generation, both in men and women',[31] whereas Versions 1 and 2 begin with an encomium on matrimony.

Two of the three versions (2 and 3) were reprinted frequently during the eighteenth century and into the nineteenth. Once the separate versions had appeared they underwent little change beyond trivial stylistic updating and a certain degree of paraphrasing and textual corruption: in an early nineteenth-century printing, the great Islamic philosopher, Avicenna, has become, rather appropriately, 'Advicene'.[32] The longevity and stability of these texts are truly remarkable, though it is understandable that publishers found it less troublesome to continue printing established manuals without rewriting or revision. It is interesting that the reading public does not seem to have demanded new views, newfangled scientific facts, or different approaches – more outspoken or more guarded? – to sexual secrets.

The exception is what will be termed Version 4, first published in the nineteenth century. In the discussion to follow in this chapter, this edition will be ignored: it will be discussed later (pp. 128–31). For simplicity's sake, the three earlier versions will now be considered collectively.

Some preliminary words may be appropriate. One of the great debts we owe to Michel Foucault stems from his emphatic denial that sexuality is a timeless constant. Our idea of sexuality, he contended, is quite distinctively modern; it must not be assumed to apply to past centuries.[33] This advice must be heeded in approaching *Aristotle's Master-Piece*. For one of the reasons why scholars have typically dismissed that work as a strange hotchpotch is precisely because few of the topics canonical to twentieth-century sexology receive any substantial treatment in it. Little is said of sexual desire in relationship to guilt or danger (medical, moral or religious). There is no inkling of the perversions or of a *psychopathia sexualis* in the Krafft-Ebing mould, nothing about homosexuality, masturbation, sado-masochism, prostitution and nymphomania, or about any dialectic of sex with neurosis. Indeed, most fundamentally, *Aristotle's Master-Piece* conveys no notion that sexual activity involves problems inherent to the psyche and expressive of unconscious predicaments of the self: sex is not seen, in other words, as a psychological category, it is barely a matter of the inner self at all.[34]

Nor does *Aristotle's Master-Piece* anticipate modern sexual therapeutics. There is no rhetoric, comparable to passages found in mid-twentieth-century works, stressing the need to transcend sexual shame, repression and guilt; no advice for avoiding unwanted pregnancies, no training in coital positions. *Aristotle's Master-Piece* merely assumes that sex is Nature's way to provide for 'the business of generation'. Its coherence derives from having as a unifying theme the subject of reproduction. This organic scheme is apparent from even a casual glance at the chapter headings. For example, the 1690 edition (Version 1)

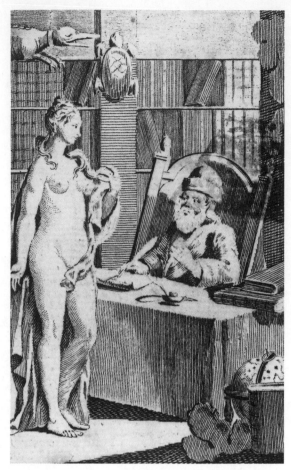

3   The sexual advice genre in a nutshell:
the naked female body spells fertility, the
male represents wisdom. Frontispiece to
*The Works of Aristotle, the Famous Philoso-
pher*, n. d. but *c.* 1810.

opens with a discussion of the correct age for marriage viewed as the
rite translating reproductive potential into social actuality; and by the
second chapter it has proceeded so far as advising couples how they may
contrive to beget, according to preference, male or female children.
Successive chapters explain why children resemble their parents.[35] This
teleology will be analysed in greater detail below, but the point here to
be stressed is that the compiler did not see his main task as to give
readers instructions in the basic performance of the sexual act itself.
That, it is taken for granted, would be teaching your grandmother to
suck eggs. There was no anticipating James Graham's later anxiety that,
in a decadent age, desire itself might leak away unless one celebrated
'the rites of Venus in a variety of ways'.[36] Instruction, according to
Version 3, was to be not just in 'the bare performing of that act'. More
was at stake, that is,

the performing it so as to make conducive unto the work of generation. And since this act is the foundation of generation, and without which it cannot be, some care ought to be taken and consequently some advice given, how to perform it well: and therein I am sure the proverb is on our side which tells us, that, what is once well done is twice done.[37]

For *Aristotle's Master-Piece* it is axiomatic that intercourse is fundamental to the grand design of the propagation of the species.[38] This notion is expressed in various ways. It is declared (perhaps disingenuously) that couples self-evidently want children. 'Though there are some that desire not to have childbirth and yet are very fond of nocturnal embraces to whom these directions will be no way acceptable,' states Version 3,[39]

> yet I doubt not but the generality of both sexes, wherein a married state, have such a desire to produce the fair image of themselves, that nothing can be more welcome to them than those directions, that they make their mutual embraces most effectual to that end.

Indeed, we are informed that anticipation of motherhood is the chief pleasure certain women take in the marriage bed.[40]

Procreation is also explained as both the end of Nature and the command of God ('go forth and multiply').[41] Only the most hardened lechers, Version 1 asserts, could pretend to be ignorant 'to what end they were created Male and Female, which was to beget children and propagate their kind';[42] and all versions set the reproductive history of mankind in context of a panorama of 'the plastic power of Nature',[43] viewed as *natura naturans*, a great creating Mother, in the 'dark recesses' of whose 'womb' fresh creations are constantly coming to fruition.[44] And if Nature be the eternal Mother, instilling mankind with the generative instinct, the Lord is the Father who commanded Adam and Eve (and through them all successive generations) to people the Earth. In His third person, God is also the Holy Ghost, the fecundating agent in the divine fiat. As both Father and Spirit, the Lord made the cosmos fruitful:[45]

> It plainly appears in Holy Writ, that this glorious Universe, bespangled with gaudy Fires, and everywhere adorned with wonderful objects, proclaiming the Wisdom and Omnipotence of the Great Work-Master who in six Days Erected all Things for his pleasure, was at first drawn out of Nothing, or at most a Formless Chaos of Confusion; no Fruits nor Pleasure, no creature that hath breath, had being in the place this lower World possesses, till GOD out of the Abundance of his Goodness, sent forth his Holy Spirit, who Dove-like,

with mighty outspread Wings, sat brooding on the Vast Abyss, and made it pregnant: Then Light put Darkness soon to slight, and all the glorious Lamps of Heaven appeared, all Creatures soon had being, and every Plant, Tree, Herb, or Flower of fragrant Smell, sprung from the Verdant Earth, rais'd by Command above the Waters; every thing of life having Seed in it self, that no second Creation was needed.

Subsequently every coupling has been a sacramental love feast, commemorating the Creation; according to Version 3:[46]

The natural inclination and propensity of both sexes to each other, with the plastic power of Nature, is only the energy of the first blessing, which to this day upholds the species of mankind in the world.

The subject of *Aristotle's Master-Piece* is *reproduction*. That both men and women will long to copulate, that passion will not prove delusory or destructive, that there is an esteem and respect between the sexes which transcends brute lust – all these are taken for granted, requiring no special pleading, syllogisms or learned footnotes. Mutual sexual attraction is assumed to be unproblematic. No chapter deals with loss of libido; no mention is made of homosexual desires or practices,[47] of bestiality or buggery, of erotic mania,[48] or even of that new eighteenth-century bugbear, masturbation.[49] *Aristotle's Master-Piece* feels under no obligation to vindicate to its readers the pleasures of heterosexual intercourse; it will merely instruct them in how to do it well.

It is not presumed, of course, that sex is all plain sailing. A woman, it is noted, has a limited child-bearing career; her cravings and her fertility will wax and wane. But that is readily explained within the humoral medical framework presupposed throughout the book: being constitutionally cooler and moister, women are less vigorous. Instructions are given to guarantee that copulation will be enjoyable and effective. Relax, the reader is instructed, cast care aside, indulge in fine wines and delicacies; for (in the words of Version 2):

When a married couple, from a desire of having children, are about to make use of those means that nature ordained to that purpose, it would be very proper to cherish the body with generous restoratives, that so it may be brisk and vigorous; and if their imaginations were charmed with sweet and melodious airs, and care and thought of business drowned in a glass of racy wine, that their spirits may be raised to the highest pitch of ardour and joy, it would not be amiss; for any thing of sadness, trouble, and sorrow, are enemies to the delights of Venus. And if, at any such times of coition, there should be conception, it would have a malevolent effect upon the child.[50]

Nevertheless, the prime concern of *Aristotle's Master-Piece* – more so than in the writings, for example, of Nicolas Venette or James Graham – lies not in overcoming anticipated amatory difficulties but in tackling hindrances to conception and in surmounting the spectre of sterility.

The solution to these problems was seen to lie in marriage. Conjugal sex was not merely moral and civilized, 'happy . . . pleasant . . . delightful', but was more likely to prove fertile.[51] Promiscuity and whoredom were not just brutish but barren as well. But marriage, for its part, was not presented as a means of taming the flesh, in the manner advocated by Defoe in his anonymously published *Conjugal Lewdness* (1727), in which he warned of the sinfulness of carnal desire unless strictly disciplined; nor was marriage endorsed as an instrument of some kind of proto-Malthusian 'moral restraint' for reining back runaway population growth through deferred gratification.[52] Marriage, it was emphasized, had been instituted in Paradise as the divinely ordained instrument for peopling the world.[53] And the pro-natalist message of *Aristotle's Master-Piece* was unambiguously in favour of early marriage and implacably opposed to all obstacles to it. It urged that women should marry while still in their teens, as soon as their bodies had ripened. The age of 18–20 was recommended – markedly below the age of marriage typical in late Stuart and early Hanoverian England, when rural custom, social retrenchment and economic anxieties had made late nuptiality the norm.[54] Parents were also urged that in no circumstances should they obstruct the connubial desires of their children – daughters especially – for reasons of family policy, matchmaking or the foolish quest for 'a large dowry'.[55] For one thing, enforced sexual abstinence caused characteristic diseases of pubescent girls like the green sickness or chlorosis.[56] But worse might follow. Hinder young people from copulating lawfully within marriage, and they will do so promiscuously. The ensuing evils, according to *Aristotle's Master-Piece*, would not merely be sin, vice, disease and social confusion, but also the frustration of Nature's intentions, for casual copulation and prostitution rarely resulted in pregnancies, or at least not in bonny children.[57] In line with that of other pro-natalist sex educators like Venette and Graham, the message of *Aristotle's Master-Piece* was that married unions would prove fertile, but irregular fornication bred sterility and disease. Pro-nuptialist as well as pro-natalist, *Aristotle's Master-Piece* thus contributed to the climate of opinion repudiating aristocratic or plebeian 'libertinism', and championing marriage as more than a prudent economic contract. It was companionable, sexually fulfilling, healthy both for the couple concerned and, along mercantilist lines, productive for the body politic. Although, bantered Version 3, 'matrimony, in the present age, is looked upon as a most insupportable yoke – wives and husbands are accounted the greatest clogs and burdens to those who give up the reins to their unbridled appetites',[58] in reality the marital knot was both blessed and enviable, 'of all conditions the happiest'.[59]

Aristotle's Master-Piece's advice to the married was that regular – though not excessive – sex was most favourable to generation:

> They that would be commended for their Wedlock Actions, and be happy in the fruit of their Labour, must observe to copulate at distance of time, not too often, nor yet too seldom, for both these hurt Fruitfulness alike.[60]

The text assumes that there is no need to detail frequencies, or offer timetables of the right hours of the day or seasons of the year to perform – niceties that would appear in Venette's *Tableau de l'amour conjugal*. It does, however, prohibit intercourse during menstruation;[61] for, reflecting both medical and popular opinion, menstrual sex was seen not just as filthy but also as liable to engender monstrous or defective children.[62] Abstinence is advised during the later stages of pregnancy, to reduce the risk of miscarriage. But the general tenor is to avoid policing sex with rigid medical or moral decrees.

The advice for sexual intercourse follows a different tack. Its chief concern is with aids to conception. In particular, it is stressed that conception is most likely to follow when the wife is aroused, not just the man:

> It is also highly necessary, that in their mutual embraces they meet each other with equal ardour; for if the spirit flag on either part, they will fall short of what nature requires, and the woman must either miss of conception or else the children prove weak in their bodies, or defective in their understanding and therefore I do advise them, before they begin their conjugal embraces, to invigorate their mutual desires, and make their flames burn with a fierce ardour, by those ways that love better teaches than I can write.[63]

Arousal of female desire, however, poses no great problems, since 'Aristotle' views women as no less libidinous than men. In this context, the compiler debated the Hippocratic conviction that conception entailed the mingling of both male and female seeds, and hence required mutual and roughly simultaneous orgasm for fecundation to occur. But this view was rejected as physiologically unsound: there was no evidence that women really ejaculated seminal fluid.[64]

Alongside this general advice for promoting conception, further hints were offered as to how to produce a boy or a girl (it being assumed that boys would be preferred). Here *Aristotle's Master-Piece* retailed the popular supposition – one repudiated by Venette from his lofty vantage point as a learned physician battling against superstition – that males will be produced if in intercourse the woman lies on her right flank, because boys are engendered on the right side of the womb. Copulating when the moon is on the wane will, for symbolically obvious reasons, produce girls.[65]

The remainder of the book spells out the biological consequences of copulation. How is a woman to know if she has conceived?[66] A choice of pregnancy tests is suggested, mainly involving urine inspection – tests largely dismissed by the superior Venette. 'If urine be put in a glass three days,' for instance,[67]

> and the woman have conceived certain live things will appear to stir in it. If a bright Needle be put in a whole night and she have conceived, divers little red Specks will be thereon, but if not it will be blackish or rusty. Nor are these imaginations, but the proved assertions of the Learned in Physick and skilful in Midwifery, who have made it their study to search into the depth of Nature's Secrets.

And then, once pregnancy is established, how is one to know if the growing foetus is a boy or a girl? Various signs are listed, with their interpretations. Boys are said to cause less painful pregnancies than girls; and it is a sure sign of a boy if it is the right side of the womb that is agitated.[68]

Subsequent chapters give tips for pregnancy management.[69] Tight-lacing is to be avoided, and charms and medicaments are prescribed to prevent or ease the swollen breasts caused by the plethora of blood during pregnancy.[70] A simple account is offered of the quickening and maturing of the foetus in the womb. Unlike the elaborate embryology presented by Venette, *Aristotle's Master-Piece* is little concerned with anatomical or physiological niceties but instead addresses the problems it believes most worry pregnant women.[71] One section addresses the old question of whether the foetus derives all its nourishment through the umbilical cord, or imbibes some through the mouth (the latter view is – wrongly – accepted). Another gives an account of the stage of development reached by the foetus in the successive months of pregnancy.[72]

The latter half of *Aristotle's Master-Piece* then looks forward to child-birth itself – a theme handled more amply in the other pseudo-Aristotelian works, the *Compleat Midwife* and the *Last Legacy*, often bound with *Aristotle's Master-Piece*.[73] The account of midwifery techniques will not here be examined,[74] though in the light of scholarly controversies about the rise of man-midwives, it is worth noting that in all editions of *Aristotle's Master-Piece* it is taken for granted that normal births will be attended by women but that male operators will deal with difficult presentations.[75] Nor will there be discussion of the bundle of

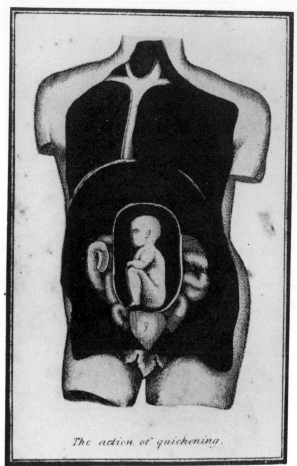

The action of quickening.

4 'The Action of Quickening', from *The Works of Aristotle the Famous Philosopher, Containing his Complete Masterpiece, and Family Physician; His Experienced Midwife, His Book of Problems, and His Remarks on Physiognomy*, n. d., but Victorian.

chapters tagged on to later editions, known as 'A Private Looking Glass for the Female Sex', which treats 'of several maladies incident to the womb, with proper remedies for the cure of each'.[76] The presence of that section in most late Georgian editions probably reflects increasing awareness of repeated and difficult lyings-in as the widespread cause of ill-health in women, and seems to give further evidence that this was a work expected to be read by women.[77]

The centrality of 'the business of generation' to *Aristotle's Master-Piece* is evident in the fact that almost all the problems addressed in the text relate not to sexual intercourse itself but to child-bearing. The problem treated most fully is barrenness – it heads the contents list on the title-page of the 1690 edition.[78] The text assumes that protracted failure to conceive will be experienced as devastating. It lays responsibility at the door of the woman – the idea is not even entertained that a man may be potent but sterile[79] – for by their nature women are less vigorous than men. Defects in the female constitution are examined – the woman may, in humoral terms, be too dry, too moist, too cold or too hot – and these excesses or deficiencies, it is suggested, may be rectified by appropriate medicaments and restoratives, recipes for which are itemized.[80] Alterations in lifestyle may also help: above all, luxurious habits are to be avoided: 'city dames that live high and do nothing, seldom have children'.[81] Relaxation and contentment are recommended as conducive to fertility, and barren couples are advised to have sexual relations neither too rarely nor too often.[82] The tone of this advice is comforting rather than worrying: barrenness is not assumed to be divine punishment for vice or sin. Rather the text reads as a constructive attempt to provide a measure of reassurance translatable into practical action, thereby helping partners to restore control over their reproductive destiny.

As well as giving explanations of barrenness and copious advice on pregnancy management, the text also tackles head on the most terrifying of reproductive aftermaths. What if pregnancy results not in a healthy live baby, but in a monstrous or shapeless lump of dead flesh?[83] The text offers physiological rationalization of these 'moles' by explaining that they have been caused by weakness either in the male seed or in the womb, which lacked due heat or spirits to generate a normal child. Sexual intercourse during menstruation was another precipitant.[84] Restoratives and tonics were recommended to prevent a repetition.

This raised the problem of the status of such abortions in Nature and under God. Were they truly human? If so, did they have souls? What did that imply about the nature and history of the soul? How and when did infusion of the soul into the foetus take place?[85] Such problems were agonizing for individual parents (was this fruit of one's womb possessed of an immortal soul?) but no less for the community at large (who was to be baptized? who buried in holy ground?). Not surprisingly, most versions of *Aristotle's Master-Piece* included a chapter on the soul. This explained, in orthodox theological terms, that souls were not engendered by the copulation of male and female, but were superadded by God to foetuses during development in the womb. For ensoulment, two criteria had to be satisfied. First, it was only independent, live foetuses with a human form which became ensouled. This excluded such shapeless accumulations of flesh as 'moles'. Secondly, only fruits of regular intercourse between male and female were endowed with immortal souls. This stipulation of course addressed the problem of live-born 'monsters', an issue prominent in most versions of the *Master-Piece*.

Being delivered of a severely malformed child was not just a ghastly trauma for the parents, it was an ominous social event, a portent or punishment.[86] Most editions of the *Master-Piece* carried horrifying illustrations of grotesque monsters – all the more conspicuous since they were often the only illustrations in the book. These included what the nineteenth century was to call 'Siamese twins', but characteristically they were grotesque – hairy, simian or black. In offering explanations for these, *Aristotle's Master-Piece* lapsed into a misogyny uncharacteristic of the text as a whole. It attributed responsibility for them to the mother, seeing them as the consequence of one of four possibilities. Perhaps the mother was suffering from a grave internal disorder; or she had copulated with an animal, bringing forth a hybrid man-beast (in which case the offspring, being sub-human, had no soul).[87] Or the woman had lain with some demon.[88] This view – scotched by Venette as a biologically absurd superstition – continued to appear in editions of *Aristotle's Master-Piece* until well into the nineteenth century, and may indicate (through its clear acceptance of incubism) the lingering of macabre witchcraft beliefs. The fourth possibility is that the monster was a product of female imagination.[89]

The doctrine that at the moment of conceiving a woman had the power to imprint whatever was in her imagination upon her conceptus was widely accepted within both regular medicine and popular culture.[90] It was challenged by the science of the Enlightenment – and indeed was rejected by Venette and eighteenth-century medical figures.[91] But it was a doctrine staunchly endorsed by *Aristotle's Master-Piece* throughout its publishing career. Its implications were extraordinarily equivocal. On the one hand, it could serve as a comforting rationalization of what was otherwise terrifying and inexplicable.[92] Why was a child born with 'port wine' stains on its skin, or with a hare-lip? Because at a crucial juncture the mother had eaten a strawberry, or her path had been crossed by a hare; no more, no less.[93] Yet it also endorsed the dangerous power of women. The future of the race seemed to depend on what chanced to be flitting through the mind of the weaker vessel, whose rationality was not thought strong (a theme, of course, central to the opening jest of *Tristram Shandy*).[94] Moreover, though the drift of the chapter on imagination was to blame women for producing deformities, it also, bizarrely, instructed them how they might commit adultery undetected.[95] If in the steamy embraces of their lover they called their husband to mind, the resulting issue (they are helpfully informed) would indeed resemble him. Thus the text fanned flames of suspicion against women, while also indirectly spelling out to them the art of foolproof infidelity.

This instance runs against the grain of the book, which is not generally misogynistic or worrying, aiming to promote better understanding and reconciliation between spouses. Male misgivings about women are allayed in two chapters. One deals with the dilemma created by the cultural fetish of virginity. If, on your wedding night, your wife does not bleed on first penetration, does this prove that she was no virgin? Not at all, 'Aristotle' reassures us.[96] For there are many natural ways for the hymen to be ruptured before the first encounter with a man: Version 3 mischievously suggests that the lady, erotically aroused, had possibly been exploring herself rather too energetically with her fingers.[97] In any case not all virgins bleed when the hymen is ruptured. Hence the brisk, no-nonsense advice:

> When a man is married, and finds the tokens of his wife's virginity upon the first copulation, he has all the reason in the world to believe her such, and to rest satisfied that he has married a virgin; but if on the contrary, he finds them not, then he has no reason to think her divirginated, if he finds her otherwise sober and modest.[98]

Secondly, if your wife bears a child just seven months after your wedding, does this mean she was premaritally unfaithful? Not necessarily. It is argued that the best medical and legal testimony shows that live births occasionally occur highly prematurely. Once again the wife deserves the benefit of the doubt.[99]

Aristotle's Master-Piece has been set in its problem world and its strategies explored. These are totally different from the sexual preoccupations of the Victorians or the post-Stopes generation. Later currents were to associate sex with danger (prostitution, perversions or overpopulation), with recreation, or with the unbiddable and mysterious drives of the psyche. *Aristotle's Master-Piece* by contrast set sex in a context that was fundamentally functional – neither tainted by sin, nor coerced by the phantoms of the unconscious. Physically embedded in reproductive biology and guided by Aristotelian teleology, sex is Nature's way of ensuring generation and safeguarding the future of the species within the wider pious purposes of the cosmos.[100]

The longevity of the work shows that it evidently chimed with the mood of its times and the needs of its readers. Indeed, as later chapters will show, other contemporary works of sexual instruction also promoted a vision of sex-as-generation. There are major differences between *Aristotle's Master-Piece* and the writings of Nicolas Venette and of later authors like James Graham and Ebenezer Sibly. Being regular physicians and writing in their own names, Venette and Sibly produced texts claiming to establish new discoveries in physiology and embryology.[101] For its part, Venette's text made a parade of book-learning. Nevertheless, those texts share with *Aristotle's Master-Piece* the assumption that 'sensual felicity' is not taboo but a natural function, at once pleasurable and health-giving when pursued within the social institution of marriage and directed by Nature towards reproduction.

Precisely how the pro-natalism of *Aristotle's Master-Piece* interacted with the outlooks of its readers is an interesting question. Historical demographers have demonstrated that various strategies of family limitation (including deferred marriage) were practised in pre-industrial times.[102] All too aware of the fate of the nursery rhyme old woman who lived in a shoe, and anxious not to produce too many infants too closely bunched together, would couples really have taken to heart the pro-natalist message of *Aristotle's Master-Piece*? It is probable that the readership of *Aristotle's Master-Piece* principally consisted of those who didn't yet have children, or didn't yet have enough, or those experiencing difficulties in producing them (and in particular male heirs). Though we have only the scantiest concrete evidence about who actually read the work in the eighteenth century, it may be illuminating that the 1690 edition advertised itself as being 'very necessary for all midwives, nurses and young married women'. It was probably newly-weds, or those about to marry, who acquired it or had it given to them, while those experiencing sterility turned to it for reassurance and guidance. The fact that its sales spanned more than two centuries suggests it had some success in meeting readers' expectations.

The profile of the readership is largely guesswork, but the book's sales were so great as to suggest a social mix. While the text is not erudite, it does not talk down to the barely literate; nor was it ever spoon-fed in abbreviated, diluted form. Though, as the quotations have shown, mostly written in plain speech ('yard' is its standard term for penis),[103] the text is also sprinkled with Latin phrases and medical terminology; it contains some anatomical technicalities, and readers are assumed to be able to take in their stride references to 'the Galenists' or Avicenna. Arguably, this display of learning was attractive to readers, in that it suggested expertise.[104] The same may apply to the lofty social atmosphere the work evoked. The putative reader was presumed to be of such social standing as to be able to switch her residence during pregnancy,[105] to have access to a lavish, costly *materia medica*, to be able to order pheasant, quinces and pomegranates as aphrodisiacs, and to sip muscatel and malaga so as to make the night right for love.[106] Readers were expected to be able to afford a wet-nurse, and to have parents who might act as marriage-brokers.[107] Presumably only a tiny proportion of actual readers fell within this social bracket, but these fantasy assumptions pandered to reader snobbery, and were an astute advertising strategy.[108] Yet the Grub Street editors may have been out of touch with purchasers: the glacial changelessness of the text over the course of a couple of centuries suggests that little care was taken to adjust it to new readers. On the other hand, the continued unchecked circulation of what in a later bowdlerizing generation must have seemed a dubious if not a dirty book was quite possibly facilitated precisely because *Aristotle's Master-Piece* was perceived to be so venerable.

How far did readers absorb a 'hidden agenda' – a broader ideological freight – along with the facts of life? Did *Aristotle's Master-Piece* aim to induce the common reader to abandon traditional (folk) beliefs about the mechanisms and morality of sex and to defer instead to the 'opinions of the learned'?[109] How far was a new sexual discipline being instilled? It does not seem that *Aristotle's Master-Piece* was trying to enhance the mystique of science; rather it proclaimed a democratic epistemology, which promised to unfold to the readers the 'secrets of generation',[110] asserting that sexual information should not be withheld from anyone, man or woman.[111] Admittedly, it passed itself off as the teachings of the incomparable Aristotle, praised his wisdom to the skies, and decried 'vulgar errors'.[112] Yet it also admitted that the Ancients were far from infallible as oracles – indeed their anatomical teachings were mostly wrong![113] In citing the 'learned' as authorities, it generally *confirmed* popular lore, reassuring rather than penalizing. The text instructed the sick reader to summon professional medical advice, yet it assumed that self-dosing would be the norm, and tabled self-physick remedies.[114] *Aristotle's Master-Piece* is better seen as part of the commercialization of popular sexual beliefs into print culture than as a tool crafted for the control of minds and manners.[115]

How far, it might be asked, was *Aristotle's Master-Piece* instrumental in designating and underwriting gender roles?[116] This is a complicated issue, raising deep questions regarding the cultural reinforcement of gender identity. The text was operating within a holistic medical system, derived from the Greeks, which viewed males as inherently stronger and healthier than women (being, in humoral terms, both hotter and drier). Women were more disease prone, because they were intrinsically weaker and because they suffered the diseases of childbed. It is notably the anatomy and diseases of *women* that pervade the text. As is characteristic of medical writing, maleness is taken as normal and normative, natural and healthy, hardly requiring sustained attention.

Yet *Aristotle's Master-Piece* does not deliver a crude celebration of 'macho' qualities.[117] There is no endorsement of a 'double standard', and the book is mostly free of the gross misogyny disfiguring many Renaissance texts on women and marriage.[118] Women are not portrayed as nymphomaniacs or hags, nor does the text project the ideal of women as passionless, delicate and hysterical that became so prominent in the literature of the Victorian age.[119] Men and women were indeed seen as different, and these distinctions of course embodied prejudices – for example it is assumed that a male foetus will give a mother-to-be an easier pregnancy than a girl.[120] A key aspect of this view of gender complementarity is the belief that in reproduction men supply the active component, women the passive.[121]

Yet the text also stresses female power: children, for instance, take after their mothers more than their fathers, and overall it is sexual similarities, not polarities, that are emphasized.[122] Women enjoy parity in sexual desire; female desire is not viewed as grotesque, but is rendered sympathetically, seen as contributing to the well-being of both woman and child.[123] Moreover, there are physical grounds for this parity in esteem, since, *Aristotle's Master-Piece* insists, men and women are anatomically of a piece in respect of the genitalia; there is no 'vast difference between the Members of the two sexes',[124] for the 'use and action of the clitoris in women is like that of the penis or yard in men, that is, erection'.[125] Admittedly the female genitals are inverted versions of the male, but they amount to the same in the end:[126]

> For those that have the strictest searchers been
> Find women are but men turn'd outside in;
> And men, if they but cast their eyes about,
> May find they're women with their inside out.

– a view confirmed in another piece of doggerel that appears in the third version:

> Thus the woman's secrets I have survey'd
> And let them see how curiously they're made
> And that, tho' they of different sexes be,
> Yet in whole they are the same as we.

Aristotle's Master-Piece must be understood as ratifying sexual activity within a pro-nuptialist and pro-natalist agenda. It might be suggested that this propaganda for 'sweet conjugal love' and child-bearing is an attempt to 'sell' these institutions to reluctant young folks, women especially. But this seems somewhat unlikely, in that most of what we know about life amongst common people indicates that the young were generally eager to marry and set up households, even if that eagerness largely reflected a desire to escape the tutelage of parents and – in the case of women – to avoid spinsterhood. 'Aristotle's' advice may, however, resonate with the anxiety, expressed by social commentators towards 1700, that the nation was being weakened by underpopulation.

If *Aristotle's Master-Piece* was read by those for whom marital union was both destiny and choice, that readership would surely have found its tone and advice positive and reassuring. Sex was not presented as stained with the stigma of sin, decadence, libertinism,[127] enslavement to passion or psychological disturbance. Nor did it need to be suppressed, sentimentalized or sublimated. Rather it was an agency of Nature.[128] The text's trust in Nature interweaves into a harmonious fabric the organic philosophy of Aristotle, the optimistic naturalism of the early Enlightenment discussed in the previous chapter, and the earthy realism of popular culture.[129] *Aristotle's Master-Piece* is generally relaxed about what the Christian churches had made an inflammatory subject, which goes some way towards explaining its enduring success.

Appendices to Chapter Two

1: *Editions of* Aristotle's Master-Piece

Generations of Editions

Version 1	Version 2	Version 3	Version 4
1690: London	1710 and subsequent editions: London	early 18th-c.: London, 12th edn	
		(Entirely new format in table of contents; division of material into 3 parts; divisions of chapters into sections, etc. Remains unchanged at least until the 15th edition of 1723.)	
		1749: London: 23rd edition remains identical to the format of 12th, 13th and 15th editions. New material added: *Aristotle's Compleat*	
	First part is almost		

(*Table Continued*)

Version 1	Version 2	Version 3	Version 4
	identical to chapters I–XV of the London edition of 1690. Remainder of the edition order of contents unique.	*Midwife*; *Aristotle's Book of Problems*; and *Aristotle's Last Legacy.* This publication constant up to latest editions so far found which appear to be dated early 19th century.	*Victorian editions* (dates unclear)

The table above is provisional. Most editions of *Aristotle's Master-Piece* lack a date of publication and information about the publisher. Some give an edition number, but it is dubious whether these may be relied on. The following editions have been consulted:

Version 1: *Aristotle's Master-Piece* (1690); (1694)

Version 2: *Aristotle's Master-Piece* (1710); *Aristotle's Master-Piece Compleated* (Glasgow, 1782); *The Works of Aristotle* (undated, *c.* 1810); ditto (undated but early 19th century); ditto (undated, probably early Victorian, published in Derby).

Version 3: *Aristotle's Master-Piece* ('Twelfth', undated but early 18th century); ('Thirteenth', undated but early 18th century); ('Fifteenth', 1723); ('Twenty-Third', 1749); ('Twenty-Eighth Edition', 1764); ('Thirty-First', 1776); *The Works of Aristotle* (1790); ditto (1791); ditto (1793); ditto (1796).

2: *Contents of* Aristotle's Master-Piece

The contents of the first edition of *Aristotle's Master-Piece* (London: R. How, 1690) run as follows

ARISTOTLE'S MASTER-PIECE

Or The Secrets of Generation Display'd In All The Parts Thereof.

Very Necessary for all Midwives, Nurses, and Young Married Women.

THE INTRODUCTION

Chap. I. Of Marriage, and at what Age Virgins and Youths are Capable of the Marriage-Bed, and the Reasons that prompts them to desire it; With the Signs of Barrenness, and how long a Man or Woman are Capable of having Children.

Chap. II. General and Particular Rules laid down by Learned Physicians, how to proceed in getting a Male or Female Child; and of the EMBRYO and Perfect Birth, and the fittest Season for Copulation.

Chap. III. The reason why Children are often like their Parents, and what the Mothers Imagination contributes thereto, whence grows the Kind, viz. Whether the Man or Woman is the cause of the Male or Female Child, etc.

Chap. IV. A serious discourse of the Soul of Man: That it is not propagated from the Parents, but is infused by God, and can neither dye nor corrupt; and what day of Child-bearing it is infused. Of the Immortality thereof, and certainty of the resurrection.

Chap. V. Of Monsters and Monstrous Birth, and the reason thereof, according to the Opinions of sundry learned Men, with serious consideration, whether Monsters are endued with reasonable Souls.

Chap. VI. A more peculiar and Exact Treatise of the happy Estate of Matrimony, as 'tis appointed by God, and the true felicity that redounds thereby to either Sex, and to what end it was ordained.

Chap. VII. Of Errors in Marriage, and what they too frequently are, and the prejudice that arise thereby.

Chap. VIII. The Opinions of the Learned concerning Children conceived and born within the space of seven Months, with lively Arguments upon the Subject, to prevent suspicions of incontinency, and the bitter Contests that thereon too often arise between Man and Wife. To which is added, Rules for knowing the disposition of Mans Body by the Genital parts.

Chap. IX. The cause of the Green-Sickness in Virgins, with Symptoms, and Directions for its cure: Together with the chiefest occasion of Barrenness in Women, and by what means to remove the Cause, and render them fruitful.

Chap. X. Virginity what it is, in what it consists, and how violated; together with the Opinions of the Learned in the point of mutation of Sexes in the Womb, during the Operation of Nature in framing the Body.

Chap. XI. A Midwife, how she ought to be qualified.

Chap. XII. Things worthy to be observed by Midwives, tending to their Advancement, and what they ought to avoid, etc.

Chap. XIII. Of the Genitals of Women, External and Internal to the Vessels of the Womb.

Chap. XIV. A description of the Wombs Fabrick, the preparing

Chap. XXXIV. A Tumour in the Breast, its Cause and Cure.
Chap. XXXV. The Anatomy of the Organs of Generation in Man.
Chap. XXXVI. What Women ought to marry, with what Men that they might have children.
Chap. XXXVII. A Word of Advice to both Sexes, in the Act of Copulation.

3: Contents of 'Version 2' of Aristotle's Master-Piece (taken from Glasgow, 1782, edition)

ARISTOTLE'S MASTER-PIECE

Compleated

In Two Parts

The First containing the secrets of Generation in all the Parts thereof.

Treating

Of the Benefit of Marriage, and the prejudice of unequal Matches, signs of insufficiency in Men or Women: Of the infusion of the Soul: of the likeness of Children to Parents. Of Monstrous Births. The Cause and Cure of the Green Sickness, a Discourse of Virginity. Directions and Cautions for Midwives. Of the Organs of Generation in Women, and the Fabric of the Womb. The Use and Action of the Genitals. Signs of Conception, and whether a Male or Female; with a word of Advice to both Sexes in the Act of Copulation. And the Picture of several monstrous Births, etc.

The Second PART being, A Private looking-glass for the Female Sex.

Treating the various Maladies of the Womb, and all other Distempers incident to Women of all Ages, with proper Remedies for the Cure of each. The whole being more Correct than any thing of this kind hitherto Published.

INTRODUCTION.
PART THE FIRST.

Chap. I. Of Marriage, and at what Age Young Men and Virgins are capable of it: And why they so much desire it: Also how long Men and Women are capable of having Children.
Chap. II. How to get a male or female child, and of the embryo and perfect birth; and the fittest time for copulation.

The End of the First Part

A PRIVATE LOOKING-GLASS FOR THE FEMALE SEX
PART THE SECOND.

Treating of several Maladies incident to the Womb with Proper
Remedies for the Cure of each.

Chap. I.   Of the Womb in General
Chap. II.   Of the Retention of the Courses
Chap. III.   Of the Overflowing of the Courses
Chap. IV.   Of the weeping of the Womb
Chap. V.   The false Courses or Whites
Chap. VI.   Of the Suffocation of the Mother
Chap. VII.   Of descending or falling of the Mother
Chap. VIII.   Of the inflammation of the Womb
Chap. IX.   Of the Schirrosity or Hardness of the Womb
Chap. X.   Of the dropsy of the Womb
Chap. XI.   Of Moles and false Conceptions
Chap. XII.   Of the Signs of Conception
Chap. XIII.   Of Untimely Births
Chap. XIV.   Directions for Breeding Women
Chap. XV.   Directions to be observed by Women at the time of their
falling in Labour, in order to their safe delivery, with directions for
Midwives.
Chap. XVI.   In Case of Extremity, what ought to be observed; es-
pecially to Women who in their Travail, are extended with a Flux of
Blood, Convulsions, and fits of the Wind.
Chap. XVII.   How Child-bearing Women are ordered after delivery.
Chap. XVIII.   How to expel the cholic from women in child-birth.

THE FAMILY PHYSICIAN:

Being Choice and approved Remedies for several Distempers incident to human Bodies, etc.

For Apoplexy.
A powder for the epilipsy or falling sickness.
A Vomit for Swimming in the head.
For an Head Ach of long standing.
For Spitting of Blood.
A powder against vomiting.
For a looseness.
For the bloody flux.
For the inflammation in the lungs.
Pills very profitable in an asthma.
The weakness in women.
A clyster proper in a pleurisy.

An ointment for the same.
An ointment for the itch.
For a running scab.
For worms in children.
For the Gripes in children.
Of the Judgment of Physiognomy, taken from all Parts of the human Body.

4: Contents of 'Version 3' of Aristotle's Master-Piece (London, n. p. n. d., but nineteenth century, and called 'twelfth edition')

ARISTOTLE'S COMPLEAT
MASTER-PIECE

In three parts –

Displaying the Secrets of Nature in The Generation of Man.

Regularly digested into Chapters and Sections, rendering it far more Useful and Easy than any yet Extant.

To Which is Added,

A TREATISE OF HEALTH; OR, THE FAMILY PHYSICIAN

To The Reader
The First Part Displaying the Secrets of Nature.
The Introduction

Chap. I. A particular Description of the Parts of Instruments of Generation, both in Men and Women.
  1. Of the Instruments of Generation in Man, with a Particular Description thereof.
  2. Of the Secret Parts in Women, appropriated to the Work of Generation.
  3. Of the Use and Action of the several Parts in Women appropriated to Generation.
Chap. II.
  1. Of the Restriction laid upon Man, in the Use of Carnal Copulation etc.
  2. Of the Happiness of a Married State.
  3. At what Age young Men and Virgins are Capable of the Marriage-bed; and why they so desire it.

Chap. III. Of Virginity; What it is, how it may be known, by what means it may be lost; and how a Person may know that it is so.
1. Of Virginity, and wherein it consists.
2. How Virginity may be lost etc.

The Second Part. Displaying the Secrets of Nature in the Production of Man.

Chap. I. What Conception is; what is pre-requisite thereto; how a Woman may know when she has conceived, and whether of a Boy or Girl.
1. Of Conception.
2. Of the Pre-requisites to Conception.
3. A Word of Advice to both Sexes: or, Directions respecting the Act of Coition, or Carnal Copulation.
4. How a Woman may know whether she has conceived.
5. How to know whether a Woman be conceived of a Male or Female Child.

Chap. II. How a Woman shou'd order herself that desires to conceive and what she ought to do after Conception.
1. How a Woman should order herself in order to Conception.
2. What a Woman ought to observe after conception.

Chap. III. How the Child lieth, and how it groweth up in the Womb of the Mother, after Conception.
1. How the Child is form'd in the Womb after Conception.
2. Of the Manner and Form of the Child's lying in the Womb, from the Conception to the Birth.

Chap. IV. Of the Obstructions of Conception; with the Cause and Cure of Barrenness, and the signs of Insufficiency, both in Men and Women.
1. Of Barrenness, with the Cause of it.
2. Of the Signs of Barrenness and Insufficiency in Man and Woman.
3. Of the Cure of Barrenness.

Chap. V. How Child-bearing Women ought to govern themselves during the Time of their Pregnancy.
1. Of Air, Diet, Exercise, etc.
2. Further Rules for Women to observe during their pregnancy.

Chap. VI. Directions for Midwives how to assist Women in the time of their labour; and how Child-bearing Women should be ordered in the Time of their lying-in.
1. How a Midwife ought to be qualified.
2. What the Midwife must do, when the Woman's time of Labour is come.
3. Signs by which the true time of Womens Labour may be known.

10.   Of Judgment drawn from the Teeth
11.   Judgments drawn from the Tongue
12.   Judgments to be drawn from the Voice of Men or Women.
13.   Judgment drawn from the Chin
14.   Judgment to be made from the Beard
15.   Of Judgments drawn from the Ears
16.   Judgments drawn from the Face either of Man or Woman
17.   Of Judgments drawn from the Head in general, either of Man or Woman

Chap. III.   Of Judgments drawn from several other parts of the Man's body etc.

Chap. IV.   Of Palmistry shewing the various Judgments drawn from the Hand.

Chap. V. Judgments according to Physiognomy drawn from the several parts of the Body, from the Hands to the Feet.
1.   Of Crooked and Deformed Persons.
2.   Of the divers manner of Going, and particular postures both of Men and Women.
3.   Of the common Gate and Motion either in Man or Woman.
4.   Judgments drawn from the Stature of a Man.
5.   General Observations worthy of Note.

Chap. VI.   Of the Power of the Celestial Bodies over Men and Women.

CHAPTER THREE

Doctors and the Medicalization of Sex in the Enlightenment

*A*ristotle's *Master-Piece* is a complex text. Drawing on traditional learning and folklore, it was a composite work, and became ever more so as it enjoyed a publication life of a couple of centuries. The other great sexual Bible of the age shares certain similarities. It too was being reissued well over two centuries after it was written, though the relation of the later texts to the original recalls the proverbial endlessly darned sock: few original threads remained. It too forms an intriguing amalgam of traditional medico-scientific learning with other sorts of information. Yet there were many features that distinguished Nicolas Venette's *Tableau de l'amour conjugal* from *Aristotle's Master-Piece*, not least the fact that it was written by a medical man of some standing,[1] and consequently targeted at a better class of reader. If *Aristotle's Master-Piece* was written for artisan and petit bourgeois readers, Venette's work (at least in its original form) was aimed at those possessed of some learning.

Though written in French, Venette's text is apposite for discussion in this volume because his work proved an international bestseller, and was translated into major European languages, English included. 'Il n'y a gueres de persones sçavantes en France et même en Europe qui n'ayant ce livre dans leur cabinet,' concluded his editor in 1764.[2] In the English publishing world, Venette's text was pillaged and plagiarized, diluted and reworked. It became in effect an honorary English-language work, and forms the obvious springboard for discussion of other works mentioned in this chapter.

Biographical details of the author are somewhat scanty.[3] Born in La Rochelle around 1633, Venette studied medicine, first at Bordeaux and from 1657 in the conservative Paris faculty, where he was a devoted pupil of those pillars of the medical establishment, Guy Patin and Pierre Petit.[4] In the 1660s he travelled for a time, chiefly to Portugal and Italy, returning to practise medicine in La Rochelle. His first publication was a treatise on scurvy, *Traité du scorbut et de toutes les maladies qui arrivent sur la mer* (1671). The intendant of La Rochelle, Michel Begon (1638–1710), encouraged him to write his next work, the *Observations sur les eaux minerales de la Rouillase en Saintonge, avec une l'eau commune* (1682), with a view to making improvements in the town's water supply. Venette's other published works are on a variety of topics, from nightingales (1697) and pruning fruit trees (1683) to the treatment of fevers (1693) and the generation of bladder and kidney stones (1701). In addition to the *Tableau de l'amour*, published at Amsterdam under the anagram 'Salocini, Venétien' (not very hard to crack), he prepared a translation of Petronius which remained in manuscript. He died in La Rochelle in 1698.

First published in 1686, his *Tableau de l'amour conjugal* remained in print well into this century, going through over a hundred modified editions and reprints as the standard handbook of sexual advice consulted by the French bourgeoisie and peasantry. Any attempt to assess the work's astonishing prominence in French popular culture is beyond the scope of this volume.[5] This chapter will examine how Venette framed and pitched his sexual advice, and will assess how it might have been received by its contemporary English audience.

The work defies easy summary. Some of the preoccupations that might be expected to agitate the late seventeenth-century mind do not loom large – the institution of marriage, the prohibitions of consanguinity and incest and the canon law grounds for nullity, for example, command little attention. The moral instruction of children is not covered. Venette does not enlarge upon that favourite mercantilist topic, the encouragement of matrimony, procreation, and family life to strengthen the state.[6] Nor does he play the Counter-Reformation pastoral theologian, urging sexual discipline in the name of purity, scruple, the discipline of the flesh and the advancement of the faith.

Venette's text may appear a pot-pourri. His topics range from explorations of the reproductive fibres to panegyrics upon Classical heroes who died for love and Petronian bawdy about man-eating strumpets. Some of his themes are mainstream – what is the optimum age for marriage? Others seem skittish or titillating – can eunuchs be potent? His sources move from contemporary naturalists like Regnier de Graaf back to Cappadocian Church Fathers, the Scriptures and the erotic poets of the Silver Age. His scholarship is solid, but sometimes he enjoys teasing his readers and sporting with his authorities. On occasion we are invited to read between the lines and enjoy a Rabelaisian chuckle at presumption and folly – for instance at the phenomenon of monks, who cannot possibly have any experience in the matter, pontificating upon sexual technique. Venette uses learned wit and rhetorical flights to protect himself from possible civil or ecclesiastical wrath on such a delicate subject; the authorial presence is camouflaged.

His text draws upon the diverse traditions of discourse within which sexual matters had customarily been raised. There were rich lodes of erotica, from Rabelaisian bawdy to the more highbrow pornography emerging in the seventeenth century.[7] There was a literature of seduction, an *ars amatoria* crystallized by Ovid. There was a folk wisdom of bedroom advice, recipes for herbal aphrodisiacs and prophylactics, and remedies for disease and disappointment.[8] There were practical handbooks of obstetrics, ranging from ancestral knowledge to academic physiology.[9] Long-standing scientific disciplines, dating back to Aristotle's *On the Generation of Animals*, explored the mechanics and philosophy of reproduction, explaining gender, fertility and inheritance.[10] During the sixteenth and seventeenth centuries, learned anatomy had made great strides and a sub-section of this tradition dealt specifically with defects of the genitalia, concentrating on the new scourge of venereal infections.[11] Many works offered the fruits of fresh research into the womb, the newly investigated Fallopian tubes, the testicles, the mechanisms of erection and conception. By Venette's day, embryological debates had been spurred by Harvey's investigations into the egg and by the discovery of micro-organic spermatozoa, which rekindled the vexed question of the relative contribution of male and female to reproduction.[12]

Venette's text is intriguing, but also problematic, because it incorporates all these traditions – and more. Quotations from the recently rediscovered Roman poet, Petronius, jostle with autopsy reports, pieties from St John Chrysostom come hard on the heels of purple passages about the wiles of seductresses and pharmacological recipes to 'restore' maidenheads – and all in a text capacious enough to accommodate both Cicero and outrageous sexual *doubles entendres* without too much sense of discordance.[13] A comparable mix may be found in Joannes Sinibaldus's *Geneantropeiae, Sive de Hominis Generatione Decateuchon* (1642), which was one of the prime sources quarried by Venette.[14] But it was unique in a book of manageable proportions (Sinibaldus's came to a staggering 1,050 folio columns), written in an engaging style, and in the vernacular.

Venette's medical analysis of procreation and sexual therapeutics cannot stake any great claims to scientific originality. Rather his book adds to the digests, lectures and commentaries dealing with generation produced by such Renaissance *érudits* as Plater, Fabricius and Casserio and later compilers like Freind and Tauvry, whose texts served as commentaries upon received doctrines that had changed little in essentials since originally advanced by Hippocrates, Aristotle, Galen and other fathers of Western medicine. Lack of originality in no way disqualified Venette from popularity. Arguably, it was precisely because of its breadth of topics – from the anatomy of the abdominal tubes to juicy digressions about monsters and hermaphrodites – that Venette's book succeeded in outstripping all rivals.

For whom did he write? Who read him? With what effect? By contrast to *Aristotle's Master-Piece*, the *Tableau de l'amour* was more upmarket. It is a substantial tract, running to some 400 pages, its early editions handsomely produced. It presupposes a readership capable of handling learned allusions, human anatomy expounded in technical jargon and scholastic metaphysics. It contains Latin quotations and Greek terms. It was written for the educated. In his 'Preface' Venette argued that only a 'small number of learned and judicious persons' could be expected to love the 'naked truth' he was imparting, whatever the reactions of the 'clownish multitude'. Such disclaimers were conventional devices for shelving responsibility for a *risqué* genre, yet there is little doubt that Venette pitched his work at a polite and educated audience, and at lay people rather than the medical profession.[15] Most of its advice was directed to males, some chapters addressing the question of the ideal qualities to seek in a bride, but Venette did not intend his readers to be men only. His 'Preface' recounted how women could profit from his book – everyone had something to learn, not least atheists and libertines, who would discover routes to redemption.

The *Tableau de l'amour conjugal* scored an instant success. Approved by such medical and philosophical eminences as Daniel Tauvry and Pierre Bayle, it went through eight editions in French during the eighteenth century. Despite its popularity, however, it quickly dropped out of serious medical and academic esteem. Antoine Portal labelled it 'un roman anatomique', and by the time of Pierre Roussel's *Système physique et moral de la femme* (1775), it received a solitary footnote mention.[16] Thereafter Venette's *Tableau* sank to an item of popular consumption. Why? The slide stemmed partly from the fact that even during Venette's lifetime the *Tableau*'s medical foundations were obsolescent, dependent as they were on Classical embryology and humoralism, assailed even then by the modish mechanical philosophy, by new microscopic and experimental discoveries, and a new physiology of nerves and fibres. Eighteenth-century literati did not forgive Venette his anatomical 'errors'.[17]

But there was another reason. Fashionable Enlightenment thinkers, formulating their philosophies of sexual attraction amidst aspirations to politeness, craved greater 'sensibility' – decorously titillating – than Venette had to offer. To them he seemed contemptibly low and lubricious. In their discussions of love, and in particular of femininity,[18] the *philosophes* sought to introduce sex to the salon, by refining it, stressing elevated sentiments, shunning licentious humours and gross anatomical discussion of organs and malfunctions, and indulging in lofty speculations about attraction and enticement, innocence and corruption, identity and ambivalence. To those attuned to Diderot's aesthetics, Boucher's paintings or Sterne's *Sentimental Journey*, Venette would have seemed like a suite of heavy, old furniture.[19]

This descent continued during the nineteenth century, when Venette's book became the Bible of the French peasantry and petit bourgeoisie in versions which (despite abridgements and updatings) continued to reproduce a remarkable proportion of the original text. It irked Flaubert that French public taste accepted free circulation of the lubricious *Tableau* while branding his own masterpieces pornographic: 'Do you know what books sell best year after year?' he asked his mistress: '*Faublas* and *L'Amour Conjugal*, two inept productions'.[20] Possibly the venerability of the *Tableau*, together with Venette's medical credentials, lent it a quaint respectability.

The *Tableau* was swiftly translated into Dutch (1687), German (1698), and English (1703). In all three languages its publishing history was similar.[21] It first appeared in full-length, reasonably faithful translations, subsequently coming out in cheaper, abbreviated, bastardized and pirated editions (the fate of so many books in the cut-throat publishing trade). There were at least five editions in German and eleven in Dutch, and a Spanish translation as late as 1826. The publishing history and impact of Venette's work in Britain will be considered later in this chapter.

Venette's subject is not 'sexuality' with all its modern overtones. His theme, as announced in his 'Preface', is 'the History of Generation' ('history' here connoting 'operations'). It is a field at once more circumscribed and concrete, yet also wider than 'sexuality'. Venette's focus is physical, in that his core chapters deal with the structure and functions of the sexual organs.[22] His text, especially Part I, dwells on the mechanics of sexual intercourse, how it can be efficiently accomplished, how obstacles can be overcome and defects remedied. It is about the tangible organic results of copulation (pregnancy, parturition, offspring: Part II), and their socio-legal implications (paternity, impotence, inheritance, divorce: Part IV). Venette's centre of moral gravity is more private than public, oriented towards the individual and family rather than the commonwealth. And his concern is more with *la physique* than with *la morale*. This is not to imply that Venette was preoccupied with sexual technique and positions, in the manner of Aretine's *Postures*.[23] But for him, as for many of his medical contemporaries, the psychology of erotic attraction was essentially unproblematical. Libido was taken for granted. Desire varied somewhat in intensity from person to person, according to age, experience, stamina, climate and humoral temperament – though not particularly according to gender, for Venette saw men and women as equally lascivious. Desire assumed different forms, being more tyrannical amongst women, but Venette did not feel that sexual problems were rooted in psychological inhibition or psychopathology. His discussions of impotence and fertility concentrate overwhelmingly on physical and constitutional defects (Part IV, chs 1–3); and even his 'psychological' cures – he advocated such recreations as horse-riding as a cure for impotence – are traditional wisdom rather than the result of professional expertise. Neither was he fascinated by 'sex on the brain' – erotic stimulus through suggestion, sensibility, voyeurism, imagination and fantasy.[24] An example lies in his discussion in Chapter 17 of whether it is better to marry a beautiful or a plain woman. Venette does not discuss this hoary topos in terms of individual psychological needs, unconscious wishes, fears or anxieties. Nor does he embrace the Renaissance paradox that a man is bound to regret either choice. Rather, he briskly concludes that beauty is preferable, for to choose otherwise would countermand Nature's promptings.[25]

In short, Venette's frame of reference was quintessentially physical. He opened his volume with foundational chapters on the structure and function of the male and female reproductive equipment, discussing their malfunctions, remedies, and how male and female organs could optimally be matched, canvassing Plato's and Thomas More's solution of mutual inspection, prior to marriage. This steered him to the business of generation, above all the respective roles of male and female in fecundation, and the growth and nutrition of the embryo *in utero*. Taking the individual foetus, he asked: what determines the baby's sex? Can one predict that outcome? Can one control or change it? Wider issues are then explored. How does one explain resemblances between parents and offspring? Is it through pangenesis, as had been suggested ever since the Hippocratic writings? (And if so, how can the seed derive from the entire body?) Or does the maternal imagination intervene, impressing upon the foetus the images ruling her mind at conception? Here, as ever, physical rather than psychological explanations carry the day with Venette.[26]

Venette thus wrote a treatise about the mechanics of copulation; regular performance of the act did not need to be elaborated – instinct took care of that. Yet his subject was also *love*, as proclaimed in his title.

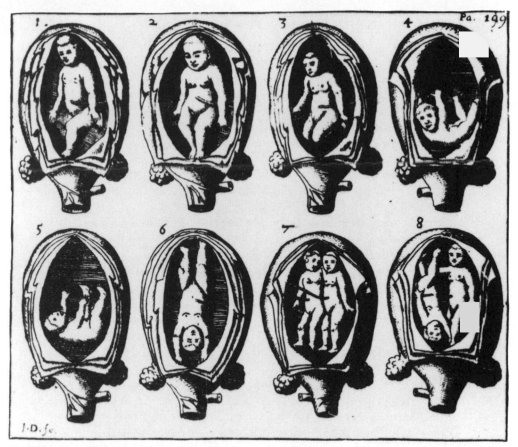

5   Different 'postures of children' in the womb, from Jane Sharp, *The Midwives Book. Or the whole Art of Midwifry Discovered,* 1671.

How love and sex would harmonize was critical. If their union within marriage seems to us the standard solution, that is partly because we are heirs to writers such as Venette. A wider historical view will help to explain.[27]

From Classical times through the Renaissance, there had been many ways of construing the intersections of love, sex and marriage, but few had been so optimistic as to meld them harmoniously together, without remainder or contradiction. After all, Christian doctrines were negative towards eroticism (preferring divine love, chastity, virginity, asceticism and mortification);[28] Catholicism was distrustful of women, and even somewhat equivocal about marriage, following the Pauline apothegm that marriage was merely preferable to burning.[29] Courtly love had gloried in romantic passion, but that flourished outside marriage. Similarly, Renaissance love poetry celebrated ardour, and *libertins* and *esprits forts* revelled in the sports of love, but independently of matrimony. By contrast, marriage remained the butt of bawdy, farce and cynicism, its mercenary and wrangling estate an endless fount of black comedy.[30]

Perhaps these literary attitudes mirrored life. For amongst the upper orders especially, traditional marriage was arranged and pragmatic, prioritizing alliance, policy, convenience, property and inheritance over love – indeed, regarding passion as a peculiarly unsuitable basis upon which to build a marital union.[31] Wives produced the heirs; mistresses supplied the eroticism. The 'long' eighteenth century, historians have argued, brought a sea-change, marked by a thaw into warmer, more companionate modes of conjugality, in which sexual attraction and tender feelings counted for more. And historians of *belles lettres*[32] have equally argued that it is eighteenth-century imaginative literature – notably the fiction of Richardson, Rousseau, Lessing and Goethe – that first saw exploration of the delights and dilemmas of romantic love *within* marriage.[33] Medico-sexual writings like Venette's provided material foundations for these original views, above all because they began to construe love as a *healthy* psycho-physiological passion, the very soul of being.

Venette's text struggles to square the physiology of sex with the narratives of love. Love's persuasiveness and power are not for him a force needing explanation or justification. The heady, heroic, but perilous sway of love is to be acknowledged, even celebrated, as a force of Nature. He writes time and again of love as 'the strongest of all passions', of 'the empire of love', or 'the violence of love'; love is 'so impetuous, that we cannot master it whatever prudence we show',[34] thanks to which people 'are the slaves of love'.[35] Love, for Venette, is unchallengeable and irresistible – yet blind, uncertain and 'disordering'. It is a fever: 'the passion of inordinate love causes such strange Disorders' – women in particular will die and destroy for it.[36] Venette provides a medical analysis of the pathos of the lords and ladies of human kind being transported by the most ecstatic and least merciful of passions. Yet he does not respond to the empire of love with fear, contempt or stoic indifference; nor does he mock like a cynic. Rather, love is ultimately noble, if often tragic, in ways that should remind us that he was the contemporary of Milton, Racine, Fénelon and Dryden.[37]

Moreover, Eros, in Venette's view, is Nature's occult *wisdom*. For the frenzied private passions are press-ganged by the hidden hand of Nature for grander designs, especially the perpetuation of the species. Libido provides initial attraction, but the problem is that Cupid is blind. It is the translation of sexual desire into the public estate of matrimony that transforms the chaos of the passions into order. Marriage bonds in their turn are given solidity and permanence by the bonds of offspring, but also by the scaffolding of civil and canon law, property, moral principles and society. Moreover, thanks to the cunning of Nature, experience proves that the most exquisite sexual pleasures are those taken moderately and regularly – that is, within settled conjugal alliances. Without marriage, Venette argued, unbridled lust would rapidly fatigue, and prove ruinous to individual health and civilized society. Yet who would accept the silken fetters of marriage without the bait of sex? Father of twelve children, Venette is frank and worldly-wise about the throb of the flesh: 'Conjugal caresses are the ties of love in matrimony . . . they make up the essence thereof'.[38]

Venette's is a pre-Enlightenment tract. This is not to say that it is exclusively Catholic in its outlook: far from it. Its spiritual and theological truths are sometimes expressed in an ironical manner that may force the reader to judge for himself.[39] Venette delights in showing that he is *au fait* with Church Fathers and Scripture, especially when their authority may be used to clinch his refutations of vulgar pieties (though prudes often condemn the private parts as shameful, Moses, he insists, called them 'holy'). Neither is he averse to casuistical sharp practice in exploiting theological support – he even recruits St Jerome, somewhat outrageously, as an advocate of matrimony![40] Yet St Augustine and other ecclesiastics who issued prohibitions that contradict Nature all received from Venette a timely rap over the knuckles. On various occasions Venette even grants himself a sly laugh at the expense of men of the cloth. Thus he notes *en passant* the taste for limber youths betrayed by a particular Archbishop of Milan, and contends that sex must be a holy subject indeed, in view of the fact that it is so exhaustively treated in Holy Scripture, citing numerous divinely approved cases of what turns out to be sexual irregularity – Thamar, Bathsheba, Hosea, etc. – that pepper the Old Testament.

Venette makes copious reference to Christian cosmology, but in his writings the Lord is habitually yoked with Nature: 'God or Nature' is a characteristic phrase. His invocations of superior powers and designs do not conjure up the God of Mysteries, the Providential miracle-worker of Revelation, but the Architect of Order. For Venette's ultimate metaphysical commitment is to the subtle wisdom of Nature, immanent in all things, producing order out of strife. Nature is constant and works by regular laws.[41]

Nevertheless, there is a pre-Enlightenment timbre to Venette's *Tableau*. It resides not specifically in any note of religious ambivalence (though one is reminded that Venette was Bayle's contemporary and that Bayle approved of his book) but in Venette's view of the elemental character of the passions. A couple of generations later, intellectuals' attitudes towards sex and feelings had grown more refined and senti- mental.[42] The *philosophes* developed conjectural histories of manners celebrating the improvement of sexual decorum and the rise from polygamy to monogamy, accompanied by a more respectful treatment of women, and they celebrated a new ideal of melting, ecstatic, exquisite eroticism.[43] They also forged myths about primitive innocence – Diderot's Tahiti – and a fashionable erotica of boudoir titillation and voluptuousness, pictorialized by Watteau and Fragonard.[44] By contrast, for Venette Venus was still an all-powerful, primeval goddess, the erotic drive was subterraneous, obscure, sublime. For Venette, the return to Nature was, in his translator's phrase, a 'mystery'.

Yet 'mystery' is a two-sided notion. It is a secret. Yet a mystery is also a craft, a knack. Harking back to the Renaissance corpus of hermetic and esoteric wisdom,[45] Venette sees love as a rite, as magic. Venette's reference point is an occult art, a bag of tricks. As author, he enjoys acting as the puppet-master or the animator of the carousel of love, or even occasionally as Prospero or Oberon waving his wand over the human comedy.

Venette is thus Janus-faced. He can denounce the tyranny of the Ancients and their idolaters, and he can doff his cap to experience. On the other hand, he knows no antagonism or demarcation between Ancients and Moderns, and certainly does not credit the Moderns with a corner on wisdom.[46] He has no inkling of what we today call the Scientific Revolution or a *terra nova* of knowledge colonized by Bacon, Descartes and the mechanical philosophy. For Venette, rather, there was a file of sage physicians stretching back to Hippocrates, and forward, through Vesalius, Falloppio, Colombo, Paré and Bauhin, to his own friends and contemporaries, supported by other philosophers such as Cicero and St Thomas. Venette's edifice was built on Hippocratic humoralism and his climatic and environmentalist doctrines on airs, waters and places, his physiology on coction and digestion. Venette backed Hippocrates against Aristotle, Galen and many of the Moderns, as well as on issues such as pangenesis.[47]

Venette was a medical conservative. His absorption in, and accept- ance of, the texts of the Renaissance and the teachings of the schools of Paris and the Italian universities was unlimited and unproblematic.[48] It was in a different direction entirely that Venette proved a polemicist. He posed as a paladin of science; in need of his protection was the damsel, Nature; and the dragons threatening her were ignorance and super- stition.[49] Venette championed solid knowledge against credulity, among which the bungling ignorance and alarmist precepts of midwives and wise-women vexed him particularly. He was derisive about magic, the paranormal and the fabulous. He scorned grotesque fables regarding sexual congress with incubi and succubi, or between witches, devils and demons – witches were not possessed but 'sick'. He recounts, it is true, the prodigious sexual feats and abnormalities recorded in the Bible and by Classical authors and poets, but generally with some distancing, sceptical phrase ('as the historian records'). His aim was to scotch folk errors such as the belief that semen from the left testicle produced girls, and from the right boys.

Moreover, Venette's Hippocratic humoralism was bonded to an Aristotelian, materialist conception of Nature. Together, they dispelled the more mystical elements of Renaissance Neoplatonism, alchemy and astrology.[50] Venette did not interpret sexual attraction in terms of higher cosmic sympathies, universal analogy, erotic symbols or metaphysics.

Venette's science of the healthy human body was essentially humoralist, concerned with the fluids rather than with the solids, and hingeing on the balance of hot and cold, dry and moist dispositions. Male and female, as we shall see, were differentiated in accordance with this grid.[51] The organs that principally concerned him were the genitals. Venette abandoned the Classical dictum, found in *Aristotle's Master-Piece*, that female genitalia were merely the imperfect, incomplete inverse of the male, outside-in as it were, a mould into which the male fitted. Yet, while rejecting the 'mirror image' interpretation so popular through-out the Renaissance,[52] he was concerned to stress the similarities between male and female genitals. As an organ of pleasure, the clitoris was, after all, a kind of penis; and both male and female produced 'seed'.[53] Venette rejected Aristotle's doctrine that the female role in procreation lay merely in providing a seedbed for male semen, offering nourishment but making no other contribution to the embryonic babe.[54] The patent fact that children commonly took after their mother exploded that simplistic idea.

Venette was writing in the early days and on the margins of what was becoming a watershed of embryology, the so-called animalculist–ovist debate, which shaded into the preformation versus epigenesis contro-versy.[55] At stake were the issues of what determined foetal formation (was its 'form' pre-existent, ready stored within the spermatozoa, or did it emerge by stages in development?); and the relative contributions of male and female – did the foetus derive principally from the semen or the ovum? Venette was familiar with the writings of the participants – he cites Harvey, De Graaf, Wharton – in what was to become a deeply significant debate within the sciences of life, but he hardly participated in it himself, being content with Hippocratic teachings, confirmed by his own observations. The male and the female, he believed, made similar and roughly equal contributions to conception. Both sexes produced seed; the intermingling of those seeds generated the living foetus. Neither male nor female was automatically paramount, though the gender and vitality of the offspring would be determined by the relative vigour of its parents.

In one respect, the male contribution was superior. In Venette's opinion, males were by nature stronger, because they were more plentifully endowed with hot and dry qualities; women were cooler and moister. The superior heat contributed by the male was needed to activate fertilization. Uncommonly virile and hot males had greater prospects of producing male offspring. If a woman were more robust than her mate, or if the climate was enervating, or if the mother had some deficiency or disease, a girl was likely to result.

Venette operated within sexual stereotypes, yet these were quite complex.[56] His vision was phallocentric (the merest glance at a penis, he reveals, will make women go wild with desire), and it was certainly man-oriented (he devotes chapters to the choice of a bride but not a husband, thereby endorsing social reality). Venette was not a harbinger, however, of the sexual division of labour destined to become medically endorsed by the nineteenth century, in which the requirements of purity in mothers and of delicacy in ladies forbade female sexual initiative, thereby making orgasm problematic.[57] It was self-evident for him that healthy women no less than men tingled with sexual desire. A young man, he writes, is a 'satyr', and 'all women are agreeable to him in the dark'.[58] But no less was this true of women, for the clitoris is 'the fury and rage of love', and women are constantly seeking 'conquests in love'.[59] No sooner is many a wife delivered of a child than she 'attacks her husband afresh and gives him an amorous battle' – and for Venette this is not 'nymphomania', nor does it sully the sacred office of the matron.[60] Nothing is so insatiable, he writes, as 'the privy parts of a lascivious woman', for 'women are naturally inclined to love'.[61]

In short, men and women share a common lasciviousness.[62] In both, libidinous fires blaze to engender transports of delight. Both enjoy and suffer from love – physically, for 'nothing ruins our stomachs, and weakens digestion more than love', but no less emotionally, for love can be a chameleon, flighty, vertiginous.[63] It is not in sexual energy but in its modes of expression that the sexes differ. Being stronger, men are blunter, more soldier-like in their conquests. More readily satisfied, males are also more readily exhausted. They love, and leave, more straightforwardly. Being weaker, women must be more subtle; they need greater wiles, are more capricious, kittenish or tigerish; they have to resort to artifice, and are more prey to jealousy, vanity, despair and revenge. For, argues Venette, endowed as they are with weightier intellectual faculties and stronger nerves, males can exercise steely self-control. Women, by contrast, live at the mercy of their desires, Venus's victims.

Venette regarded an eager libido as a barometer of bodily and psychic health, and sexual performance as medicinal:[64] 'there is nothing in the world more refreshing to those that are bilious than the caresses of women'. Copulation was a remedy for melancholy and the green sickness (chlorosis), and it mitigated hysteria.[65] In short, 'there is no surer or safer means to preserve Health and avoid a sudden death than now and then to take a frisk with a woman'.[66]

Yet he also warned of the perils of indulgence. Excessive gratification out of season could be physically damaging – not just to the parties but also to any offspring. 'Sensuality is poyson,' he insisted, and sickness was the wages of lust.[67] Joining the fray too often, at too early an age, or excessively in old age, in steamy weather or after gourmandizing – all were hazardous, while moderation in all things was the golden rule. Venette did not, however, anticipate that anxiety about enervation characteristic of many Victorian doctors, who argued that coupling needed to be whittled down to a couple of times a month.[68] When he quotes the Rabbinical rules restricting sexual congress it is quizzically, to draw attention to their teaching rather than to approve their parsimony – but men who claim to perform more than five times a night, he declares, are braggarts. Neither did Venette dwell on the Pandora's box of alleged evils, such as hysteria or what would later be called neurasthenia, consequent upon irregular or excessive sex. And he is oddly silent about venereal infections.[69]

Venette was eager to recommend remedies for sexual disability and difficulty. Some were by way of prophylaxis: couples should check before matrimony to ensure that their equipment was in good order. Others were surgical: minor operations to enlarge constricted vaginas or to remove growths from penises. Still others were pharmaceutical or mechanical: contraptions such as a cork ring to be slipped on, in case a penis were too long for the woman's comfort – though, he added, few women complained about that particular problem nowadays. He discussed various aphrodisiacs, such as opium, bengue (bang, hashish), and betel – aids to marriage, he warns, not to be misused by libertines – concluding that one of the best was water, for Venus herself was born out of the ocean.[70] Once again, his therapeutics were physical rather than psychological. For example, he tendered almost no discussion of the psychological incompatibility of partners, recommending little more subtle in the case of defective coital accomplishment than attention to the benefits of appetizing food, relaxation, air and exercise – the time-honoured non-naturals. Healthy people should not need an elaborate rule-book of love: coupling should come naturally. What they needed was the art of managing and directing love, to maximize pleasure and health.

Impotence and infertility were matters of considerable concern to Venette. He acknowledges that potency had its psychological aspect ('our privy parts are not at our nod'),[71] but by way of therapy chiefly recommended such familiar nostrums as good cheer. He dealt in far greater detail with physical impotence stemming from organic malfunctions, taking in such problems as misshapen penises and the failure of the testicles to drop at puberty. With his customary humane circumspection, Venette alerted readers to the unreliability of the impotence tests used in judicial proceedings in nullity cases, and deprecated, as humiliating, inconclusive, and hence meaningless, all public potency trials.[72]

Infertility he largely blamed on women, stressing the plethora of contributory disorders and deficiencies seated within the female reproductive apparatus, not least resulting from the fact that women were inherently cooler and moister (considerable heat was needed to produce the coction required for conception).[73] What an array of gynaecological afflictions followed from difficult labour and miscarriages![74] Yet Venette had few remedies to offer, except to remark that the craving for magical infertility 'cures' was no more rational than blaming enchantment or possession.

Certain anatomical and therapeutic problems seized his attention. One concerned the topography of conception. Venette pointed out that the traditional belief that the womb itself was the site of conception was fallacious – rather it was the 'horns of the womb', the Fallopian tubes. This location explained gender, the right horn being responsible for male, and the left for female children. Here was an instance, according to Venette, in which the new anatomy validated time-honoured advice – the belief that for producing a son, the best coital position was one with the female lying on her right side.

Signs of pregnancy were also treated. Venette sifted the conventional ragbag of symptoms, some behavioural (women allegedly shudder when they conceive and subsequently look confident and happy), some physiological (a pregnant woman will generally be 'drier'), some visible (varicose veins often appear). He suggested a number of medical preparations as pregnancy indicators, but dismissed uroscopy.[75] Yet, here again, as in all matters relating to the delicate moral and personal implications of generation, Venette cautioned of the fallibility of all tests.

*   *   *

What moved Venette to write? Following Horace's *sapere aude*, he made much of his commitment to the value of all manner of knowledge, intellectual and carnal alike. Knowledge was too important to be stifled, left to chance and ignorance; yet it was a 'two-edged knife', lethal in libertine hands. In this matter, he was himself above reproach: 'I have no other design in writing than to instruct the reader in virtue'. Properly used, *prudentia carnis*, by counselling moderation, would lead to optimum satisfaction.

It is Venette's pride as an enlightened *honnête homme* to parade free-spirited contempt for vulgar errors, inane credulity and superstition ('*Odi profanum vulgus et arceo,*' he predictably quotes from Horace);[76] he nails his colours to Nature's mast, all good and all wise. 'Nature is wonderful in all its works, and produces nothing without design,' he claims, or, quoting Hippocrates, 'Nature is always constant in its action'.[77] Nature, moreover, is fecund: 'The world is full of productions,' he writes, 'even in the very entrails of the earth.' 'Follow Nature' should be the doctor's maxim.[78]

Venette does not deny that Nature produces occasional still-births, abortions and monstrosities.[79] But these were exceptional and never the product of Satanic intervention. He would have no truck with explanations in terms of diabolism, witchcraft or sorcery.[80] Witches he regarded as crazy crones, more in need of hellebore than of the Inquisition.[81] The experience of incubus in nightmare was not a matter of objectively being ridden by a hag but a natural breathlessness brought on by lying prone; sufferers should sup sparingly.[82]

Superficially, Nature displays disorder. Yet to the discerning, a deeper harmony is visible, orchestrating what might seem the blind and arbitrary pipings of Cupid. Thus Nature has determined physically optimal times for marriage and child-bearing, and has stipulated a proper term for gestation (birth normally occurs at the commencement of the tenth month). The art of generation involves discovering Nature's laws and shunning what is 'contrary to Nature'.[83]

Scholars argue that in medico-scientific writings 'Nature' has served as a normative category and often as a coercive moral rule.[84] In sexual advice literature, 'unnatural' often carried a profound 'anxiety making' censure;[85] and Venette is no exception, painting, for example, lurid caricatures of the pains, premature decay and senility consequent upon the unbridled expression of 'unnatural' lust. But that is not the general tenor of his work. For one thing, Venette did not present Nature principally as akin to a corpus of judicial law, perceived by the elite through reason, delivered in judgement upon the common people and reinforced by physical punishments; rather Nature speaks through the instincts of the flesh. 'This treatise,' Venette can write, with a puckish touch, 'was not made to bring the work of generation or action of the genital parts, into a method. . . . That has been done before by the strength of Nature alone.' Expel Nature through the door, and it re-enters by the window. Hence Venette's manual does not thunder Levitical prohibitions; neither does it stir trepidations about such bug-bears of later ages as premature ejaculation. Venette was relatively liberal on matters like sexual postures. He noted, for example, that the normal coital position was *Venus observata* (the 'missionary'). But inter-course *more canino*, doggy-fashion, had much to be said for it, it being easier, not least, for fat men and pregnant women. Moreover, he suggested, it was good for conception, as the seed was less prone to dribble out.

On many matters upon which the Church and folk tradition roused misgivings and condemnation, Venette's medical gaze enabled him to play the relaxed, sceptical man of the world, laying ghosts and permitting individuals to find their own levels.[86] Is sexual intercourse permissible during menstruation or pregnancy?[87] It is, he responds, a matter of individual decision, need, desire and health: look, after all, he suggests, at the varied sexual mores of different civilizations, which show Nature's uniformity and culture's diversity. The Phoenicians honoured the custom of debauching maidens before marriage.[88] Its function was to minimize the pressures of the marriage night, partly by removing vexatious questions which beset modern Europe (is she really a virgin?). It had its own wisdom.

Sex was Nature's device for the preservation of the species: desire was co-opted for grander purposes. But in the individual case, writes Venette, the father of twelve children, it was also an engine of personal pleasure that 'surpasses all others'.[89] A constant refrain in his writings is not the moral, religious, familial and social *duties* of reproduction, but its *pleasures*, when taken in measure: 'Our health would be more perfect if we used the pleasures of love with prudence.' Venette prized coitus as a personal and private affair. He was indignant when private lives became unduly subject to public scrutiny, as in the obscenity of judicial potency tests. He wished to teach 'the pliantness of Love for their diversion'.

Scholars, and in particular feminist critics, have seen physicians as stokers of sexual anxieties fanned by rumour and tradition.[90] This hardly seems true of Venette's text (unless one believes that to offer advice upon a subject is *ipso facto* to establish webs of stigma and con-trol). Preoccupation with such charged issues as the virginity of brides and proof of paternity stemmed, he believed, from outmoded notions of honour that thwart Nature's purposes. The compassionate doctor urges charity and tolerance. In any case, no tests of paternity, legitimacy,

chastity, virginity and pregnancy are infallible. If your bride hasn't
a maidenhead, that could be for many reasons – hymens are easily
ruptured by horse-riding. If she does not shed blood on her wedding
night, do not fear: many virgins do not bleed. Venette is even prepared
to give brides-to-be advice on simulating virginity: abstain for a while
and use styptics, and the vagina will contract. Indeed he tells how brides
can trick husbands, using dried blood inserted into the vagina on the
wedding night. If it secures family peace and promotes marriage, he
inquires, 'might it not be allowable?' Supremely aware of mankind's
follies and foibles and their heedlessness of Nature's dicta, Venette sees
his job as to coax and cajole them back on to Nature's blissful path.

What impact did Venette's work have in England? It was quickly translated, though it is not exactly clear how many editions were published in
English translation. The following have been traced:

(a) *The Mysteries of Conjugal Love Reveal'd* (1703). No copy of this has
     been located.
(b) *The Mysteries of Conjugal Love Reveal'd* (1712). This claims to be
     the third English edition, taken from the eighth French edition.
(c) *Conjugal Love Reveal'd*. Published around 1720.
(d) *The Pleasures of Conjugal Love Explained*. Published around 1740.
(e) *Conjugal Love, or the Pleasures of the Marriage Bed*. Published after
     1774.

Conjugal Love, or the Pleasures of the Marriage Bed claims to be the 'twentieth' edition, but this is probably an idle boast or should be taken to
mean that it was lifted from the 'twentieth' French edition – which itself
could be yet another idle boast. It is difficult to be confident of the
accuracy or completeness of this publishing history, because few individual copies have survived – were they 'read to death', one wonders, or
did owners keep them off their bookshelves and out of their library
catalogues? In England none of the major eighteenth-century institutional libraries – Oxford and Cambridge colleges or the medical
corporations – seems to have acquired a copy, perhaps indicating that
it was regarded not as serious scholarship or medical inquiry but as a
work of private instruction or amusement.

How should we interpret the publishing record of the original
English version of Venette, *The Mysteries of Conjugal Love Reveal'd*? First,
it is worth noting that, while all concerned in the publication of this
edition took the prudent precaution of anonymity, it provoked neither
prosecution nor public outrage. Legal suits against 'obscene' publications were no more than sporadic in Enlightenment England, and most

seem to have exploded when personal or political vendettas were at stake, as with the prosecution of John Wilkes for his *Essay on Woman*, or when particular practices touched a nerve – for example the presentation of homosexuality in John Cleland's *Memoirs of a Woman of Pleasure*.[91] Yet an indictment was brought at Queen's Bench in 1709 against the surgeon John Marten for his *Gonosologium Novum*, a medical work highly derivative from Venette. 'Being evil disposed and wicked,' Marten, the accusation alleged,

> intending to corrupt the subjects of the Lady the Queen and seduced by cupidity, published and sold a scandalous book entitled Gonosologium novum, or a new system of all the secret infirmities and diseases natural accidental and venereal in men and women . . . written by way of appendix to the 6th edition of his book of the venereal diseases lately published and done with the same letter on the same paper, that those who please may bind it up with that.[92]

In the event, the charge was dismissed.

The Mysteries of Conjugal Love was not prosecuted; but neither did it sell in England as hotly as in France. Why? It may have been because the English market was contested. At the superior end, new home-grown publications closely resembling Venette's were also on sale, including the aforementioned and derivative *Gonosologium Novum*. And with the common reader, *Aristotle's Master-Piece* and its offshoots succeeded in wiping up the market.

It may say something about English Grub Street perceptions of how to present and sell a *risqué* work that, unlike the *Tableau de l'amour conjugal* in France and its original English translations, Marten's *Gonosologium Novum* portrayed sex as a rather filthy and degrading business, in need of convoluted apology.[93] So unbecoming was it as a pursuit for rational man, argued Marten, not a little disingenuously, that had not God prudently made it so exquisitely pleasurable, no one would stoop to perform it – indirectly echoing Sir Thomas Browne's disdain for 'this trivial and vulgar way of coition' two generations earlier ('I should be content that we might procreate like trees, without conjunction'),[94] and the ancient trope of classing orgasm as a minor epileptic fit. It may form a relevant coda that Daniel Defoe anonymously published in 1727 a work whose very title seems deprecatingly to echo Venette: *Conjugal Lewdness*. Defoe warned even married couples, in the Augustinian manner, that it was sinful to copulate with the carnal enjoyment clients derived from whores. The next generation's most popular middlebrow how-to-do-it book of generation, John Armstrong's versified *The Economy of Love* (1736), was highly idealized, and spoke in flowery periphrasis, without anatomical details.[95]

What was the English readership of *The Mysteries of Conjugal Love Reveal'd*? We do not know for sure. The first edition of the translation sold for 6 shillings, which sets it into the medium price bracket. The abbreviated later versions were somewhat downmarket – one sold for a shilling. No edition attracted review or a flurry of public pamphlets. No listings have been seen in private library catalogues or sale catalogues, nor have any private letters, or jottings in diaries and commonplace books been found referring to it. Certain medical popularizers plundered Venette's text when cobbling together their own compilations. Marten's *Gonosologium Novum* (1709) closely followed Venette in subject matter, arrangement and examples, and also in a number of passages reproduced his text almost verbatim.

Two editions of Venette's work survive that derive quite closely from the faithful 1703/12 translation, though some errors and vulgarization are introduced. The former, claiming to be the 'seventh edition' and plausibly dated in the British Library catalogue at about 1720, bears the title *Conjugal Love Revealed*.[96] In broad terms it reprints the first two books of Venette's text (those dealing most directly with the act of copulation), omitting the latter two. The translation is essentially that of the 1712 edition, but in many places the text has been paraphrased or simplified, and Venette's parade of learning has been pared down. The result is a book which much more closely resembles a practical and functional 'sex manual' than Venette's literary and scientific text with all its quirky charm and personal touches.

The second of these parasitic translations, entitled *The Pleasures of Conjugal Love Explained in an Essay Concerning Human Generation*, and tentatively dated about 1740, is basically a reprint of the above.[97] A few errors are corrected, some new ones introduced, and the translation diverges at various points – possibly indicating that whoever prepared the text for the printer had access to a French edition. The general impression given is that the publisher was grabbing the opportunity of reprinting a work that might turn a quick penny amongst a wider audience. The 'third' edition had sold for 6 shillings, whereas the later *Pleasures of Conjugal Love Explained* was priced at a shilling. What is noticeable about both these editions is the omission of the latter portion of Venette's text. Venette had written his work in four books. Part I tackled the anatomy and physiology of the genitals, their mechanics and malfunctions and remedies for defects. Part II broached larger questions of the nature of sexual desire and love, discussing compatibility and the optimal frequency of lovemaking, and giving recommendations for the best diet, hour of the day and season of the year for copulation. Part III examined reproductive physiology, adjudicating between rival embryological theories. And the final part debated the wider social, legal and religious issues arising out of love, sex and the family – including divorce on the grounds of impotency,[98] the supposed effects of witchcraft upon sexual capacity, heredity, monsters,[99] hermaphrodites, and so forth. The emphasis seems to be on the popular and the practical.

The final edition we possess, *Conjugal Love, or the Pleasures of the Marriage Bed*, represents a major departure.[100] It is considerably later, containing an internal reference to William Hunter's classic text on the human gravid uterus, a work not published until 1774. Moreover, the text bears only an indefinite resemblance to Venette's original. A duo-decimo of under 200 pages, *Conjugal Love, or the Pleasures of the Marriage Bed* not only completely omits many of Venette's original topics, but also, unlike the two truncated texts just discussed, contains far less verbatim translation from the *Tableau*. It is less a translation than a reworking. And, uniquely to this edition, alien (non-Venettian) material is for the first time introduced. The publisher or editor evidently felt it a selling point to retain Venette's name and the skeleton of his text; yet by the latter part of the century a substantial part was clearly judged inappropriate for reprinting – whether because it was out of date, or too recondite, or inappropriate in tone for the anticipated readership. It is difficult to pronounce with confidence on this matter. When we look at *Conjugal Love, or the Pleasures of the Marriage Bed*, do we see essentially a scissors-and-paste job, a patchwork of original text and modifications which will not bear close scrutiny as a whole? Or is it a carefully crafted unity?

Much of the sexual information purveyed in *Conjugal Love, or the Pleasures of the Marriage Bed* was digested from the *Tableau*, or from the works of John Marten. Sections like Chapter VIII, 'How many times may one amorously caress one's wife in a night?', or Chapter XIV, 'Whether women are more constant in love than men, and why', reproduce Venette's views. In many of its details, the sexual lore derives directly from Venette – as for example on the differential sexual seasonality of the male and the female:

Men are most apt for the company of women in winter and in spring; women most desirous of commerce with man in summer and autumn; and this proceeds from the contrary complexion, in respect both to the times and person; which complexion is nothing else than the different mixtures of warmth with cold, and moisture with dryness.[101]

The intonation of the original has mostly been preserved. For instance, sexual gratification is still presented as natural and valuable. Though this edition must date from around 1780, there is no sign of an 'evangelical backlash', no prudery or descent into euphemism. *Conjugal Love, or the Pleasures of the Marriage Bed* perpetuates the fundamental rendering of coitus as a healthy discharge:

> There is nothing in the world more refreshing to those who are bilious than the caresses of women. . . . All constitutions find benefit by it, the action warming the phlegmatic gently, and exciting the sanguine. The melancholy become gay, and by this means drive away their sadness and timidity. . . . Indeed, the pleasures we take with women cure our melancholy sooner, and have a better effect than all the hellebores of physicians. The very thought of love enlivening and strengthening us, by augmenting our heat, and dispersing the black and thick splenetic humour.[102]

The text merely cautions in favour of moderation and prudence: 'Forbear the mercenary harlot, and think of the joys which await you in the arms of a mistress or a wife.'[103]

Yet much has changed since Venette's original text. The graphic anatomical depictions of the organs of generation, so prominent in the 1712 edition and still conspicuous in the two subsequent editions, have largely been excised. In the post-1774 text, for example, there is no mention of the physical incompatibility of men's and women's genitalia; no discussion of surgical and other means to remedy defective organs, restore lost 'maidenheads' or stiffen 'flaggy' penises. Perhaps a hint of delicacy has intruded here; but we may be witnessing something more subtle, a shift in the core subject-matter of sexual advice literature. Examination of the teachings of medico-sexual authors first appearing during the latter decades of the century – James Graham, Ebenezer Sibly or A. M. F. Willich, for example – suggests that attention was shifting away from an earlier preoccupation with the physico-mechanical dimensions of sex towards a more psychological orientation.[104] Even Graham, more concerned than most with revitalizing the nation's sexual energies, had almost nothing to say about the mechanical operation of the genitals, concerning himself rather with emotions, foreplay and emotional arousal. This final edition of Venette's text is quite possibly evidence of a shifting centre of emphasis.

Conjugal Love, or the Pleasures of the Marriage Bed does not betray the generous confidence in Nature shown by Venette's original; it is not 'repressive' in tone, anxious or leering about sex. It is, however, notably more earnest, spiritual and elevated in its voice. It is perhaps illustrative of its new didacticism that its sections are called not 'chapters' but 'lectures'. Venette's raunchy jokes, double meanings, ironies, innuendoes and sly asides have disappeared, and *Conjugal Love, or the Pleasures of the Marriage Bed* condemns debauchery more sternly than earlier versions – not just the excesses of profligacy but even immoderate coitus within marriage, in ways that echo Defoe more than Venette:

> For nothing is more certain, than that unbounded licentiousness in the conduct of the marriage bed, is the ruin of many thousand couples. And let this assertion be remembered by every man, which is recorded by one.[105]

The spiritual purposes of marriage are stressed in this edition in high-flown sentiments foreign to Venette's original pitch, but perhaps now echoing Protestant piety. Or take the following account of ill-health as the inevitable consequence of immoderate venery amongst women:

> But to speak with regard to the conduct of the Marriage Bed. We often see women, who while they were maids (that is to say, before they knew man) were the most lively and alert imaginable, that afterwards became the direct opposite, grew thoughtful, and dronish, their hair becomes thin, and their complexion yellow. They are at a loss to account for this extraordinary change, but let them ask their own hearts: Have not they given too great a loose to their desires in conjugal embraces? Have not they tasted too freely of the nuptial pleasure? They have: by which means the animal spirits are exhausted; the fibres too much relaxed; and they fall a victim to their own wantonness.[106]

Venette's *Tableau* contains no equivalent to this: the Frenchman had generally advocated intercourse as the answer to female problems like green sickness and the 'whites'. And probably not unconnected with the new moral earnestness is the insertion of a more didactic Christian element into *Conjugal Love, or the Pleasures of the Marriage Bed*. Venette's original text was peppered with religious references, but he deployed them with studied ambiguity. Whatever equivocal game Venette may have been playing, *Conjugal Love, or the Pleasures of the Marriage Bed* was unambiguously didactic in its deployment of Christian teachings. In a sober Protestant manner, the editor introduces biblical warrant for its sexual advice, underpinning it with a Latitudinarian natural theology familiar to the uplifting godly writings of the Georgian age, as is conspicuous right from the most un-Venettian opening sentence:

> The benevolent Author of our being, when he placed our first parent in his happiest situation, 'saw that it was not good he should be alone'; therefore he created him a partner after his own image; but

sweeter, softer, and fairer, and endowed with more graces than Adam.[107]

Venette, by contrast, had launched his work with a sentence about the penis – a quite different author of our being! Whereas Venette had spoken of the wisdom and sufficiency of Nature, *Conjugal Love, or the Pleasures of the Marriage Bed* is at pains to emphasize the divine origins of marriage:

> Marriage being instituted by God in the Terrestrial Paradise, sufficiently shews his will and pleasure therein. Adam in his state of innocency stood in need of a helper, as the scriptures signify: And why should we be unhappy in such an alliance as rendered our first father happy?[108]

Not least, the presuppositions of a natural theology emphasizing divine design pervade *Conjugal Love, or the Pleasures of the Marriage Bed*. Venette had seen the relations between men and women, sex and society, as precarious, heroic, even tragicomic. *Conjugal Love, or the Pleasures of the Marriage Bed* by contrast drew attention to preordained harmonies, and depicted sexuality in a more sententious manner. Harmony is ensured by the 'Wise Disposer of all Things':

> The wisdom of God appears not more in any part of the formation of man, than it does in the construction and fitness of that portion of the human system, ministering to the propagation of the species; for considering their union proportion, figure, and action, and also the spirits that are fluent in those regions, the pleasure that resides there, and the exquisite texture of the whole, we must admire and adore, and own, the 'hand that formed us is divine'.

The most substantial alterations, however, follow as a result of a distinct sort of editorial addition: the introduction of new sexual dicta absent from Venette's original. What determines whether a baby is to be a boy or a girl? *Conjugal Love, or the Pleasures of the Marriage Bed* answers that boys are produced from seed emanating from the right testicle, girls from the left:

> The male child, as I have already mentioned, according to the opinion of many learned men, is conceived on the right side of the womb, and the female on the left: but though it is quite proper that a woman should pay some regard to this doctrine, yet, let me say, that the conception of a male, or female child, does not so much depend on the side of the womb on which it is engendered, as from the testicle that sendeth forth the seed; from the right testicle cometh the male, and from the left, the female: besides, the seed coming from

the right testicle, is more conducive to generation, and diffuses a greater delight all over the body. I knew a soldier who, having lost his left testicle in an hospital at Antwept [sic], had afterwards six-and-twenty children, all boys; and, being willing to make an experiment of the contrary kind, I cut the right testicle from a dog, and making him often line bitches, I do aver, that the puppies were all of the female gender.[109]

And then: what determines the appearance and features of a newborn baby? It is whatever thoughts or images were in the mother's imagination at the instant of conception:

Certain it is, that if the woman be young, and, in the act of copulation, be mindful of her husband, or some other friend, the child shall resemble that person then thought on: the truth of which has been proved a thousand times.[110]

Furthermore: what determines the shape and size of a baby? It is, states *Conjugal Love, or the Pleasures of the Marriage Bed*, the dimensions of the original seed as it comes into the womb:

But to be a little more particular upon this head, if the seed be ejected lengthways into the womb, the child will be lean and tall, if otherwise, it will be thick and short. This sperma, or seed, is the *materia prima*, of the first matter, in the creation of an infant. It is, as I said before, the noblest part of the blood of man or woman, which is, by agitation, converted into a white clammy substance; and this being more light and more active than the part remaining doth therefore ascend.[111]

Additionally: why are some babies sickly ('leprous')? It is because of their mothers' infections, their 'flowers':

For if there be nothing of these flowers in the cell of the womb, the act of copulation, as to conception, is not effectual. As on the other hand, if the womb too much abounds with them, the child, at that time begotten, will be leprous, and of a very weak and sickly habit of body, during its infancy at least, if not for the whole course of its life. However, I must observe, that children so conceived, seldom come to maturity, and therefore parents should be very cautious how they offend against the delicacy proper to be observed in this point.[112]

And, one final example: what explains the periodicity of menstruation? *Conjugal Love, or the Pleasures of the Marriage Bed* deems it is the moon:

The monthly terms in a woman are regulated by the wax and
wane of the moon, and the influence which that planet has upon
the sea.[113]

It is worth citing these instances at length to note that not merely are
these *not* Venette's views, but they are opinions that he had quite explicitly attempted to scotch. He regarded certain of them – for example
the power of maternal imagination – as factually untrue. But he also
viewed all such beliefs as the tip of an iceberg of sexual superstition
which was not merely erroneous but positively anxiety-creating and
victimizing (as, for instance, the notion of the polluting effects of
menstrual blood, which Venette disputed but *Conjugal Love, or the Pleasures of the Marriage Bed* reintroduced).

The story of the successive English translations of the *Tableau de
l'amour conjugal* poses an enigma of 'relative time'. *Conjugal Love, or the
Pleasures of the Marriage Bed* may be dated at around the 1780s. But it is
a debatable matter in what sense it is really contemporary with other
sexual texts of the last decades of the eighteenth century, such as the
prolific outpourings of James Graham, including his *Lecture on Generation* (1780), Ebenezer Sibly's *The Medical Mirror* (1794), and A. M. F.
Willich's *Lectures on Diet and Regimen* (1799). These latter works are
themselves quite liberal by contrast with much of the sex advice literature of the Victorian age; but by the standards of Venette's original, they
may be seen as sowing the seeds of an new anti-sensualism, and propagating sexual anxiety and guilt. Graham and Sibly thundered against
the evils of masturbation, while, for his part, Willich weighed up the
medical advantages of regular sexual outlets against the dangers to
health and morals concomitant upon them, and concluded, from both
medical and moral viewpoints, that it was highly dubious whether sexual
activity were really a blessing. All three were terrified of the debilitating
effects of excessive expenditure of semen, Willich being of the opinion
that 'the emission of semen enfeebles the body more than the loss
of twenty times the same quantity of blood', and warning that 'the
frequent loss of it cannot but weaken the nerves, the stomach, the
intestines, the eyes, the heart, the brain – in short, the whole body,
together with the mental faculties'.[114] Contrast the much lighter and
merrier tone of the pseudo-Venettian *Conjugal Love, or the Pleasures of the
Marriage Bed*:

There is no pleasure swifter or greater than that of love: it exhilarat-
ing all the body in an instant, and filling the soul with transport. We
need no instructions, nor means to learn to love, Nature having
implanted in our hearts something, I do not know what, of loving,
which is cultivated by degrees, as we grow up; and when it incites us

to caress a woman, it is hardly expressible how many ways there are to please us: the approaches of love being as delicious as the enjoyment itself.[115]

The implications are clear. No exclusive strand of sexual teachings was threading its way down the generations in Georgian England; no single debate was being waged. There were multiple and even clashing views on offer; and a curious dialogue was being conducted in England in the name of the supposed writings of a Frenchman who had died at the beginning of the century.

CHAPTER FOUR

Masturbation in the Enlightenment:
Knowledge and Anxiety

A book such as this on the making of sexual knowledge cannot decline a crucial challenge thrown down by Michel Foucault. Foucault argued that it was false to picture history as a shift from silence (or the silencing of sex) during the long centuries of Christianity, to emancipation (delayed till the present century) when speech was finally possible. He argued for a history not of silence but of garrulity; 'this is the essential thing,' he wrote; 'that western man has been drawn for three centuries to the task of telling everything concerning his sex; that since the classical age [that is, the seventeenth century] there has been a constant optimization and an increasing valorization of the discourse on sex.'[1] Hence the 'repressive hypothesis' – the idea that sex was rendered taboo, unspeakable – was false. And in certain crucial ways Foucault was right. The mere existence of the works just discussed like *Aristotle's Master-Piece* and the *Tableau de l'amour conjugal* refutes without further ado the repressive hypothesis in its crudest form: authors did not find such texts too abominable to write, magistrates did not automatically outlaw them, or did so only rarely, and customers bought them. Yet naturally things were not so simple; censorship and repression operate in subtle as well as grossly punitive ways. Purchasers may not have handled their sex manuals in the same way as other books. 'Away to the Strand to my bookseller's,' Samuel Pepys wrote in short-hand cipher in his diary,

> and bought that idle, roguish book, *L'escholle des Filles*; which I have bought in plain binding (avoiding the buying of it better bound) because I resolve, as soon as I have read it, to burn it, that it may not stand in the list of books, nor among them, to disgrace them if it should be found.[2]

If magistrates did not make bonfires out of erotica, perhaps that was because buyers' consciences were already doing their work for them –

or at least feeling the need to mouth such pieties to the confessional of their journal. Carnal knowledge was evidently an ambivalent thing, dangerous, desired, denied. And readers enjoyed playing with fire.

In the post-Gutenberg centuries, anxieties were ceaselessly voiced over the act of creation: authorship.[3] These anxieties applied with special force to questions of sexual discourse, its legitimacy and diffusion. Since the Fall, carnal knowledge had been original sin; could its propagation then be proper, or must it be kept under wraps? The shame cloaking sexual knowledge within the Christian grand narrative meant, at the very least, that such publishing could not be as unproblematic as the broadcasting of agricultural tips. Above all, the potential role of the medical profession in spreading carnal knowledge could readily come under suspicion. Especially in the guise of the man-midwife, physicians and surgeons were open to derision as a type of voyeur, pornographer or adulterer, gaining erotic kicks out of medical practice.[4] Yet, as Foucault implies, the game of testing the taboo, speaking the unspeakable, prompted sly and devious pleasures. Defining, denying and defiling the conventions of writing sex perhaps afforded *frissons* equivalent to delineating and defiling the conventions of sex itself. And money must have talked. As popular culture grew commercialized in the Grub Street era, all manner of sex books became profitable. Sex was prostituted in printed pornography; and as with phone sex today, sex discourse developed delights of its own, independent of coitus itself.[5]

The period after 1660 saw an enormous increase in printed erotica all over Europe.[6] Mostly, however, this was produced in limited editions for aristocratic and affluent audiences; in various ways it was erudite, recondite and coded, and had a restricted circulation. Up to a point, such elitist writings, however shocking, threatened nobody and so caused little social fuss.[7]

But the unprecedented surge of sexual writing targeted at a wider and indefinite readership triggered far greater anxieties. An integral aspect of early sex manuals consists of controversy conducted within their pages about the legitimacy of sex literature itself. There were plenty of objecting voices – both real and fantasized – taking the view that sexual discourse (the 'writing sex act', so to speak) was indecent and noxious. These protests had to be rebutted, both 'really' and ritualistically. In the rhetorical counter-arguments set forth, professions of serving the public interest loomed large. Authors appealed to social need and popular demand to justify bursting into print on such delicate matters.[8] The nation, such apologetics argued, was suffering sexual miseries and afflictions: impotence, infertility, venereal diseases – all were on the increase. Such troubles were the outcome of ignorance, or, worse still, misinformation from false friends, overconfident

confidantes or rapacious quack doctors. 'How many married Men and
Women have complain'd to me of Seminal and other Weaknesses,
Gleets, &c. to their depriving them of having Children?' demanded
John Marten in his *Gonosologium Novum: Or, A New System of all the Secret
Infirmities and Diseases, Natural, Accidental, and Venereal in Men and Women*
(1709). 'How many totally defective or incapable of performing the
Conjugal Duty, being wholly abridg'd of that pleasing Sensation, and
that from Venereal as well as Natural and Accidental occasions, is almost
incredible to consider?'[9] Such victims solicited advice, *deserved* advice,
retorted the obliging authors: sufferers should not die of ignorance. So
long as vulgar errors were endemic and quacks were puffing erroneous
opinions, responsible authors were duty bound to counter lies with
verities. He had been driven to write on delicate matters, apologized the
same assiduous Marten in his *Treatise of all the Symptoms of the Venereal
Disease, In both Sexes*, 'that no Persons therefore for the future may be
drove to the Necessity of Ship-wrecking their Bodies, Purses and Repu-
tations upon those Rocks of Destruction, (I mean those wretched
Ignoramus's QUACKS, MOUNTEBANKS, and ASTROLOGERS that
swarm in every Corner, imposing on the too credulous World their
peddling insignificant *Remedies*)'. Critics judged this a classic case of the
pot calling the kettle black, since Marten himself was widely regarded as
an empiric, not to say swindler.[10]

For medical writers who needed to vindicate themselves for launch-
ing into print on sex, it was fortunate that false views were apparently
ubiquitous and endemic. A couple of generations later, the Scottish
medical popularizer William Buchan denounced the widespread 'truth'
that a man could be cured of venereal disease by deflowering a virgin:

> Many absurd opinions still prevail concerning this disease, which lead
> to very improper practices. Such opinions generally die away as the
> public mind becomes more enlightened; but as that is by no means
> the case, with regard to medicine, we shall mention a few of them
> only to shew how little foundation they have either in reason or
> common-sense.
>
> One of the most absurd notions that ever entered the mind of man
> is, that a disease may be cured by communicating it to another. Yet in
> most countries this has been believed, and is at present in this, with
> regard to the venereal disorder. We might as well suppose that one
> mad-dog, by biting another, would receive a cure; or, that the wretch
> expiring under the plague, would recover by communicating the
> disease to those around him.
>
> It would be difficult to say whether an attempt to obtain a cure by
> communicating the disease to another, is more wicked or absurd.[11]

A
TREATISE
Of all the
Degrees and Symptoms
OF THE
𝕲enereal 𝕯iſeaſe,
In both SEXES;

Explicating *Naturally* and *Mechanically*, its *Cauſes*, *Kinds*, various *Ways of Infecting*; The Nature of *Hereditary Infection*; *Certainty* of knowing whether *Infected* or not; Infallible way to *prevent Infection*; *Eaſineſs* of *Cure* when *infected*; *Reaſons* why ſo many miſs of *Cure*; How to know when, and when not, in Skilful Hands for *Care*, and the *Uſe* and *Abuſe* of *Mercury* in the *Cure*.

Neceſſary to be Read and Obſerv'd by All Perſons that *Ever* had, (many other Diſeaſes being occaſion'd by the *Venereal Taint* and *Mercury*) *Now* have, or at any time *May* have, the Misfortune of that Diſtemper, in order to prevent their being Ruin'd by *Ignorant Pretenders*, *Quacks*, *Mountebanks*, *Impoſtors*, &c. whoſe Notorious Practices are clearly evinc'd.

To which is added,

The Cauſe and Cure of Old *Gleets* and *Weakneſſes* in *Men* and *Women*, whether *Venereal* or *Seminal*, briefly deſcribing the *Uſe* and *Abuſe* of their *Genital Parts*, and why *Gleets* (as ſometimes they do) hinder *Procreation*, cauſing *Impotency*, &c. in *Men*, and *Barrenneſs*, *Miſcarriages*, &c. in *Women*. With ſome remarkable Caſes of that kind inceited.

The whole Interſperſ'd

With peculiar *Preſcriptions*, many pertinent *Obſervations*, *Hiſtories*, and *Letters* of very extraordinary *Cures*.

The like, for general Advantage, never Publiſh'd by any *Author*, Ancient or Modern, ſince the *Diſeaſe* came firſt to be known in the Worᵈ.

By *JOHN MARTEN*, Chirurgeon.

The Sixth Edition *corrected and enlarg'd, with a copious Index to the whole.*

LONDON:
Printed for, and ſold by S. *Crouch*, in *Cornhil*, N. *Crouch* in the *Poultry*, J. *Knapton*, and M. *Atkins* in St. *Paul's Church-yard*, P. *Varenne* at *Seneca's* Head in the *Strand*, C. *King* W. *ſminſter-hal*, J. *Iſted* againſt St. *Dunſtan's* Church *Fleet-ſtreet*, Bookſellers, and at the Author's Houſe, the further End of *Hatton Garden*, on the Left-hand beyond the *Chappel*, *John Marten* Surgeon writ over the Door. Price Bound 4 ſ.

6 John Marten was one of the most self-publicizing medical writers of the early eighteenth century, boasting of infallible cures for venereal diseases.

The only way to scotch such 'absurd opinions', he argued, was through popular education, and it was for this public-spirited reason that he had penned his *Observations Concerning the Prevention and Cure of the Venereal Disease* (1796), maintaining that 'these hints' would 'conduce to put the young and unwary on their guard against the direful consequences of this insidious malady'. It was necessary for responsible doctors to be bold, in view of the fact that the venereally infected found it expedient to 'conceal' their conditions.[12]

In favour of publishing there was thus the argument from necessity. There was also an assertion of right. After all, this was the age of Enlightenment. If by no means all *philosophes* trumpeted the rights of man in a democratic fashion, there was at least unanimity about the rights to truth and toleration. Following the Horatian injunction, *sapere aude*, many authors proclaimed the sovereignty of truth and the basic

right to knowledge about one's own body and its functions. Keeping
people in the dungeon of ignorance was, it was argued, the pernicious
ploy of princes and priests; knowledge ought to be democratic and
liberating. 'While men are kept in the dark,' proclaimed Buchan, 'and
told that they are not to use their own understanding in matters that
concern their health, they will be the dupes of designing knaves.' So the
thirst for knowledge could be vindicated, not in the name of idle
curiosity or some dubious *libido sciendi*, but as integral to the human,
humane and humanist quest for self-knowledge.[13] 'There is nothing
human nature is more desirous of knowing,' contended Venette's
English editor,

> than the origin of their being; which is explained in this little treatise;
> the admirable order of nature in the production of man, is exactly set
> forth for the satisfaction of every Reader. A young man may know, by
> this book, what constitution he is of, and whether he is disposed for
> continency or matrimony. He may learn at what age he ought to
> marry, that he may not be enervated in his younger years, and pass a
> considerable time of his life without pleasure.[14]

The mysteries of generation were the key to the innermost secrets of
one's being.

Necessity? Yes. Entitlement? Maybe. But surely hazards too. For – and
this was the objection that was always raised – might not trumpeting
sexual techniques imperil the innocent? Would not the provision of
information about cures for venereal disease spare the guilty? Indeed,
might not the corruption of virtue actually be the diabolical, if surreptitious, motive of authors perversely inflamed by the *libido scribendi*?
Innocents, some would argue, no more needed to read sex handbooks to comport themselves properly than, in the eyes of the
post-Tridentine Church, it was necessary to scan the Bible to be suffused
with grace.

Apologists for publishing had their rejoinders at the ready. True
innocence, they protested, would never be corrupted;[15] and it was a
wicked world anyway, which sooner or later would profane and deprave
simplicity itself. 'It is impossible to prevent every thing that is capable
of sullying the imagination,' argued one author. '*Dogs* in the Streets,
and *Bulls* in the Fields may do mischief to Debauch'd Fancy's, and it
is possible that either Sex may be put in mind of Lascivious Thoughts,
by their own *Poultry*.' In such circumstances, surely it was preferable
to buttress modesty with knowledge than wait until other 'Causes of
Uncleanness in general, such as *Ill-Books, Bad-Companions, Love-Stories,*
Lascivious Discourses, *and other Provocatives* to *Lust* and *Wantonness*'
undermined unwary vulnerability.[16]

In works like Venette's that purported to instruct the married and the
betrothed in the arts of marital love, the risk of corrupting innocence
was not perceived as a fatal stumbling block. Heterosexual coitus was,
after all, an act which, it was assumed, every adult would wish to perform, indeed, by Nature's promptings and civic responsibility, *ought* to
perform. The business of instruction manuals was purely to specify the
right parties, times, circumstances and postures; for

> Constitution, age, climate, season, and our way of living, influence all
> our caresses. A man at twenty-five, of a hot complexion, full of blood
> and spirits, who lives in the fertile plains of Barbary, and in easy
> circumstances, is better able to kiss a woman five times a night in the
> month of April, than another aged forty of a cold constitution, who
> lives on the barren mountains of Sweden, and gets his bread with
> pain and difficulty, can once or twice a night in the month of
> January.[17]

Once works such as the *Tableau de l'amour conjugal* had stipulated that
they were intended solely for the married, there was little (at least in the
pre-Bowdler age) it could be indecent to mention.[18] Indeed, scanning
them nowadays, we may find them notably anatomically explicit in their
descriptions of sexual equipment, and matter of fact in the mechanics
of foreplay.

Considerations of the protection of innocence, however, weighed
infinitely more heavily in the case of masturbation. Signalled by a
succession of publications from the anonymous *Onania* (1710) through
Tissot's *Onanism* (1760)[19] and beyond, there was rising public concern
about the supposed spread of self-abuse. This is not the place to explore
historians' different interpretations of the cause and meaning of this
grande peur,[20] though the question will briefly be addressed in the next
chapter. The special feature of masturbation is that it was a sex act
portrayed in the advice and warning literature as entirely pernicious –
a vice doubly dangerous because it could so easily be savoured in secret
with the aid of nothing but a lurid imagination and perhaps some
stimulus material. Since it was assumed to be a failing principally of
unmarried men and women, books against onanism were targeted at
the young and single. Such individuals had no legitimate business
having a sex life at all: was it not, therefore, needlessly provocative to
put into their very hands the means for finding out about forbidden
practices? Was not the danger, critics thundered, that writings against
self-abuse like *Onania, Or the Heinous Sin of Self-Pollution, And all its
frightful Consequences, in both Sexes, Consider'd with Spiritual and Physical
Advice to those, Who Have Already Injur'd Themselves by This Abominable
Practice. And seasonable Admonition to the Youth of the Nation, (of both Sexes)*

ONANIA;
OR, THE
HEINOUS SIN
OF
𝖘𝖊𝖑𝖋=𝕻𝖔𝖑𝖑𝖚𝖙𝖎𝖔𝖓.
AND

All its Frightful Consequences, in both SEXES,
Consider'd,

WITH

Spiritual and Physical Advice to thofe, who
have already injur'd themfelves by this abominable Practice.

And feafonable Admonition to the *Youth* of the
Nation, (of both SEXES) and thofe whofe
Tuition they are under, whether *Parents*,
Guardians, Mafters, or *Miftreffes.*

The EIGHTH EDITION, Corrected, and Enlarg'd
to almoft as much again, as particulariz'd at the
End of the P R E F A C E; and are all the
ADDITIONS, that will be made to this BOOK,
how often foever it may come to be Reprinted.

And ONAN *knew that the Seed fhould not be
his: and it came to pafs, when he went in
unto his Brothers Wife, that he fpilled it on
the Ground, left that he fhould give Seed to his
Brother.
And the Thing which he Did, difpleafed the* LORD:
wherefore he Slew him alfo. GEN. 38, ver. 9. 10.

LONDON: Printed by ELIZ. RUMBALL,
for THOMAS CROUCH, Bookfeller, at the
Bell in *Pater-Nofter-Row,* near *Cheapfide,* 1723.
[Price Stitch'd Two Shillings.]

7   The anonymous *Onania* was the best-selling anti-masturbation tract of the first half of the eighteenth century, and served to create the scare about self-abuse.

and Those Whose Tuition They Are Under, Whether Parents, Guardians, Masters, or Mistresses would instruct youngsters in a crime they had never even contemplated: would such works not serve, in other words, as schools of vice?

It was an objection all authors condemning the secret vice felt obliged to confront and rebut. To speak or hold one's tongue? The anonymous author of *Onania* had his riposte. It was precisely because masturbation was a 'heinous sin', he claimed, that it was crucial that the admonition be broadcast not just to *habitués* but also to adolescents who had 'never contracted this guilt'.[21] Unfortified innocence was unlikely to prove impregnable to temptation, so 'forewarned is forearmed' was the best philosophy. *Onania* enunciated a robust policy to refute

those who are of Opinion, that notwithstanding the Frequency of this Sin, it never ought to be spoke of, or hinted at, because the bare mentioning of it may be dangerous to some, who without it, would never have thought of it.[22]

A little reading about sex would not prove a dangerous thing, the Preface argued, so long as what was read was proper – that is, not fiction or titillating, tantalizing *belles lettres* but *Onania* itself and similar pious, improving works. Of course, the line between the uplifting and the inflammatory was a fine one, but *Onania*'s author felt confident that it could and should be drawn. He was, he declared, 'fully persuaded, that there are very few Sentences throughout [his] Book, which do not more or less tend to the Mortification of Lust, and not one that can give Offence to the chastest Ear', even a female one.[23]

Not all, the author conceded, would be so readily convinced. In the 'Preface' to the seventh edition he disclosed that, whilst in earlier versions he had 'taken all imaginable Precaution against every Danger of raising impure Thoughts, even in the most Lascivious', he had, nevertheless, found to his 'sorrow, that some People, not only are Deaf to all wholesome Advice, but likewise will misconstrue and pervert the most candid Meaning' – indeed he was amazed to discover that 'some have accused me of writing obscenely and forwarding the Corruption of Manners'.[24] Hence, oozing wounded virtue, he had been led to ponder whether it might not be better to omit 'several Words and Passages, against which I know that Exceptions have been made'.[25] In other words, *Onania*'s advocacy of candour was vulnerable from the start: might not plain-speaking be obscene, if not in intention at least in effect? And the matter would not rest there. At the opening of the first chapter, like a dog to its vomit, the author returned to the problem that was fretting him:

> It is almost impossible to treat of this Subject so as to be understood by the meanest Capacities, without trespassing at the same time against the Rules of Decency, and making Use of Words and Expressions which Modesty forbids us to utter.[26]

At this point, the writer seems to be somewhat changing tack, emphasizing that his goal was less the promulgation of naked truth than the upholding of morality:

> As my great Aim is to promote Virtue and Christian Purity, and to discourage Vice and Uncleanness, without giving Offence to any, I shall chuse rather to be less intelligible to some, and leave several things to the Consideration of my Readers.[27]

For 'by being too plain', he might, he acknowledged, 'run the Hazard of raising in some corrupt Minds, what I would most endeavour to stifle and destroy'. He would thus, he confided, say rather little on the evil of women masturbating with dildos, because 'it would be impossible to rake in so much Filthiness, as I should be oblig'd to do, without offending Chastity'.[28] Indeed, even this much had to be said under cover of Latin: '*cum Digitis & aliis Instrumentis*'.[29] Moreover, as will by now be clear, the anonymous author, by a curious strategy, had been informing readers precisely what it was too inflammatory for them to be told. This is not, *ipso facto*, to adjudge him guilty of bad faith and the promotion of voyeurism; it is merely to point out the predicaments inherent in talking the taboo at a time when, and under circumstances in which, the boundaries of legitimate truth were being challenged by the revolution in popular print.[30]

The ultimate tactic lay in deflection, disavowal and offloading of responsibility. 'It was reasonable to think,' the author excused himself, 'that in the beginning of the Second Chapter, I had taken all imaginable Precaution against every Danger of raising impure Thoughts, even in the most Lascivious.' Not so:

> But as I found to my sorrow, that some People, not only are Deaf to all wholesome Advice, but likewise will misconstrue and pervert the most candid Meaning, I would in the 4th, 5th and 6th Editions, and likewise in this *Seventh*, to shew the integrity of my Intention, have omitted several Words and Passages, against which I know that Exceptions have been made.[31]

So he would have happily gone in for self-censorship. But he didn't – 'this, I say I would have done, had not some Gentlemen of great Piety as well as Penetration, diswaded me from it by this Argument': that an author 'ought never to be blamed for relating Facts as they are stated'.[32]

He had been persuaded by higher authority – these upright gentlemen – that the author was not answerable for his opinions. Indeed, in such professions of highmindedness, batteries of higher authorities, especially the dead, were frequently invoked. Venette justified his frank talk about matters sexual by contending that the Bible and the church Fathers had set wholesome precedents. And, in his turn, playing the martyred innocent, John Marten cited the *Tableau* on this very matter. '*Venette* tells us,' he noted, deploying a double denial of responsibility,

> if modestly speaking of affairs of the *Secret Parts* be blamable, neither St. Austin, St. *Gregory* of *Nice*, nor *Tertullian* should be perus'd, who all speak of Conjugal Affairs in such terms, as he durst not Translate. And by the same rule, one would suppress the Book of *Secrets of Women*, wherein he sets forth a great many things to provoke to Love.

And in fine, the Books of Physicians and Anatomists ought not to be seen, if the Complaints above recited were just and reasonable.[33]

Friends and other authors (preferably dead) were thus ultimately to blame for any alleged lewdness. As also were the readers. For the bottom line, claimed the author of *Onania*, was that purity or prurience lay in the reader's mind. 'Therefore, as I shall be forc'd to make use of some expressions in this Chapter,' he explained in his second chapter,

> which tho' spoke with a Design the most remote from Obscenity, may, working by the reverse, perhaps furnish the Fancies of silly People with Matter for Impurity; therefore I say, I beg of the Reader to stop here, and not to proceed any further, unless he has a Desire to be chast, or at least be apt to consider whether he ought to have it or no.[34]

Caveat lector: but, one might respond, what surer come-on could be issued than an invitation to the reader to 'stop here'? A parallel might be seen in the disclaimer-cum-prompt offered by Venette, whose 'Preface' insisted that his work was intended only for the 'small number of learned and judicious persons' who could be expected to share the pure love of 'naked truth' he was imparting: which reader, at that point, would exclude himself?[35]

Thus the heart of the matter: if the heinous sin of self-abuse arose from mischievous knowledge, was not any information liable to be misused? *Onania* nailed up a pious warning: 'every Body, who would write profitably against any sort of Uncleanness whatever, and not do more Harm than Good by his Endeavours, ought to be very careful and circumspect as to this particular'.[36] The writer's final ploy was to insist that his own stance was at least franker and more effective than that adopted by others. In particular he castigated 'the Learned *Ostervald*', author of the *Traité contre l'impureté*, published in 1707 and translated into English in the next year as *The Nature of Uncleanness Consider'd . . . to which is added A Discourse Concerning the Nature of Chastity and the Means of Obtaining it*.[37] Jean Frédéric Ostervald's book, accused *Onania*, had, 'through an Excess of Modesty', completely omitted all discussion of masturbation. By passing 'over this abominable Sort of Impurity in Silence', or by muttering about 'it in such general Terms, blending it with lesser Trespasses of the Uncleanness', the mealy-mouthed Osterwald had 'failed of Representing the Heinousness that is in it'.[38]

Interestingly, Ostervald had admitted as much himself. In his 'Preface' he had granted that, 'being too scrupulously modest', he had remained silent upon 'many particulars', whereon he had been 'forc'd to be defective'. He conceded that certain points should have been more enlarg'd upon; and some Objections more particularly consider'd; but this would have necessitated me to touch upon some Things, which Decency forbids. There are also divers Things, which I am oblig'd to express only in general Terms; others which I dare but just hint; and others again that I am forc'd totally to suppress.[39]

Ostervald here put his finger on the problem. It was all very well for handbook authors to protest that their writings could do no hurt. Venette, for example, disavowed that his work entailed any danger by insisting that he was merely enunciating what comes naturally. 'We need no instructions . . . to learn love,' Venette somewhat disingenuously insisted. *His* teachings were harmless, because they were *Nature's* promptings. 'Nature has taught,' he claimed, 'both Sexes such Postures as are allowable; and that contribute to Generation; and Experience has shown those that are forbidden and contrary to health.' His treatise 'was not made to bring the work of generation or action of the genital parts, into a method. . . . That has been done before by the strength of Nature alone.' Yet such blather begged all the questions. For if it were natural, why teach it in the first place? If disseminating carnal knowledge had no tendency to corrupt, how could it purify or fortify? Venette and others seemed to have entrapped themselves in self-contradictory denials of the efficacy of the medium through which they had chosen to express themselves. If not precisely duplicitous, the apologia could hardly be clinching.[40]

These were problems – when to speak, when to be silent – that did not go away.[41] They loomed large in the work of the most significant writer on self-abuse in the second half of the eighteenth century, the Genevan physician, Tissot, author of *Onanism or a Treatise upon the Disorders Produced by Masturbation*.[42] Unlike the anonymous author of *Onania* whose prime idiom was moral and religious, Tissot, as befitted a physician, focused largely on the physiological and pathological evils (barrenness, wasting disorders) supposedly consequent upon self-abuse. Tissot explicitly distanced his text from *Onania*, condemning the English work as 'a real chaos . . . one of the most unconnected productions that has appeared for a long time'.[43] Nevertheless, he adopted many of the same positions regarding speech and censorship as *Onania*. What was the proper language for sexual discourse? 'I have not neglected any precaution,' Tissot insisted,

> that was necessary to give this work all the decency, in point of terms, that it was susceptible of. . . . Should such important subjects be passed over in silence? No, certainly. The sacred writers, the fathers of the church, who almost all wrote in living languages, the ecclesiastical

writers, did not think it proper to be silent upon crimes of obscenity, because they could not be described without words.[44]

Like Venette, Tissot grounded his title to speak on 'indecent' matters upon the Fathers – in the process enhancing his own prerogative to pontificate in a quasi-religious tone, and contributing to a fascinating dialogue between the medical and the religious modes of authority.[45]

Emphasizing how 'desirous' he was, in the public interest, of 'rendering this work of a more general utility',[46] Tissot made a point of noting that he had written in French rather than Latin; the consequence, he lamented, was that he had thereby landed himself in the 'difficulty of conveying ideas, the terms and expressions of which are indecent'.[47] He stressed, however, that in such cases of potential indelicacy, he 'must be allowed the expression; the subject authorizes such licences'.[48]

More reticent about what was licensed was the late eighteenth-century British physician Thomas Beddoes, a prolific medical writer of politically radical views, ferocious in his condemnation of the gagging of free speech by reactionary British ministries during the French Revolution.[49] Beddoes was assured of the evils of masturbation.[50] Yet, despite his championship of free speech, he found it impossible to mention those dangers except through bombastic periphrasis.

Commonly begun at boarding-school, self-pollution was subsequently, Beddoes argued, encouraged by the sedentary habits of high-society teenagers, who were allowed to loll on sofas reading lubricious romances: 'novels render the sensibility still more diseased,' he accused in a passage that got to the bottom of the anti-masturbation movement; 'they increase indolence, the imaginary world indisposing those, who inhabit it in thought, to go abroad into the real'.[51] Their imaginations being thus inflamed, the results were dire, for self-abuse led to debility and disease. Onanism was a disorder caused, or at least exacerbated, by the suggestive, seductive power of language. Not least, Beddoes believed, masturbation had been the cause of Jonathan Swift's premature senility, leading to 'loss of associative power' and attendant 'nervous complaints', culminating in the 'madness of misanthropy'.[52]

One wonders how many readers of Beddoes's *Hygëia* (1802), the book that levelled these charges, actually picked all this up from the text? How many gathered the force of this crucial warning? For the fact is that nowhere, throughout the numerous pages devoted to the subject, did Beddoes use any term whatsoever – be it 'onanism', 'self-abuse' or 'masturbation' – that identified the practice. His entire account was veiled in circumlocutions and generalities. Indeed, throughout his many popular works of medical advice, on the occasions when he felt moved to address matters sexual, Beddoes took refuge in the decent obscurity of a foreign or a learned tongue. At one point, discussing female libido, he printed wholly in French a passage about '*fureur érotique*';[53] elsewhere he broke into Latin, to broach the topic of seminal emissions, stating that a particular person had had a 'debilitating' night, and adding in a footnote '*hoc nomine designatur pollutio nocturna*'.[54] Elsewhere he discussed dizziness as a symptom of sexual irregularity, in a page of Latin, 'to avoid giving offence'.[55] He further stated that he would desist from mentioning one of the causes of hypochondria by name, wishing to 'avoid scandalizing the overdelicate among my readers'.[56]

Regarding Swift's complaint – Beddoes clearly believed that Swift had brought on premature ageing and dementia by his own hand – Beddoes beat about the bush by saying that the Dean's mental condition 'scarcely admits of any but a physical solution', and contending that literary critics, 'not being professional men, [had] failed to develope the mystery fully'.[57] In other words, even in a work explicitly committed to breaking the magical, and pathological, power of deceptive pseudo-medical terms, Beddoes found the pressures too powerful to permit straight talk.

While Beddoes 'resolved' his 'mystery' in a most unsatisfactory, and (if one wishes) prurient, manner, by pretending transparency while creating tantalizing smokescreens, the author of *Onania* had tried a slightly different tactic, warning the reader not to proceed with reading his tract *unless* – unless 'he has a Desire to be chast'. By allowing the reader to close the book, he thereby divested himself of responsibility for the consequences of exposing the naked truth about masturbation. But, thanks to *Onania*'s stratagem, all self-regarding readers were morally obliged to read on. It became the moral duty of the man or woman in the street to opt for knowledge over ignorance, even while the author was warning that he was running grave risks of 'intrenching upon Modesty'. As in so many contemporary texts – *Tristram Shandy* would be the precise fictional parallel – the author cunningly secured the reader's collusion in his *jeux interdits*.[58] From *Onania* to *Hygëia*, the author embroiled himself and the reader in a rhetorical seduction.

The dilemmas of speaking of forbidden pleasure in the sex-advice literature of three centuries ago raise various issues of general relevance for understanding the rise of a masturbation literature and, more broadly, of discourses of sexual knowledge. In the light of all the best insights of the '*livre et société*' school of historians, in particular the history of reading techniques pioneered by Roger Chartier and Robert Darnton, and similar studies of chapbooks, fairy tales and other popular writing, we must be alert to the diverse possible uses of sex literature – not merely practical but mythic, ceremonial and rhetorical.[59] Early texts within this domain should not trustingly be taken at face value. A great merit of the critical literary theory of the last twenty years has been its insistence upon the need for subtler techniques with texts, and this is patent in the case of the handbooks here under consideration. They were often anonymous or pseudonymous, and they were revised, by publishers' hacks, through successive scissors-and-paste editions. We often know nothing at first hand of the author's intentions (a perfect case of the 'death of the author'). Equally, because of the somewhat shameful nature of their subject-matter, we know little about how they were actually read or used, beyond the bare fact that some of them sold and sold and sold, so must have answered *some* want in the public.[60]

As this chapter has attempted to explore, we must be sensitive to ambiguities, to conspiratorial and collusive double meanings and double readings, to ways the texts may not directly be saying what they mean or meaning what they say. Unlike much of the erotica being produced during the 'long eighteenth century', these works protested their highmindedness: they claimed to be educational, informative, admonitory.[61] But were they written as smut? sold as smut? Were they read as smut? Did they trade on the taboo? Such has been argued by Peter Wagner, who in a discussion of *Onania* has contended that this genre of work had a hidden agenda and should be construed as concealed pornography: 'the hidden aim in every case,' Wagner argues, 'was the sexual stimulation of the reader'. In other words, anti-masturbation literature, as with *L'escholle des Filles* for Pepys, was literature to masturbate with.[62]

By a parallel ploy, it may be argued that much of the advice literature was meant to be read, or at least *was* read, via an exercise in reversal: instruction manuals were handbooks in the forbidden. Angus McLaren has observed the unusually helpful interdictions that fill the texts. *Aristotle's Master-piece* cautioned husbands not to withdraw too rapidly; women were advised not to move after coition, and to avoid sneezing. Why? Because all such acts would hinder conception. Venette listed the coital postures to be avoided because they were unlikely to lead to pregnancy. Was not all this, it may be suggested, veiled contraceptive guidance? Were not these works the devil's manuals? The questions are crucial, but we can hardly expect clear and distinct answers. For we are confronted with a profound problem.[63]

Print culture brought sex books into prominence. Thereafter people (as before) had sex, and people (unlike previously) had sex books. Some had one, some had the other, some had both. The relations between writing sex books, reading sex books, and having sex – sex in the body, sex on the brain, thought and action, use and abuse – are profoundly enigmatic and subject to Shandyesque regressions.[64]

Foucault was only half right in his demolition of the 'repressive hypothesis'. In its crude form, the hypothesis is false; there was, precisely as he stressed, ever more writing about sex, writings that were rarely wholly banned. Nevertheless, Foucault was misleading on another issue. For, in a certain regard, sex was indeed comprehensively silenced, or at least muffled. Despite all the coitus going on, despite all the copies of erotica in circulation, our hard evidence about the sexual lives, thoughts and feelings of Europeans in 1650, 1750 or 1850 remains pathetically meagre, because it was a domain of life that was furtive and shameful, as was the body itself, whose fragmented past is only now being pieced together. Hundreds of British working-class autobiographies survive from these centuries, but hardly any mention sex, let alone masturbation.[65]

On the positive side, we do have the texts discussed. We must never mistake texts for people. But texts, properly read, can illuminate. And on the potentially positive side, modern scholarship has a subtle programme of topics recovering sexualities long hidden from history. Over the last generation, social historians have been rediscovering the history of the silenced, the micro-realities of the dynamics of gender, of parents and children, family and household, masters and servants, probing the interpersonal complexities of struggle and collusion, duplicity and complicity, control and resistance, individuation and stereotyping, socialization and difference. Richer histories of private life, of popular culture, of lifestyle, of representations, are being constructed, histories from below that avoid the trivialities of traditional social history – history with the politics left out – and assume significance by being alert to culture and gender conflict, the construction of the self, the production and reproduction of power relations, and, not least, the capacity of language and symbols to define reality.[66] One dimension this new social history can reclaim is sexuality. Works like the anti-onanist literature are signs of, yet also constitutive of, such developments.

CHAPTER FIVE

Quackery and Erotica

Rival readings of the sexual history of England during the 'long eighteenth century' confront us. Some see liberty; others the creation of anxiety. Many historians have drawn attention to the 'libertarian' aspects – the century's eroticism and pornography. Others reply that pornography betrays fear and hate, offering a revisionist outlook that presents a darker picture: a more ferocious male libertinism, intensified exploitation of vulnerable servant women, teenage prostitutes, the excitation of new sexual fears about masturbation, nymphomania, hysteria, enervation.[1]

Both pictures have their truth. The mistake is to present them as mutually incompatible rather than as concomitants. The Georgian sexual economy was public and permissive in its fashions, its street life, gossip, and not least in its erotica.[2] This point is confirmed by its popular medico-sexual literature. As has been seen, in such treatises as *Aristotle's Master-Piece* the keynote is not the blessings of chastity or restraint, but the joys of sex, so long as they were experienced under appropriate moral, personal and medical circumstances.[3] The assumption of Georgian medico-sexual writings is that heterosexual erotic activity is and ought to be pleasurable and healthy.

It was a culture setting great store by erotic appearance. All manner of cosmetic and medical preparations were marketed for heightening sexual attractiveness, most beauty preparations being targeted at glamorizing the ladies. As part of a profound and ambiguous transformation in social status and power of women, being female was becoming equated with 'femininity'; increasingly treated as sex objects, women were expected to subscribe to eroticized norms in appearance.[4] As a consequence, the market was flooded with preparations claiming to cleanse women's skin, improve the complexion, remove, or conceal, spots, expunge scurf and other blemishes, and rid women of facial hair and body odour. The 'young look' came into fashion amongst the late

Georgians, though – by contrast to the twentieth century – it did not lead to a preoccupation with slimming preparations.[5]

Quasi-medical commercial preparations contributed to the selling of sex. Many also conveyed the promise of fecundity. Amongst the constant refrains in quack bills during the 'long eighteenth century' was the promise to cure infertility (it was typically assumed that women were to blame) by restoring the courses.[6] Should we here be reading between the lines? For one way of 'removing obstructions' or 'restoring the courses' is, of course, procuring abortion. Are all the advertisements promising to 'remove obstructions' selling not fertility but abortifacients? Some medicines for women deliver explicit warnings that they are *not* to be taken by women 'with child' – surely a broad hint. Likewise, what do we make of it when Samuel Solomon states that, thanks to his Balm of Gilead, 'ladies at any time of life may by this medicine, be freed from one of the most afflicting disorders incident to the sex, and at a certain period, it is most highly useful'?[7]

But certain preparations for 'women's diseases' genuinely seem to have been targeted at ladies wishing to conceive and be fruitful (rather than those seeking to terminate pregnancy). And why not? It was a medical commonplace that the fecund woman was the healthy woman, ignominy was attached to the wife who failed to produce heirs, and barren women commonly visited spas and drank medicinal waters in hopes of conceiving.[8] A 'Doctor of Physick' advertising 'The Private Cure' played upon the common association between women's diseases in general and barrenness in particular, by promising to be able to cure all at a stroke, including

> Fits of the Mother [hysteria], Vapours rising up to the Throat, Passions or Tremblings of the Heart, Obstructions, Convulsions, Green Sickness, Weakness, and Pains of the Back, [He also] makes Fruitful, takes away the cause of Barrenness or impotence in men or Women, which secret preserves youth and prolongs life.[9]

Georgian culture associated sexuality with health, happiness, beauty and fertility, and quack medicine pledged to promote these ends, though there was a darker side: venereal disease.[10] Usually, there was no beating about the bush. One bill arrests the reader with the headline: 'An Herculeon Antidote Against the POX' (the public-spirited advertiser promises that so as not to 'give Incouragement to vice' he will not breathe a word about the ingredients used in his remedy).[11] Another bill, put about by John Case, announced in bold type, 'A Most Infallible, and Sure Cheap Secret Safe and Speedy Cure for a Clap',[12] and 'Dr Rivers' headed a poster 'The True Symptoms of a Clap or Pox with its

Cure', stating he was available for consultations at the Golden Ball in Three Kings Court on Ludgate Hill, where he had 'a light at the door in an evening'.[13] Another bill, headed 'Venus Deceiv'd or An Account of the Seat, and Nature of a *Clap*', sold a cure, a mere 'seven' doses of which would do the trick (a hint, surely, of a magic number?)[14] Quackish promotion of potency, fertility and VD cures traded on fantasies about sexual knowledge.

Venereal disease remained a fertile seedbed for quackish practices, performed no less by doctors who in many respects were impeccably 'regular', because it was shameful: secret diseases bred secret remedies.[15] John Marten's *Treatise . . . of the Venereal Disease* (1708) was perhaps the lengthiest exposé and denunciation of the villainy of clap quackery. Yet Marten's is a comprehensive work of self-advertisement, his boasts being no less grandiloquent than those of the quacks he vilifies; and he was himself a prime target of Spinke's *Quackery Unmask'd*.[16] Medical quackery treated sex as a straightforward system of desires. It offered beauty preparations to heighten female sex appeal, and 'pick-me-ups' to rejuvenate rakes and roués. And it purveyed pills to the poxed. Yet the Enlightenment also regarded sex as more than coitus – as culture; in other words, the focus shifted from *sex* to *sexuality* in ways pregnant with possibilities, not least for quackery. Above all, an influential rhetoric emphasized that sexual desire must be treated not as a given biological, physiological and pathological drive but as psychosocial. Sexuality, Enlightenment thinkers argued, was inseparable from sensibility, and hence was a function of the nervous system and the imagination. The head was the organ of arousal,[17] and sexuality was a state of mind. Opportunities arose for quack writers to set themselves up as the 'sexperts' of their age, precisely because of the special insights their trade gave them into the techniques of seduction.[18] If, to the Enlightenment mind, the secret of sexual power lay in persuasion, who better than quacks to teach that art? The avatar of this late Enlightenment merger of quackery and sexuality was James Graham, whose medico-sexual theories encapsulated key Enlightenment convictions and who briefly proved a major cultural catalyst.[19]

Born in Edinburgh in 1745, Graham studied medicine at his home university. In 1770 he married and settled in Pontefract, subsequently migrating to America, where he practised physic, specializing as an oculist and aurist, met Benjamin Franklin, and became an enthusiast for medical electricity. Travels in Europe were followed in the late 1770s by medical practice in fashionable Bath. Success encouraged him to try his fortune in London. Opening his 'Temple of Health' ('Templum Aesculapio Sacrum') in 1780 at the fashionable Adelphi, just off the Strand, he combined lectures and multi-media spectacle with a practice privileging electrical therapy. Here he first unveiled his Celestial Bed, hired out at £50 a night as a specific against impotence and   sterility.

Graham shortly quit the Adelphi (probably because of debts), removing to the less salubrious Pall Mall, where his 'libidinous' lectures on generation kept him in the public gaze. Forced to sell up in 1783 by his creditors, Graham put his doctrines and cures on the road, and modified his views and his style in the 1780s. He called himself 'born again',[20] preaching an idiosyncratic evangelical Christianity, which wedded passionate defence of the divinity of Christ to a cosmology glorifying the spiritual unity of the Creation. He grew ardent for medical simplicity, advocating the healing power of Nature and trusting to therapeutics of water and air.

Both impresario and fanatic, Graham won notoriety thanks to the Celestial Bed, 'whose magical influences', so he apostrophized,

> are now celebrated from pole to pole and from the rising to the setting of the sun. [The Celestial Bed] is 12ft. long by 9ft. wide, supported by forty pillars of brilliant glass of the most exquisitive workmanship, in richly variated colours. The super-celestial dome of the bed, which contains the odoriferous, balmy and ethereal spices, odours and essences, which is the grand reservoir of those reviving invigorating influences which are exhaled by the breath of the music and by the exhilarating force of electrical fire, is covered on the other side with brilliant panes of looking-glass.
>
> On the utmost summit of the dome are placed two exquisite figures of Cupid and Psyche, with a figure of Hymen behind, with his torch flaming with electrical fire in one hand and with the other, supporting a celestial crown, sparkling over a pair of living turtle doves, on a little bed of roses.
>
> The other elegant group of figures which sport on the top of the dome, having each of them musical instruments in their hands, which by the most expensive mechanism, breathe forth sound corresponding to their instruments, flutes, guitars, violins, clarinets, trumpets, horns, oboes, kettle drums, etc.
>
> At the head of the bed appears sparkling with electrical fire a great first commandment: 'BE FRUITFUL, MULTIPLY AND REPLENISH THE EARTH'. Under that is an elegant sweet-toned organ in front of which is a fine landscape of moving figures, priest and bride's procession entering the Temple of Hymen.
>
> The chief principle of my Celestial Bed is produced by artificial lodestones. About 15 cwt. of compound magnets are continually pouring forth in an everflowing circle.[21]

The bed was presented to the late Georgian fashionable world as a fertility shrine, available for hire on a nightly basis. 'Should pregnancy at any time not happily ensue' from the regular course of conjugal love, promised Graham,

> I have the most astonishing method to recommend which will infallibly produce a genial and happy issue, I mean my Celestial or Magnetico-electrico bed, which is the first and only ever in the world: . . . Any gentleman and his lady desirous of progeny, and wishing to spend an evening in the Celestial apartment, which coition may, on compliment of a £50 bank note, be permitted to partake of the heavenly joys it affords by causing immediate conception, accompanied by the soft music. Superior ecstasy which the parties enjoy in the Celestial Bed is really astonishing and never before thought of in this world: the barren must certainly become fruitful when they are powerfully agitated in the delights of love.[22]

Thus Graham's much-bruited *chef d'œuvre.* He clearly intended it should make money, since he charged £50 a night for its use. It provided him with vast publicity, being the subject of smutty lampoons such as *The Celestial Beds* (1781), seemingly a self-satire penned by Graham – evidently a believer that all publicity is good publicity – which depicted jaded couples flocking in, as if to a new ark, to repopulate the species:

> Libertines and debauchees
> Thither haste with knocking knees;
> Genial and prolific fires,
> Shall wake your pulse to new desires;
> Tho' your embers should be dead,
> Stretch on his celestial bed;
> Soon you'll feel the vital flame,
> Rushing thro' your icey frame!
> Fann'd by agents all divine!
> Who condescend with him to dine.
>
> Barren Does in crouds resort
> To the Quack's imperial court;
> Sweeter, lovelier you'll seem,
> When you get a touch from him;
> In your husband's doating eyes
> You shall prove a precious prize;
> His magnetic influence
> Ev'ry hour new joys dispense.

Was this prototype king-size, as contemporaries insinuated, a hotbed of debauch and prostitution? Graham insisted that the bed was not for dissipated voluptuaries but for sterile couples desiring heirs, and that it was guaranteed to overcome flaccidity by 'an electrical stroke or two';[23] moreover, it would secure, he assured the public, the 'propagating of Beings rational, and far stronger and more beautiful in mental as well as in bodily endowments, than the present puny, feeble, and nonsensical race of probationary mortals, which crawl, and fret, and politely play at cutting one another's throats for nothing at all, on most parts of this terraqueous globe'.[24] London had no shortage of brothels and classy bagnios boasting buxom bed-mates, so it is unlikely that Graham's sentiments about sexual rejuvenation were solely a pious front for libertinism or commercial sex.

As with all astute physicians, Graham's practice had made him acutely aware of the psychology of malaise and recovery, and specifically of 'the influence of imagination in the affairs of love'. 'Strong impressions' and 'amorous stories' were crucial in stimulating the libido. Voyeurism worked:

> An old woman at Norwich, who had no teeth, sitting in the market selling greens, saw a horse copulating a mare; when she first observed the horse, she happened to have a shilling between her gums; her whole soul was fixed on the motions of the horse and mare, she was so violently agitated that she bit the shilling in two!

And, Graham insisted, it was proper to excite 'the passions by all decent means'; he told the tale of

> an Edinburgh hair-dresser, who had been married to a healthy woman some years, but had no children [who] was sent for to dress a fine beautiful young lady; when performing the operation, he was so captivated with her beauty, he found himself so animated, that he could no longer contain; he made a trifling excuse, ran home in a desperate hurry, and got his wife with three children at once. . . .

The Celestial Bed would evidently kindle the flames of desire through seductive suggestion – its subtle lighting, textures, colours, décor, and soft music. Graham's aim, in short, was to encourage sexual fulfilment – he did not 'talk of a critical moment, but of a critical hour' – and to do so even by *risqué* means, such as the use of pornographical prints or unorthodox postures: 'a certain lady of quality in this country,' he reported, 'makes no scruple to say in company, that she could not be got with child without riding St George.'

Yet, typically orthodox, Edinburgh-school medicine, his therapeutics gave pride of place to organic aetiologies and somatic treatments, and he betrayed no sign of regarding his own medical apparatus and medicines as mere stage-prop placebos, effective only through suggestion. He never contended that sexual difficulties were primarily rooted in the mind – or, as we might say, in the unconscious. He never systematically set out to deploy psychological healing strategies.[25] Graham's regimen for restoring virility gave priority to the physical, albeit in a wider social context.

Graham was, perhaps, a wizard showman flourishing in the lubricious twilight world of sex aids, yet he was neither a pander nor a pornographer. His erotic apparatus and therapies were part of a wider medical philosophy. What exactly, then, did Graham think of sex? And how did his views relate to contemporary carnal knowledge?

For Graham the key to sex was *health*, understood personally, biologically and socially. In a tradition which Foucault has traced back to Antiquity, he aimed to demonstrate that proper eroticism would enhance organic well-being. This had a psychological dimension, but Graham principally thought of sex in a hygienic-organic context. The touchstone of well-being, he claimed, was healthy eroticism, indeed the drive to propagate the species. Fulfilment of the urge to procreate, multiply and perpetuate mankind is the message of his pamphlet, *Lecture on the Generation, Increase and Improvement of the Human Species*, and is a theme handled more broadly in his later cosmological writings, where he conjures up a vision of the economy of Nature endlessly renewing itself, teeming with self-sustaining and perpetuating life-forms. 'Gentlemen,' Graham would confide to his audiences,

> the most important business of everything in the animal creation, is to propagate the number of its *species*; this is an object of the greatest consequence, so great, that the attention of the philosopher and men of science have [*sic*] been directed to consider with care, and endeavour to find out the real cause of generation.[26]

The healthy creature, he insisted, is the sexual creature, and sexual energy the acid test of physical well-being: or, put bluntly, 'The genitals are the true pulse, and infallible barometer of health.'[27] His remit, he claimed, was 'the health, beauty, vigour, happiness and security of the human species, and . . . the happy prolongation of human life'.[28] 'The *Propagation* of the human species is the subject of our attention.'[29]

Sexual instinct and its gratification ought to be an unproblematic, natural urge for men, and equally for women, for the fair sex was no less libidinous: 'Were we to be made acquainted with the real sentiments of sex,' he insisted,

even the chastest, coldest, most reserved, and least amorously com-
plexioned woman in the world, we would find her to be precisely of
the same taste, with the bishop's lady, who very frankly declared that,
for her part, she liked to have a GOOD THING in the house, or in the
bed by her, whether she made use of it or not.[30]

But, gazing at his audience, Graham espied only a 'moving hospital'
of weaklings catastrophically failing to reproduce itself. Civilized man
had rendered himself an endangered species: 'We are told by political
writers' – he perhaps had 'Estimate' Brown or Richard Price in mind –
'that the inhabitants of this island have decreased amazingly, and every
succeeding generation becomes more and more weekly [sic]; tho' these
are alarming circumstances, and call loudly for a remedy, yet it is totally
neglected.'[31] Graham's fears of depopulation, that endless lament of
contemporary moralists, were, of course, grotesquely mistaken, and it is
ironic that, little more than a decade later, Malthus would prove no less
terrified of the superfecundity of the masses.[32] The point, however, is
that Graham's anxiety was not a cranky idiosyncrasy.

This failure to reproduce stemmed from languishing libidos; and this
in turn was rooted in decrepit personal and social health. Doom lay
ahead, for

> the degeneracy and imbecility of body and mind, so prevalent in this
> country, not only destroys the state, but likewise the peace and happi-
> ness of individuals; for no man can have felicity in the hymeneal state
> when his wife is barren. Indeed, health and children are as necessary
> to the prosperity of mankind, as the genial rays of the sun are to
> enliven and cherish the fragrant plants.[33]

Graham's sexological strategy was to recuperate individual and social
health by reinvigorating vital energies, and thereby restock the nation.[34]
High society undermined wholesome sex. Graham called for social
mores which would treat desire with *less* permissiveness, maintaining
that sex could be healthy and ecstatic only within marriage. Reversing
the views expressed earlier in the century by Bernard Mandeville,
Graham claimed that sexual vibrancy could be enhanced at a stroke by
outlawing licentiousness: 'The first step towards the encouraging of
matrimony, would be to suppress all public prostitution.'[35] The heart of
the matter was that advanced society was enfeebling generative urges
because it rendered people weak and emasculated. By this Graham did
not primarily mean sick in the head but *physically* degenerate: moderns
were becoming the puny brood of 'luxury, folly and dissipation'.[36] The
pleasures of procreation were on the wane because the nation was unfit;
sexual appetite was flagging because *other* appetites went uncurbed. The

profligate gourmandized and guzzled foreign tea, coffee, 'fiery liquors' and narcotics, sometimes mistaking them for aphrodisiacs.[37] They kept late hours, indulging in 'midnight racketing', stifled themselves in stuffy rooms, and slept on feather beds, which destroyed muscle tone. Such decadent living not only sapped sexual drives, but also resulted in sickly and malformed offspring.[38] 'It is incumbent on us,' Graham insisted,

> to restore that manly firmness and vigour, which, from the depravity of human nature, by means of luxury and dissipation, has for more than a century been lost: this has brought on diseases which have enervated and debilitated the human race. The great author of our being, has, by the strongest ties, bound us to temperance and sobriety: but we, regardless of that authority or our own peace and felicity, have brought on diseases, and are so interwoven in our constitutions, which renders us totally unfit for the noble office of producing a vigorous and healthy offspring.[39]

Living clean and decent, by contrast, following the 'plain and simple laws of nature',[40] promised good health, sexual energy, sturdy offspring and long life. (Follow my advice and live to 150, boasted the man who died at 49.) Like Erasmus Darwin, Graham believed that honouring Venus meant abandoning Bacchus – and hot beverages as well – cold milk and water were more tonic. He advocated dietary discipline and a frugal food intake: macrobiotics were better than meat.[41] The raw was purer than the cooked (raw eggs were aphrodisiac). Vegetarians made the best lovers. 'What is it,' he asked, 'that makes the Irish ladies . . . such excellent companions in bed? They run in the open air, and eat of good mealy potatoes broken down in milk.' A bracing atmosphere, wide-open windows, fresh air, hard beds and early hours, and obedience to the Wesleyan golden rule of cleanliness – all were imperative, especially 'bathing every night and morning, if not the whole body and limbs, at least the *genitalia* and fundament, with very cold water'.[42] Men were repulsed by female slatternliness: if gentlemen preferred whores, it was because professionals had to keep themselves sweet smelling.[43] Yet he held no store by cosmetics and aphrodisiacs, deploring cantharides in particular, while urging bathing the genitals in icy water as a stimulant.[44] Above all, Graham argued that family tranquillity provided the perfect setting for rapturous coupling: 'Domestic music, gentlemen! little family concerts, and especially singing together, or in turn, trifling as these may appear to some, I strongly recommend,' he told his listeners,

> and still more strongly, regular worship, and sentimental, philosophical, and religious conversations and intercourses. For, gentlemen,

after the souls of an amiable couple have been softened, harmonized, illumined, and filled with approving peace, by duties and amusements so rational and delightful, when they return to an early bed, sober, serene and healthful! their bodies and their souls rush sweetly together! with the fullest, purest, intensest, and most celestial transports![45]

Healthy sexuality would arise spontaneously from wholesome social habits. But it also required *self*-discipline. In a familiar litany, Graham instructed that 'early venery' – fornication begun at too raw an age[46] – or overindulged in old age, or, indeed, too frequent coition at any age, all weakened performance and stamina, and so were short-sighted sacrifices to Eros.[47] The goal must be to 'exalt and prolong the pleasure of the marriage bed'.[48]

For Graham, as for many of his ilk, the evil of evils was masturbation.[49] Why this phobia? Self-abuse was the enemy of generation, wasting semen and sapping vigour. Graham helped develop the popular vitalist theory which saw semen as the elixir, the principle of universal vitality, a 'true and inconceivably powerful stimulus', an 'exquisitely penetrating seminal liquor' – well-nigh the world-soul: 'The seminal principle, or luminous, ever-active balsam of life, is the grand staff, strength, all-animating vital source and principle of the beauty, vigour, and serenity, both of body and of mind.'[50]

Graham was dubious of the preformationist embryological view that the 'type' of future generations lay exclusively in 'homunculi' stored in the semen. Nevertheless he believed that the seminal fluid carried the 'vivifying elementary fire', which enlivened the foetus. As the sacred torch-bearer of vitality, it was a precious liquor, whose waste spelt danger and desolation. Though nature 'be in raptures during the discharge of this matter,' he noted, 'yet when that is past, she grows sad for the loss of it, as well as for the damage done to the individual'.[51] Semen was not to be squandered by masturbation. Bathe your genitals *post coitum* in cold water, Graham told his audience, to stop dribbling emissions.

In the interests of spermatic economy, Graham demanded severe sexual self-discipline. Old lechers must heed: 'The frequent use of venereal pleasures is hurtful to all men whatever, but especially to such as are old.'[52] But above all, youth needed to be warned:

The young man who lives in the world, soberly, regularly, usefully, and perfectly continently, without ever once having known what any seminal emission is till he arrives at his twenty-first – or even to his twenty-fifth year; and is married – that young man is a hero indeed – an Hercules – an Angel – a God! I had almost said, in point of health, strength, beauty, and brilliancy, of body and of mind; when compared to those poor creeping tremulous, pale, spindle-shanked wretched creatures who crawl upon the earth, spirting, dribling [sic], and drawing off, alone, or with their vile unfortunate street trulls, or other mates, in what is called the natural way, at twelve, fourteen, sixteen or eighteen years of age; As for my part, gentlemen, if you will pardon this breach of politeness, I seriously declare, that had I my time to live over again, and were I possessed of the same knowledge I now have, I would be, I believe, thirty or forty years of age, before I would know any at all, from personal experience, about these matters.

Abstinence was proper during menstruation and pregnancy (at such times, copulation was 'rank lust'): 'Long and peaceful inter-regnums, gentlemen! at certain monthly and strawbed periods; and by all means two beds in the same room, or rather in the adjoining apartment.' Moderation was the magic word: 'There is no body so strong, that Venus is not able to weaken and overcome.'[53]

Graham thus saw semen as an 'exquisitely penetrating', 'precious' and 'nutritious' liquor, the spirit of vitality.[54] This view reflected his visionary cosmology, which regarded all the animating and vivifying powers of Nature as finding expression in vital fluids, celestial fire, electricity, magnetism, and, of course, semen. A delicate balance had to be maintained. Enough semen had to be released for procreation, but sufficient retained for reanimating the male body:

for believe me, gentlemen! that the procreation of the species, is but at most a secondary purpose of which nature prepares the seed: the chief use of this balmy – spiritous – vivifying essence, is after it has been thoroughly concocted and exalted in the seminal and gener-ative organs, to be pumped up again or exhaled into the general system, and intimately blended and churned, as it were, with the blood and all the juices, bedewing every fibre, bracing and sheathing every nerve, and animating with light, strength and serenity, the whole frame! in order that all those secretions, circulations and absorptions, upon which good bodily health and celestial tranquillity of mind depend, may be more properly carried on. For without a full and genial tide of this rich, vivifying luminous principle, continu-ally circulating in every part of the system, it is absolutely impossible that either man or woman can enjoy health, strength, spirits, or happiness.[55]

Of course, Graham's identification of semen with the vital principle made his view of the human economy phallocentric. As the human sperm-bank, the male was the higher, livelier and more spiritual gender. The female principle, by contrast, was essentially lower, earthy, womb-like, passive and receptive. Partly for this reason, most of his advice was directed to men; he recommended, for example, they pick good stock: 'In the choice of a woman . . . Hysteria, and all the said train of hysterical gloomy melancholy are carefully to be avoided';[56] Graham's phallocentric viewpoint on human reproduction chimed with his wider philosophy. For in his organic cosmology, Nature was understood through complementary male–female dichotomies, with the male being the more active and spiritual:[57] 'I may be indulged with the liberty of drawing the whole of what I have said to one point of view,' he pronounced,

> and farther to represent our World or System, as a Creature of an *ambiguous* nature, and as partaking of *both Sexes*. The *higher* part of our system, namely the Celestial, being active and *masculine*; the *lower*, or more gross *elementary* part, of the passive and *feminine* nature. As the globe of the earth then is the wondrous and capacious womb, in which the all-engendering seed of Heaven is eagerly received and faithfully *kept* for innumerable, most kind and most obvious purposes: – I may finally be allowed to remark, that as from the upper masculine part proceed the Light, Serenity, Life and strength of our System, so, from the lower or female part, (as, alas! from too many *other* female parts) do issue fires and Aetean or Vesuvian furors, corruptions, diseases, discords, desolation, and Death.

Graham was in many ways *sui generis* and enigmatic. His sexology cannot simply be slotted into some general schema. But his *ideas* should not be neglected as a farrago of slogans slung together to create eye-catching, money-spinning, cheap thrills. His sexual ideas resonate with the convictions of the Enlightenment. For Graham, Nature grants the body sexual pleasures in abundance, while also laying down objective norms of conduct and hygiene whose rewards are health and happiness and whose sanctions are disease. The discourse of sexual health is Nature's decalogue for ensuring a stable, family-based, physiologically sound community. Graham held a fine line between Nature as instinct, and Nature as normative; asserting the physical 'naturalness' of libidinous sexuality, while sermonizing and even legislating to restrain its misuse.[58]

Graham's attitudes towards sex defy pigeon-holing. He promoted it, but also sowed the seeds of fear. He was instrumental in magnifying one particular sexual fear, the dire consequences of self-abuse – a phobia which, if not precisely created by Georgian quacks, was at least largely publicized by them.[59] If late seventeenth-century quacks cashed in on fears of venereal disease – fears they in part created – a century later, quacks stirred sexual anxieties no less, but by then the focus of the fears had largely changed. 'As to certain solitary practices or bad habits,' warned Graham, which boys, &c. ignorantly fall into at schools, &c. and which, if persisted in, infallibly cheque the growth, and debilitate the bodies, and it is to be feared, damn the souls of boys and girls, or of the young men and young women, whom the Devil or their vicious companions seduce into them. Let me solemnly assure them, in the sacred name of God! – of nature, – of truth, – and of happiness, – that every such selfish and solitary act, yea, even every act of fornication, or of amorous commerce between unmarried persons, is expressly for-bidden by God, and is a stroke from the hammer of death and condemnation, to everything that virtuous, wise and human beings ought to cherish and hold sacred.[60]

The worst of all possible evils, his auditors were warned, was self-abuse:

Were I now speaking before an assembly of the young, profligate, or thoughtless of both sexes, instead of a manly, rational, and highly respectable audience! I would assure them in the name of *Posterity!* in the name of HEALTH AND HAPPINESS – in the name of GOD himself! would I assure them that every seminal emission out of nature's road – I must speak plainly, gentlemen! every act of self-pollution, and even every repetition of natural venery, with even the loveliest of the sex, to which appalled or exhausted nature is whipped and spurred by lust, habit, or firey unnatural provocations; but especially every act of self-pollution; is an earthquake – a blast – a deadly paralytic stroke, to all the faculties of both soul and body! striking on an irrecoverable chip from the staff of life; blasting beauty! chilling, contradicting, and enfeebling body, mind and memory! cutting off many years from the natural term of their life! Rather than begin, or continue this vile, soul and body destroying practice – this rebellion against, and murdering of nature, I would advise young persons to anything . . . indeed, I would seriously advise them at once, to put an end to their existence! for this horridly unnatural – this infernal – this all-blasting practice of self-pollution, and drunkenness, are the inlet to, or the aggregate of all the vices and curses, of soul and body, of time and eternity – bound up in one damning – one more than diabolical bundle.[61]

How did these fears arise? Public hysteria about the evils of onanism, accused Thomas Beddoes, the late eighteenth-century Bristol physi-cian, was the fault of the quacks; in particular he denounced the 'alarm engendered by quack advertisements'. Graham's outburst shows how, as Beddoes alleged, quacks helped create the panic over masturbation. Yet Beddoes's thrust was at best half true. For regular doctors no less than quacks played their part in creating the self-abuse scare. The anonymous *Onania* (1710) had been augmented by the *Onanism* of the ultra-respectable Swiss physician, Tissot, quickly translated into English in 1769, which attributed most lethal wasting diseases to masturbation. Indeed, Beddoes was guilty of a certain hypocrisy.[62] For in his lengthy essay on the 'Grand Source of Unhealthiness in the Male Sex' he expatiated at enormous length, though in veiled language, upon the gross evils of premature sexual arousal and masturbation, which (he claimed, in tones resonant of Graham), 'must blast every hope of the enjoyment of health'.[63]

Why the shrill denunciations of the evils of masturbation fell on prepared soil is altogether a more difficult question. It has been suggested that the Georgian dread of auto-eroticism was a response to the prolongation of childhood and the intensification of parent–child relationships within the domestic family, which brought with it greater desire to 'protect' children from waywardness and vice by overseeing and suppressing juvenile sexuality. It has also been argued that it was a rationalization of a bourgeois-capitalist ethos of 'saving' and avoiding – or deferring – 'spending'.[64]

Quack writers pandered to, and stirred up, guilty anxieties in the public mind that 'nervous conditions' had some root in darkly hinted sexual malpractices. Often advertisements mentioned nothing so vulgar as poxes and claps but rather a malaise, or a web of them, far more insidious, dangerous and worrying, suggested by such terms as debility and exhaustion. A conspiracy of silence often binds sufferer and quack together: the 'sufferer' knows he must be suffering from the condition to which the writer is alluding; the writer's polite restraint spares the sufferers.

Various late eighteenth-century quack writers fed off people's talent for convincing themselves that they were suffering from nervous disorders of sexual origin: aside from Graham, the most prominent included Ebenezer Sibly, Edward Senate, William Brodum and Samuel Solomon.[65] They made the pill-vending side of their trade play second fiddle in their self-presentations. Above all, this cohort of quacks principally aimed to sell their *opinions*, backed by the voice of science, scholarship and authority. They assiduously pursued the printed healing word. Graham himself, in a great spurt in the early 1780s, published at least fourteen different pamphlets and short books. Sibly produced his full-length *Medical Mirror* (1792) and other publications; and Samuel Solomon's *Guide to Health* sold like hot cakes. Later editions of this 200-page book assured readers that it had gone through over sixty editions and sold more than 120,000 copies.[66] Such figures may be taken with a pinch of salt, but the abundance of surviving copies with high edition numbers show that Solomon's claims were not mere pie in the sky.

Sibly especially addressed the disorders of youth. He made much of the green sickness amongst adolescent girls, implying that physical debility and emotional lability were two sides of a single coin, and suggesting their interlinking in the emergent hysterical sexual imagination (or even practices). Whereas an earlier tradition (evident in Mandeville) had been disposed to the jaunty view that adolescent disorders would melt away with sexual fulfilment in matrimony, Sibly was far more perturbed by the sexual malpractices – above all, masturbation – of adolescence, hinting that they might do long-term harm.[67]

It was, however, William Brodum and Samuel Solomon who manipulated the sexual scares of the age of sensibility. Brodum's *Guide to Old Age, or Cure for the Indiscretions of Youth* stressed the horrors of unspecified sexual disorders in a tone both lugubrious and insinuating. Without his book, he claimed, both young and old offenders would be utterly lost, on account of the catastrophic consequences of 'irregular propensities in both sexes'. His book indicated 'the proper mode of relief' for 'menstruation – chlorosis, scrofula, excess of libidinous indulgence – baneful effects of such indiscretions, especially among youth – Venereal disease'.[68]

The Liverpool quack, Samuel Solomon, produced the *Guide to Health, or Advice to Both Sexes in Nervous and Consumptive Complaints, Scurvy, Leprosy and Scrofula, and on A Certain Disease and Sexual Debility, in which is added An Address to Boys, Young Men, Parents, Tutors, and Guardians of Youth*, which supposedly reached its 64th edition by the early nineteenth century. Solomon built upon the presumed relationship between nervous disorders, consumption (wasting conditions) and furtive sexual practices, already forged in earlier anti-masturbation literature like *Onania*.[69]

The Guide to Health was a cornucopia of classical mythology, anecdotes, warnings, tales of the trials of young love and of love melancholy (Burton's *Anatomy of Melancholy* was pillaged for stories), advice on the control of 'wild imaginations' and 'extravagant fancies', indices of the symptoms of the nervous diseases consequent upon self-abuse (for example 'the eyes are clouded'), name-dropping of the heroes of medicine – Rhases, Galen, Montanus, etc. – all spliced with quotations from Shakespeare, and improving items – on the true essence of a good prose style, for example. Solomon evoked the image of the frustrated youth as his target reader, now pining, now a volcano of frustration, suffering melancholy, idleness, solitariness – and with fatal results. 'O blessed health,' he apostrophized, quoting Sterne, 'thou art above all gold and treasure' – yet how often it was flung away in vice and folly![70]

Solomon hardly needed to tell his readers outright that they were suffering from unmentionable sexual disorders, involving 'involuntary emissions', back pains, weak memory, dejection or poor eyesight:[71] this was almost a secret shared between his readers and himself. But he made sufferers feel in good company – they were linked by association with the great names of history and literature: poets, writers, geniuses, heroes. And he left them in no doubt of their duty to have immediate recourse to *his* medicine: the 'patient must be comfortable and content to be ruled by his physician'.[72] Above all, Solomon orchestrated a kind of confession by proxy. 'How many are there,' he boomed, 'that have perished because they dared not reveal the cause of their illness!'[73] Thankfully, many did: Solomon informs us of the mailbags of letters he had received from culprits confessing their sexual 'degeneracy' and 'depravation', and testifying to the power of his books and medicines in expediting recovery.

Immature sexual desires were thus the roots of disease; excessive venery led to 'lassitude, weakness, numbness';[74] yet, at the other extreme, 'continued celibacy generally loads the glands, retards the circulation, and occasions fulness and stagnation in the vessels'.[75] Worst still, celibacy led to bad habits, and eventually *habitués* became 'addicted to Onanism'.[76] Physiologically speaking, this was an evil because – for Solomon as for Tissot and Graham – it resulted in a 'waste of semen', whose consequence was constitutional weakness[77] because 'this seminal liquor is of vast importance to the human frame'.[78] This in turn was catastrophic, because such interconnected 'nervous and hypochon-driacal complaints' resist 'all remedies' – 'except the famous and highly-exalted medicine, the Cordial Balm of Gilead'.[79]

In high-flown rhetoric Solomon presented himself in the guise of a medical philosopher reflecting upon the human condition. He chose to make almost romantic play of his marginality: 'it is an incontrover-tible fact,' he boasted, 'that the most considerable improvements in medicine have been made by persons who were not regular and system-atic professors of the art'; and he championed the paramountcy of 'experience'. Yet he also insisted that he was 'regularly graduated'.[80]

Quackery helped contribute to the culture of sexuality, and indeed sexology, by providing a lively focus for formulations on a subject upon which regular biomedical science was sometimes unwilling to speak.

Part II

THE VICTORIANS AND BEYOND

Introduction: Towards Victoria

The first part of this book has surveyed the development of bodies of sexual knowledge from the second half of the seventeenth century until the close of the Georgian era. It has argued that no single, definitive, all-embracing sexual discourse dominated – there was no public consensus, no enforcement agency – nor can one discern a clear-cut arrow of change in sexual teachings. There were notable differences between upper- and lower-class formulations about sex and reproduction; when examining publications it is necessary to be aware that some authors wrote to save lives, others to save souls; some to win scientific fame, others to turn a penny. Sexual discourse in eighteenth-century England was shaped by powerful social pressures and by climates of opinion. The politico-religious upheavals of the 'century of revolution' and the urbane ideology of Enlightenment made for outlooks on sex that were secular in tendency and increasingly adapted to the notion of erotic enjoyment. Mercantilist doctrines underlining the national desirability of populousness, the new cult of motherhood, ameliorating economic prospects, and an emphasis on the family as the linchpin of the community all encouraged the institution of matrimony and promoted the notion that happy, fruitful sex within marriage was a personal blessing and a social cement. Against a swirling, kaleidoscopic background of sexual precepts and practices, sexual writings during the 'long eighteenth century' adopted as their central dogma a belief in the pleasures of procreation – the idea that the sexual drives should be fulfilled and would best find release within conjugal relations in circumstances likely to produce offspring.[1]

The virile man and the buxom, fertile woman were celebrated in the corpus of literature of the time. By contrast, other modes of sexual activity were frowned upon – and were condemned with increasing intensity. The eighteenth century brought the first great anti-onanist panic. The enhanced value attributed to conjugal ties and the nuclear family resulted in a growing stigmatization of what may anachronistically be called 'male homosexuality'. Homophobia reaffirms regular heterosexuality.[2]

The eighteenth century produced a string of texts expressive of such views. Some achieved prominence and longevity, notably *Aristotle's Master-Piece* and the works of Venette. Others made a temporary splash, including the writings of Marten early in the century, those of Graham and Solomon in later decades, and certain texts on midwifery and women's diseases.

There is no such simple thread to follow in the early decades of the nineteenth century. For reasons that may be purely fortuitous, no new hegemonic texts appeared in the same mould as those of Marten or Venette.[3] Odd though it may seem, it appears that versions of *Aristotle's Master-Piece* remained throughout the Victorian period the bestselling works spelling out the 'facts of life'.

Sexual doctrines became integral to the monumental cultural wars being waged in Britain (and, of course, throughout Europe) from the 1790s. Amongst the British ruling classes, two opposing movements were locked in struggle. The accident of the Regency, the character of the Prince Regent, and the militarization of high society produced by two decades of war led to a new and almost unprecedented era of aristocratic debauchery.[4] Noblemen, army officers and Regency bucks indulged in conspicuous libertinism. Its finest exemplars were also its finest critics, notably Byron.[5] The significance of aristocratic excess was not that it laid down new sexual norms but that it provided an instance of the Establishment itself cocking a snook at Establishment values, thereby creating targets for criticism and provoking new idioms and frameworks within which to redefine sexual standards.

Two counter-movements arose. One grew amongst the respectable and responsible elements of the propertied classes, who, seeking bourgeois moral authority, began to cultivate a new moral and sexual earnestness, often under the banner of Evangelicalism.[6] The more idiosyncratic aspects of Bowdlerism and Grundyism have offered targets for the chortles of later historians.[7] Whether we feel much sympathy for the earnest Evangelicals and their Victorian successors is neither here nor there; what is clear is that the changes in moral and social climate which one may associate with Evangelicalism helped shift the sexual debate away from the Georgian 'pleasures of procreation' in the direction of a new emphasis on public character and civic probity, a reidealization of love over sensuality, of the moral law over personal impulse or the vertigo of sensibility.

As the copious writings of Francis Place demonstrate, it was not only the propertied who aspired in the first decades of the nineteenth cen tury to sexual ideals and conduct that renounced 'Old Pleasure', the lax old ways of their fathers and grandfathers. Permissiveness, promiscuity, illegitimacy, drunkenness, swearing, obscenity, bawdy – all these were viewed by many early nineteenth-century artisan and working-class figures as symptomatic of a popular culture that had lacked self-discipline and respect, that had failed to be progressive and to seize control of its own destiny.[8]

But by an ironical twist, the plebeian leaders seeking enhanced sexual self-respect were closely associated with radical movements dedicated to using anarchic sexual ideas to expose elite hypocrisies and to put the case for a more just, egalitarian or free social order grounded in basic material realities, such as sexual drives. In ways familiar since Rabelais, and graphically expressed in the cartoon tradition, sexual satire was once again the great debunker and leveller, toppling the pretensions of the mighty and the 'moral'. Radical publishers, libellers and print-makers used sex and sexual satire as tools for unmasking corruption in high places and suggesting carnivalesque alternatives.[9]

The Prince Regent was the butt of butts: corpulent, lecherous, profligate, conceited – he and his cronies offered endless possibilities for radical attack that were exploited with panache. But there was a more serious target, a more dangerous foe, a figure who came to overshadow sexual discourse early in the nineteenth century: Parson Malthus. First published in 1798, Thomas Robert Malthus's *An Essay on the Principle of Population* achieved exceptional publicity by problematizing sex in a new way.[10] The value system of the eighteenth century had concerned itself with the encouragement of sexuality, within certain designated frameworks. Malthus's *Essay* put a stop to that. It was Malthus's argument – and it proved immensely influential – that human sexual instincts were so inexorable that the only issue worth addressing was the discovery of ways to bridle them before the inevitable consequences of immoderate procreation – famine, disease and war – did their cruel worst. Couched as an argument about the limiting of pauperism and the curbing of Poor Law expenditure, Malthus's *Essay* (which over time underwent many modifications of emphasis but no fundamental change of message) in effect rewrote the agenda of sexual debate. Plagued by fears of overpopulation, moralists swayed by the Malthusian arguments no longer saw the slightest reason for advertising the pleasures of procreation; instead they emphasized the irresponsibility and immorality of procreation and hence of sex except under the most stringent conditions (moral principle, financial security). The long shadow of Malthus made dissemination of traditional sexual advice rather akin to toying with a loaded pistol. What the young needed was not sexual knowledge but sermons in temperance and alternative mores – the pleasures of domestic affection, companionship, self-improvement, education, thrift, character-building and piety. Sexual self-restraint now became a central virtue in a new kind of often explicitly religious, anti-sensualist matrimonial advice manual.

Not everybody, of course, accepted Malthus. Powerful radicals saw in him not an objective social statistician but an ideologue of reaction, seeking justifications for an assault on the customs of the people in the name of natural law. One major anti-Malthusian claim was that if the risk of excessive births was indeed a social problem, the solution lay not in sexual (or 'moral') restraint, as urged by Malthusians, but in birth control. Thus the early nineteenth century brought a new – though officially vilified – branch of sexual discourse: the case for contraception.[11]

A glance at publications in the first half of the nineteenth century shows that birth-controlling voices were a tiny and precarious minority.[12] Instead there was a growing body of tracts of a medical or pseudo-medical nature concerned to spell out the pathological aspects of sexuality. In particular, female sexual desire came under scrutiny and suspicion; and, in ways to be explored in the following chapters, associations were increasingly drawn between 'abnormal' or 'excessive' female sexual urges and physiological maladies or psychiatric disorders, notably 'hysteria'. As Foucault has emphasized, the first half of the nineteenth century brought the 'hysterization' of women.[13] In numerous respects, sexuality became more suspect.

At the same time, positive new ideals were broadcast in the Malthusian milieu, highlighting the moral value of marriage to the disparagement not merely of pre- or extramarital sex but of excessive marital sex. This is most clearly signalled in the transformation that *Aristotle's Master-Piece* underwent in the nineteenth century. Early eighteenth-century versions of *Aristotle's Master-Piece*, it was suggested in Chapter 2, were rather frank and forthright in their sexual discussion. But in a new version that first appeared in the Victorian era (in this book it is called Version 4), explicit references to the physical aspects of sex were removed; a greater stress was placed on marriage as distinct from mere 'unions'. Bawdy language and references were excised. Victorian editions were produced for readers who were assumed to be altogether more reticent and reserved than heretofore; the aim of these later editions was to uphold and dignify such restraint.

Though retaining the original title and reproducing much of the advice about women's diseases contained in Versions 1–3, the Victorian version of *Aristotle's Master-Piece* is a fundamentally different work. Above all, the plain discussion of sex has disappeared. In the Victorian version there is no anatomy of the genitals, no tips for creating the soft-lights-

and-sweet-music atmosphere for lovemaking, no advice on how to conceive a boy or a girl – none of the elements of making love and making babies which dominate all earlier versions. The drift of this version is captured by a chapter heading that does not appear in any other variant: 'Words of Warning'.[14] Addressed primarily to young men, it has become a moral tract, designed to open their eyes to the perils of that 'foolish infatuation'[15] youths may so readily contract for flighty belles or even for 'unfortunates', women of the street:

> You find some men indulging their vicious inclinations by following the 'strange woman,' the street harlot, to her den of guilt and shame, or by alluring some simple girl by promises false and heartless to sin in that transgression which society forgives in a man, but never forgives in a woman: that sin which is unpardonable in the deceived, but venial in the deceiver.[16]

Such practices were treated as highly suspect:

> Look at the first of these two cases. 'A young man void of understanding,' associates with unfortunate women, and wastes his precious vigour in criminal pleasure. The period of youth is the glory of nature, and the healthful development of all the resources of strength in our nature is the glory of our youth.[17]

It stresses that men need to be on guard against rashness and weakness; they must recognize that 'eager pursuit of sensual gratification disqualifies for the exercise of the loftier powers',[18] and must instead cultivate 'self-command' and 'abstinence':

> Life, which is regulated by reason, prudence, and benevolence, is sure to be virtuous, but when the passions hold the mastery, they lead to every sort of excess. Rules which we approve and to which we adhere in our calmer moments are utterly violated under the influence of passion. Therefore one of the most necessary qualifications for man or women to cultivate is self-command.[19]

Virtuous men should choose not flighty ladies but innocents, whose goodness would ennoble their partners, for

> A woman's sensibilities are quicker and deeper than those of man. A woman knows better how to sympathise with others than man does. Her light always burns with a clear and steady radiance. Those qualities, intellectual and emotional, which man needs, woman supplies. There is that heroism of endurance which is unknown to man. Her love possesses an irresistible power, and her weakness is her greatest strength.[20]

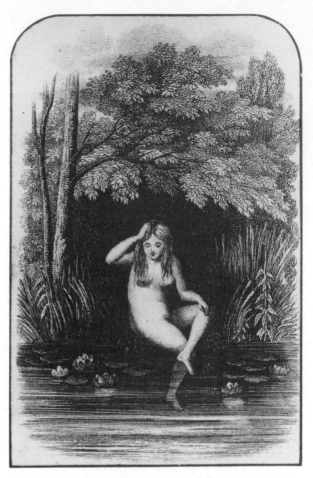

8 and 9 Frontispieces to *The Works of the Famous Philosopher Aristotle, Containing his Complete Master-Piece and Family Physician, His Experienced Midwife, His Book of Problems and Remarks on Physiognomy. To the Original Work is Added. An Essay on Marriage; its Duties and Enjoyments.* n. d., but Victorian. These Victorian editions were much more decorous than their earlier equivalents.

Young ladies for their part must learn the folly of flirtatiousness; the 'La Traviatas' will go down the road to moral and physical ruin in the end.[21]

Marriage is the true goal for the virtuous, for 'Marriage is a divine institution', and

> Marriage was peculiarly adapted to the position of the human race. It was necessary that man should have a companion, a friend, a wife; and thus it was ordained that a man should leave his father and mother, and cleave to his wife, and they twain shall be one flesh.[22]

But even then the stress must be on its 'obligations' and 'duties'[23] (though, as a slightly grudging-sounding concession the text adds, 'there is nothing debasing in connubial love').[24] Not least, as a Malthusian note, marriage must be deferred until the husband has 'adequate means of support'.[25] The pursuit of erotic pleasures that

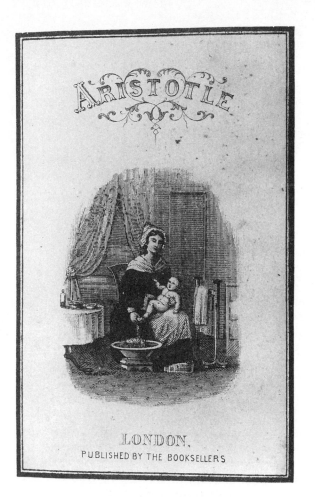

figures so largely in earlier versions has given way to prudence in respect to pounds and pence, desire has been unveiled as danger, and sex has been replaced by the higher ideals of 'family affection' and sentimental companionship.[26] This is *Aristotle's Master-Piece* for Charles Pooter. The following chapters explore the reformulation of sexuality within this new moral framework in the Victorian age and onwards.[27]

CHAPTER SIX

The Victorian Polyphony, 1850–85

The Victorians and sex have been exhaustingly, if not exhaustively, written about.[1] Assumptions about Victorian respectability and hypocrisy, about the rule of the sexual double standard, are still widely prevalent even though recent historians have demonstrated that the reality, summed up in the title of Mary Poovey's excellent study *Uneven Developments*, was complex and multilithic; all rules had many exceptions, any generalization was readily contradictable.

The 1850s and 1860s superficially appear the apogee of the double standard enshrined in legislative action. The Divorce Law of 1857 laid down that mere adultery in man, as opposed to wife, was no matrimonial crime unless exacerbated by other offences. The Contagious Diseases Acts (1864, 1866 and 1869), aimed to solve the problem of venereal disease rife in the armed forces by policing female prostitutes. Yet other evidence could be adduced to characterize these decades not as triumphant but as defensive, with these enactments emanating from paranoid fears rather than confidence, as the forces of sexual respectability saw themselves beleaguered by swirling tides of unchastity and disease.

The triumph of the respectable Victorian male was far from obviously assured. Under the 1857 Divorce Law women might petition for the dissolution of marriage, even if on unequal terms, and as James Hammerton has indicated in *Cruelty and Companionship*, many did.[2] There were proposals to extend the franchise to women, for the rights of married women to property, and to have custody of their children in matrimonial disputes, with demands for wider grounds of judicial separation, if not divorce.[3] Were vocal assertions of female difference and inferiority attempts to establish threatened male superiority upon a scientific foundation, desperate efforts to cling to a pinnacle increasingly under siege? The period was one of contradictions, overt and covert, spoken and silent, and of unexpected grounds of agreement between the apparently diverse.

In the 1850s unrespectable sex was highly visible. Harlots of all ranges paraded in public places, offering outrageous 'displays of incessant indecency', leading to 'familiarity of the young with depraving influence and conversation'.[4] Attempts to sweep 'the vicious offal of libertinism' out of sight into 'a conglomeration of . . . impurity' in such specific venues for the traffic in sex as the Argyll Rooms, so that 'the eye of the respectable was not offended', gained little credence.[5] Even if wives and children could be sheltered from these prevalent activities of the market for sex, accounts of its existence entered respectable homes in the pages of the press. Press sensationalism and prurience included extensive reporting of actions for 'crim. con.' (criminal conversation) and subsequent to the 1857 Act, of divorce cases: 'sex in high society, and . . . murder' were staples of the yellow press, but even *The Times* gave extensive coverage to murder and divorce cases.[6] Respectable homes which the more lurid journals never entered might contain reports from philanthropic organizations – preventive, punitive and reformative – engaging with problems of prostitution and other sexual vice.[7] It was hotly debated whether prostitutes themselves were frail victims of society or healthy entrepreneurs moving in and out of the profession, and whether prostitution was capable of eradication, or an eternal problem which in the interests of hygiene and civic order ought to be regulated.

The 'Social Evil' was thus a major, much discussed source of Victorian anxiety, a high-profile media issue, with the notorious letter from 'One More Unfortunate' (and the correspondence generated by it) appearing in *The Times* itself.[8] Discussions ostensibly deploring the prevalence of 'vice' could be prurient and titillating, with salacious accounts of foreign prostitutes imported to service wealthy debauchees of the upper ten thousand. An 'elderly MP', a 'Lord A——' and similarly pseudonymous aristocrats were said to have their 'peculiar fancies' indulged by French wantons at 'a well-known foreign house in Gerrard Street'.[9] Alleged swarms of foreign prostitutes parading about St James Parish in November 1858 were 'a festering sore in the midst of the metropolis of the first nation in the world'.[10] Compared to foreigners, it seems, even English prostitutes were simple creatures, 'covetted [*sic*] by foreign debauchees . . . because in the "worst" there is something to teach'. Foreign prostitutes had 'nothing to learn; even the "best" come here as teachers', as 'professional impures' offering 'special continental vices'.[11] Similar nationalistic prejudice was found in the report of

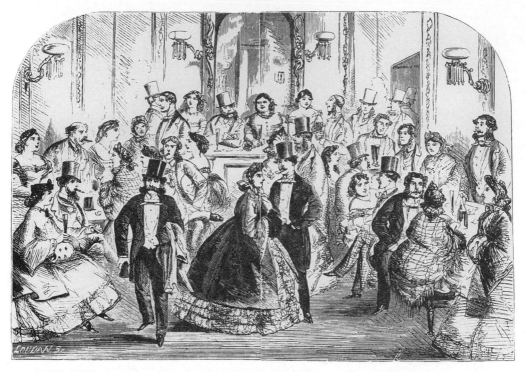

10 'A Night House – Kate Hamilton's': the smart end of the mid-Victorian prostitution market (from Henry Mayhew, *London Labour and the London Poor*, vol. iv, 1861–2).

'Seduction of English Girls in Paris'[12] and accounts of the divorce of Mrs Pulley, 'a Frenchwoman' of extravagant habits and a violent temper, who after separation from her husband committed adultery with a French army officer.[13] The implicit salaciousness of all things French was also found in the highly discreet advertisement for 'Preservatif contre les Maladies Secrète – Mons. A. Sureté supplies F.L.s' (i.e. French Letters).[14]

Another aspect of the question was, of course, the transmission of venereal diseases. The *Lancet* suggested that 'for the broad-cast dispersion of venereal disease ... nothing more perfect than our present system could be devised'.[15] But compared to the vociferous debate on prostitution, specific discussion of sexually transmitted diseases was muted. The classic 'Victorian' statement on the subject by the President of the Royal Medical and Chirurgical Society, Sir Samuel Solly, speaking in the 'official' context of a government inquiry into the problem of venereal diseases in the armed forces, was that syphilis was 'intended as a punishment for our sins and we should not interfere in the matter'.[16]

Venereal diseases and those who suffered from them (regardless of gender) were stigmatized. Subscribers to voluntary hospitals were unwilling to contribute for treatment of a self-inflicted and justified penalty for sexual immorality, so most voluntary and teaching hospitals banned venereal patients,[17] while treatment available under the 1834 Poor Law varied locally from the punitive to the neglectful, in the absence of any general policy. Hospital record-keeping tended to be deliberately or carelessly inaccurate about admissions for VD, Poor Law Commissioners' Reports were silent concerning venereally diseased paupers.[18]

Treatments available were of dubious therapeutic benefit, and savoured of the punitive. Salivation with mercury, leaving the lingering symptoms of heavy metal poisoning, was a 'cure' many perceived as worse than the disease, unpleasant, long-drawn-out, and causing noticeable physical stigmata. It was employed indiscriminately by some physicians, even for gonorrhoea, which tended to be taken less seriously than syphilis. Treatment consisted of the instillation of powerful caustics into the urethra, and the resort to cauterization in acute cases, with some gentler, if no more efficacious, lotions and potions. Cures were pronounced on the disappearance of external symptoms. Ignorance was rife and there was little attempt to dispel it. British doctors shrank from emulating the scientific investigations into venereal diseases taking place on the continent: even such diagnostic aids as the microscope and the speculum (the latter generating much debate and many moral reservations, as Moscucci has shown)[19] were not part of standard practice. Some discussion of venereal disease was initiated in medical periodicals, and textbooks were published in increasing numbers, but continuing stigma hindered the incorporation of venereal diseases into the standard medical curriculum and common medical practice.[20]

Interest in them was regarded as marking the quack. When Sir James Paget praised William Acton because he 'practised honourably in the most dangerous of specialities . . . wrote decently on subjects not usually decent, and . . . never used the opportunities which his practice offered for quackery or extortion',[21] he indicated the norm from which Acton deviated. One elderly man wrote to Marie Stopes about being treated for 'a clap' around 1880:

> The doctor . . . strongly advised me to drop masturbation. He even suggested certain houses where I might meet women of a better class, and advised the use of sheaths or injections. . . . The doctor even advised women as a lesser evil than the risk of disease in masturbation.[22]

One would like to know more about the status of this doctor; his connection with 'certain houses' may suggest the reason why reputable doctors preferred to have nothing to do with practice in sexually transmitted diseases.[23] It is possible to hypothesize a medical underworld, eluding or ignoring the strictures of the General Medical Council, of 'pox doctors' and abortionists.[24]

Given the incapacity of the medical profession and the enduring sense of moral stigma associated with the disease, many were driven to quacks or patent medicines. Quacks offered 'delicacy and secrecy', without 'confinement or hindrance of business', rapid cure (a couple of weeks at the outside) 'without indiscriminate use of mercury', even 'No Charge unless Cured', and postal advice.[25] Patent remedies, often advertised as not including mercury, were unlikely to resemble the painful local orthodox treatments, such as the brutally severe instillations for gonorrhoea which could result in stricture.[26] Those who sought such treatment were not necessarily infected: 'advertising quacks' adeptly drummed up anxiety to stimulate trade.[27]

Because of the contorted moral agenda around venereal disease, the question of preventive measures, even in the context of sanitary reform, was highly problematic. If the disease was just punishment for a moral lapse, was it appropriate to seek to prevent it? If, however, becoming venereally infected was an understandable (if regrettable) by-product of male human nature, was it not advisable to make provision for the better containment of the disease in the public interest? Class, religion, medical and social theories influenced the plethora of views on the subject.[28] Though current theories of transmission implied the efficacy of ablution after intercourse, it is unclear whether this was much advocated, given the prevalence of attitudes such as Sir Samuel Solly's quoted above.[29]

The passing, motivated by anxiety over the fitness of the country's armed forces, of the Contagious Diseases Acts of 1864, 1866 and 1869 brought the assumptions generated by questions of venereal disease control into glaring prominence. Official concern at the rising syphilis rate in the forces (by 1863 one-third of sick cases was venereal) had been increasing, and establishment of lock hospitals in naval ports was encouraged.[30] 'Rapacious and licentious soldiery' were detached from normal domestic ties, a mere 6 per cent permitted to marry 'on the strength', though attitudes to Her Majesty's troops as 'the scum of the earth' were gradually becoming modified. Barracks, quite apart from their hygienic defects, were often appallingly squalid and denigratory to any kind of human dignity,[31] but the Royal Commission on the Health of the Army recommended in 1857 that periodical genital examination of soldiers ought to be discontinued as deleterious to self-respect.[32] Unthinking assumptions about male licence under-pinned governmental attitudes and parliamentary debate on the subject.

The initial 1864 Act, inspired by the regulationist systems of continen-tal Europe, was supposed by many (including, allegedly, Queen Victoria herself) to deal with veterinary rather than human disease, and passed late at night in a very thinly attended house. It applied for an initial three years in eleven port and garrison towns (increased to eighteen in 1866), and was never in force outside these 'designated districts'. Suspected prostitutes in these localities could be arrested, examined without consent, and if venereally infected, forcibly hospitalized until 'cured'. This was intended to ensure a healthy prostitute population to service naval and military forces.[33] The Acts bore almost exclusively upon women of the working classes, and, Walkowitz has persuasively argued, by imposing preconceptions about prostitute identity on a much more fluid situation, were responsible for the definition and stigmatization of a distinct prostitute class.[34]

An organized campaign of co-ordinated opposition was slow to get off the ground, although religious opinion as well as a range of interest groups from civil libertarians to early feminists were profoundly offended by the assumptions behind and the implications of the Acts. Meanwhile exuberant advocates of the Acts agitated for their wider extension.[35] However, even the medical profession and sanitarians were divided in their opinions on the efficacy of these measures – the leading sanitarian of the day, and medical officer to the Medical Board of the Privy Council, John Simon, was extremely dubious about them and strongly resisted their extension to civilian areas.[36]

Though the statement of the 1871 Royal Commission on Venereal Diseases:

> there is no comparison to be made between prostitutes and the men who consort with them. With the one sex the offence is committed as a matter of gain; with the other it is an irregular indulgence of a natural impulse.[37]

has often been cited, this opinion should not be taken as uncontested. The Acts were regarded at the time as giving the sexual double standard the force of law by setting up a system to provide clean prostitutes for members of the armed forces, and opposition did not come from one sex alone. Men too, on grounds of moral outrage as well as the protection of civil liberties, complained against this state regulation of immorality; not only the middle and educated classes but working men.[38] Support in Victorian Britain for a double standard of sexual morality, under which prostitution was a necessary social evil to be granted official legal recognition, was far from monolithic. In spite of early claims of success, and agitation for their wider extension, the effectiveness of the Acts was and is highly questionable.[39] Yet they did provide one of the major sites where conflicting Victorian views on sexuality were both expressed and generated.

While the Contagious Diseases Acts assumed a 'natural impulse' theory of male sexuality, and opponents argued that men as much as women should observe a high moral standard of premarital chastity and continence within marriage, there were other, less articulated discourses concerning male sexuality. Throughout the later nineteenth century medical journals repeatedly attacked purveyors of quack pamphlets and remedies.[40] These appealed to those who already suspected they had a sexually transmitted ailment, but their clientele was not confined to those already diseased or with guilty reason for believing they were. The quacks, living by them, perhaps knew better than the average medical practitioner what sexual anxieties bothered the man in the street; aware of what would sell, they advertised their wares. The medical profession might be exhorted to give counsel to the sexually distressed,[41] but it was not suggested that they should publicize this service. Doubting that sexual problems would be sympathetically dealt with by a regular doctor, patients continued to turn to quacks, who drummed up trade by disseminating notions about 'Generative Debility, Seminal Weakness, etc.', and their identification.[42] Under the heading 'Nervous and Physical Debility', Robert J. Brodie, author of *The Secret Companion*, advised readers that he could be consulted in Queen Anne Street on all cases of nervous and physical debility and the cause and cure of premature decay.[43]

A more oblique approach was the appeal to prurient curiosity of wax 'anatomical' museums. These included models of freaks of nature, representations of women (and detached organs), often with exposed foetuses in various stages of development, curiosities ('the head of a New Zealand chief'), exhibits showing the evil effects of masturbation usually suggestively alongside those on the ravages of venereal disease. Typical juxtapositions were a 'Hermaphrodite photographed from life' with a model of the abdominal muscles of a man demonstrating the ravages caused by 'onanism', followed by '37 models . . . portraying secondary symptoms of syphilis' ('Some of these diseases have been greatly aggravated by the use of MERCURY'). Other parts of the body and their ailments (including 'The Dreadful Effects of Tight Lacing') were dealt with. Proprietors might claim to treat other ailments, but probably few visitors were drawn by exhibits on human nutrition or the muscles of the eye.

Museums offered for sale works such as J. T. Woodhead of the Liverpool Museum of Anatomy's *Golden Referee, Or Guide to Health*, which paid particular attention to the avoidance of 'Youthful Follies'.[44] Dr Kahn's museum off the Haymarket (open daily to gentlemen only) offered half-hourly explanations of the models and lectures on 'The Philosophy and Physiology of Marriage', 'The Great Social Evil, its Real Cure', 'Dangers of Youth' and 'Rocks of Advanced Age'. The one-shilling admission fee included a copy of Kahn's *The Shoals and Quicksands of Youth*. Panaceas such as De Roos's 'Great European Remedy for Nervousness, Relaxation and Exhaustion' and 'Compound Renal Pill' for 'The Victims of Their Own Follies' were offered (Madame de Roos would attend ladies in 'the most honourable secrecy' – possibly an allusion to abortion?).[45]

Most quack and patent remedies seem to have been milder in their operation than those of orthodox practice. The widely touted 'electrical belts' and other therapeutic electric devices, for example, seem to have operated by faith in the magical all-healing power of 'electricity' rather than by, for example, giving the sufferer electric shocks upon erection.[46] Not all remedies sold by quacks, however, were harmless placebos (if encouraging belief that a course of sugar pills had cured a venereal disease can be considered harmless). Some of them dealt in severer prescriptions: 'The American Remedy' consisted of 'a ring of common metal, with a screw passing through one of its sides, and projecting into the centre, where it had a button extremity' for application to the 'part affected' at bedtime, recommended as 'an infallible cure'. The device, which presumably had some physical effect in preventing nocturnal emissions, was apparently 'extensively used'.[47]

Such implements were not necessarily imposed – as has often been suggested in sensational discussions of the Victorian horror of masturbation – by doctors upon victimized patients, or by anxious or punitive parents upon their children. The horror associated with deliberate self-abuse and even involuntary seminal emissions was widespread, and such ferocious remedies, savouring of the punitive, may even have been acceptable because they fed into the sexual guilts of 'victims'; they seem to have been self-applied by mature male sufferers.

Representatives of fringe and unorthodox beliefs like phrenology, medical herbalism and hydropathy promulgated similar fears to those exploited by commercially motivated quack writers. Rarely was spermatorrhoea proclaimed factitious or masturbation innocuous. The prolific American phrenologist O. S. Fowler, whose works were widely

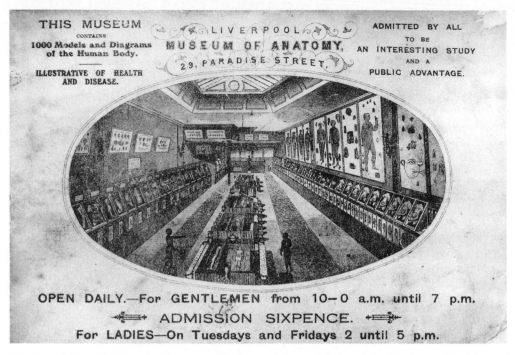

11   A rare view of a Victorian 'anatomical museum' (from the *Descriptive Catalogue of the Liverpool Museum of Anatomy*, 1877).

distributed in the United Kingdom, promoted the importance of mutual conjugal delight,[48] but was as ferocious as any in his condemnation of self-abuse. 'Masturbation outrages Nature's ordinances more than any or all the other forms of sexual sin man can perpetuate': it was a positive plague – 'Millions are ruined by it before they enter their teens.'[49]

T. L. Nichols, an American hydropathic practitioner who moved to Britain and the author of *Esoteric Anthropology*,[50] is considered by Cominos to be one of the most stringent of Victorian writers on sex.[51] The 1873 and subsequent British editions of *Esoteric Anthropology* omitted the condemnations of marriage and its abuse, and the free-love rhetoric, of earlier American editions.[52] Havelock Ellis believed that *Esoteric Anthropology* had been 'considered a respectable source of information on these secret subjects', though in most families it was 'kept locked up in a bedroom drawer'.[53] The judge at the 1886 trial of Adelaide Bartlett, accused of poisoning her husband with chloroform, however, dismissed it as 'garbage',[54] and the Bartletts' possession of the book and Adelaide's loan of it to a neighbour, were not felt to reflect well upon the couple, whose relationship had already been revealed not to accord with received Victorian notions of ideal Christian matrimony. (Although Adelaide Bartlett was acquitted, a considerable doubt existed and still does as to her actual innocence.) For Nichols, masturbation was both the cause of disease, and a disease in itself. Although the loss of semen was admittedly exhausting, the 'artificial, unnatural excitement of the orgasm, without reciprocity, compensation, or use' was the prime cause of evil results.[55]

The anxieties so productive of revenue to quacks were not unknown to the orthodox medical profession. The problematization of woman within Victorian thought and medical practice has already been extensively demonstrated by historians.[56] Although perhaps not theorized to the same extent, at the clinical level the male and his sexuality were also perceived as problematic, or at least as productive of difficulties and subject to dangers. Far from dismissing 'spermatorrhoea' as a factitious ailment, so reputable a journal as the *Lancet* published a series of essays on the subject by J. Laws Milton in 1854.[57] Further 'Contributions to the physiology, pathology, and treatment of Spermatorrhoea' by Marris Wilson appeared during 1856–7,[58] expressing Wilson's hope that

See 143

By directing inquiry to the mysterious agencies which have hitherto surrounded this most terrible moral and physical disease, much will have been accomplished, both for the science of medicine, and for the benefit of the unfortunate victims.[59]

The *Lancet* favourably noticed Wilson's monograph *On Diseases of the Vesiculae Seminales and their Associated Organs, with Special Reference to the Morbid Secretions of the Prostatic and Urethral Mucous Membrane.*[60]

So it was not remarkable that the *Lancet* should greet with an accolade William Acton's *The Functions and Disorders of the Reproductive Organs in Youth, Adult Age and Advanced Life,* on its first appearance in 1857. Such a 'scientific and conscientious practitioner', by 'openly taking . . . under his own charge' conditions among the 'most important functional ailments affecting humanity', rescued them 'from the grasp of the most disgusting and villainous quackery' with 'benefit to the patient'.[61]

There has been considerable controversy about the typicality of Acton's views about sexuality. Steven Marcus's assessment of his significance in *The Other Victorians*[62] has been subjected to a good deal of revisionism, as have accepted notions of the sex life of the Victorians.[63]

It has been argued that Acton was recognizably on the lunatic fringe,[64] and that his ideas were far less influential and much less typical of the medical profession than the more humane and tolerant views of Sir James Paget.[65] Such revisionist work does valuable service in eroding ancient polemical stereotypes of 'Victorianism', but, while it is important to recognize that not all Victorian women closed their eyes, opened their legs, and thought of England, nor did all husbands inform their wives that ladies did not move, there is a risk of setting up new and equally misleading generalizations. Widespread sexual anxieties and inhibitions should not be minimized.

Acton's importance has largely been either promoted or dismissed by engaging with evidence both for the factual basis of his statements concerning mid-Victorian bourgeois female sexuality, and for the general acceptance of such statements. In his view (happily for both society and the men they were married to) decent women seldom desired sexual gratification for themselves, submitting to their husbands' demands only in order to achieve motherhood and for conjugal harmony.[66] Certainly contrary beliefs were to be found in contemporary medical literature, and the existence of desire in individual Victorian females is well attested, but to prove that the Victorian woman was neither a sexless 'angel in the house', nor expected to be, deals with only a small corner of the Actonian agenda.

Acton, as Marcus indicated, problematized the male: it was the male's control over his own sexuality which Acton perceived as the crucial problem and not, or only incidentally, keeping all but an excluded pariah class of women chaste for motherhood. Male sexuality in the Victorian era cannot be simply dismissed by allusions to the double standard and its presumed prevalence. Acton discussed female response in order to reassure males anxious about the sexual demands of marriage; female frigidity assisted avoidance of marital excess (to Acton just as deleterious as solitary excesses), since 'reciprocity of desire' was 'necessary to excite the male'.[67]

Sex in the male, to Acton, was a dangerous force to be kept in check; enslavement in sensual habits, morally bad and physiologically dangerous, was the potential outcome of any indulgence. This was not merely because a man might get into the habit of consorting with prostitutes more likely than not to be venereally diseased. Acton also wrote on prostitution and on sexually transmitted diseases, and was an advocate of the Contagious Diseases Acts, but in spite of his professional experiences with the venereal infections, what principally worried him (and other medical men) was waste of the vital spermatic fluid. Even in legitimate marriage overindulgence could lead to the husband wasting away through the dreaded spermatorrhoea.[68] Acton did argue that self-abuse to gratify sensual urges would undermine moral self-discipline, leading to weakness in the face of other temptations, but he laid heavy stress on the physiological harm wrought by seminal losses. Sexual pleasure itself was debilitating in its intensity, comparable to an epileptic fit, and was not to be experienced too frequently.[69]

Even so, the healthy normal man with his natural healthy urges would find that continence also had its problems. Acton was ambivalent about nocturnal emissions: 'once in every ten or fourteen days' they might be 'in the nature of a safety valve, and even conducive to health in persons who do not take enough exercise, and live too well' (already a hint of pathology appears). However, should they 'occur repeatedly and leave symptoms of prostration with other ill consequences' they required medical attention.[70] Acton suggested that even this unconscious and infrequent relief could and should be controlled, by eschewing any possible sexual stimulus that might affect the sleeping mind, and by the afflicted individual training himself to awaken before emission.[71] Similar ambivalence was expressed in Milton's 1854 *Lancet* articles on the treatment of the disturbing problems of day and night discharges, and imperfect secretion of semen. But 'perfect absence of seminal emissions at night' was by no means 'compatible with health and continence'; only those occurring 'to such a degree as to weaken the powers and impair the health' were to be eradicated.[72] (There is little evidence that quacks or doctors dealt with anxieties arising from the non-existence of nocturnal emissions in the male.)

A condition approximating as far as possible to sexlessness – in which not only was sexual activity limited but as far as possible the slightest arousal was to be avoided – was not required of Victorian womanhood alone, but was the most desirable state for the man. His desires, ideally, were to be expressed either unconsciously and infrequently in sleep, or consciously, only under his will, in legitimate marriage for the purposes of reproduction. Were these opinions of Acton's really, as F. B. Smith has suggested, out on the lunatic fringe?[73] Peter Cominos was inclined to regard Acton as positively moderate,[74] given Acton's expressed opinion that sex within marriage (quite separately from its reproductive aspect) could be

> conducive, when well regulated, not only to increased happiness but long life. . . . The moderate gratification of the sex passion in married life is generally followed by the happiest consequences to the individual.

Indeed, marriage was 'the best and most natural cure for sexual suffering'.[75]

Was Acton the representative of Victorian medical orthodoxy which generations, from Havelock Ellis to Steven Marcus, have made him out to be? His views had considerable and enduring circulation: Copland and Acton were cited as authorities upon the deleterious effects of self-abuse by the *British Medical Journal* in 1881.[76] (Dr James Copland in his general guide, the *Dictionary of Practical Medicine*, 1858, deplored 'Pollutions', particularly from 'manustupration', which reduced life expectancy and caused greater morbidity among the unmarried.)[77] Jeanne Peterson has suggested that Sir James Paget's views on sexuality actually predominated among the Victorian medical profession.[78] Paget's clinical lecture on 'Sexual Hypochondriasis', presumably, as she argues, based on lectures to medical students given earlier, was not printed until 1875, nearly twenty years after the appearance of Acton's *Functions and Disorders*.

Paget, though insisting on the necessity for continence and the doctor's duty to refuse to prescribe fornication, was emphatic that masturbation did no more harm than any other indulgence, or only if it was carried to excess, and certainly did not lead inevitably to the lunatic asylum. He wished that worse could be said of 'so nasty a practice; an uncleanliness, a filthiness forbidden by God, an unmanliness despised by men'. However, Paget's *Clinical Lectures*, of which 'Sexual Hypochondriasis' was only one, went into no more than two editions.[79] Acton's *Functions and Disorders* enjoyed greater success, achieving several editions, some posthumous.

Some other contemporary writers were inclined to regard even Acton as somewhat sanguine in his views on spermatorrhoea. In *On Spermatorrhoea: Its Results and Complications* (1872), John Laws Milton contended that the ailment was highly prevalent and extremely deleterious, and that Acton's lack of misgivings about its curability were 'quite at variance' with his own experience. Milton had no truck with current opinion that a 'few emissions in youth do good' or that an occasional emission was Nature's relief – while he admitted them to be natural he so circumscribed the concept that hardly any emissions would qualify. In Milton's gloomy view a continent man could 'hardly reach twenty-six without becoming partially, if not wholly, impotent'. In his eyes, 'a greater expulsion of semen than is compatible with the maintenance for a healthy condition of the organs of generation' was the natural concomitant of celibacy. Not that he recommended marriage, even 'connexion', as a cure; cure had to precede, not follow, marriage. If Milton had a conception of what a healthy sex life might be, it does not come through in the pages of *On Spermatorrhoea*.

As a preventative for emissions and masturbation Milton advised (as well as sedatives, tonics and changes in regimen) various spiked and toothed rings, 'a light wire cage' over the genital area, and an ingenious

device whereby erection set off an electrical alarm to awaken the
sleeper before emission took place.[80] Even more brutal Victorian remedies for self-abuse and spermatorrhoea were certainly commended to
the profession. 'Slight soreness of the body of the organ . . . sufficient to
render erection painful' would 'guard the penis . . . against improper
manipulation'; and cauterization might be generally advised for 'over-
sensitivity' of the organ.[81] It should be borne in mind that some quack
remedies were equally gruesome; see the 'The American Remedy' mentioned above (p. 139).

At this period the profession appears to have been hyper-sensitive about
drawing the distinction between quack and doctor. Acton's *Functions
and Disorders* cannot have enjoyed sales comparable to Samuel La'mert's
*Self-Preservation: A Medical Treatise on Nervous and Physical Debility,
Spermatorrhoea, Impotence and Sterility*, which went into numerous editions
during the 1850s and 1860s. La'mert, a licentiate of the Society of
Apothecaries and an MD of the Royal University of Erlangen in
Bavaria,[82] was legitimately entitled to appear on the Medical Register
and to be snooty himself about 'unqualified empirics';[83] until struck off
in 1863 for publishing this 'indecent and unprofessional treatise', and
claiming a medical degree he did not possess.

La'mert's self-published volume, with its numerous testimonials from
grateful patients, does not convince the reader that his rhetoric about a
dangerous conspiracy of silence and the risks to the reputation of a
doctor dealing with problems of sex, was allied to disinterested devotion
to the relief of suffering ignored by the profession. One of the charges
against La'mert was that he falsely associated his son, a licentiate of
the Royal College of Physicians of Edinburgh, with *Self-Preservation* by
publishing his name as joint author. Lima Abraham La'mert, who held
the more highly reputed Edinburgh degree, was apparently anxious to
dissociate himself from his father's dubious practice.[84]

'Advertising imposters who publish books full of *secrets*',[85] however,
were not necessarily promulgating very different messages from 'men
of honour, probity, and intelligence', such as Acton. The latter was
praised for 'his readiness to deal with the diseases of the reproductive
organs in all their most questionable forms and social relations', and his
identification 'with all the aspects of the sexual question' was lauded for
its 'honesty, boldness, and manifest good intent'.[86] Yet La'mert argued
for 'moderation in the enjoyment of the highest physical pleasure',
advocating 'a very prudent and well-regulated amount of intercourse'.[87]
Like Acton, he cautioned against perilous overindulgence in these
pleasures in the intoxicating days of early wedlock. But he was doing so

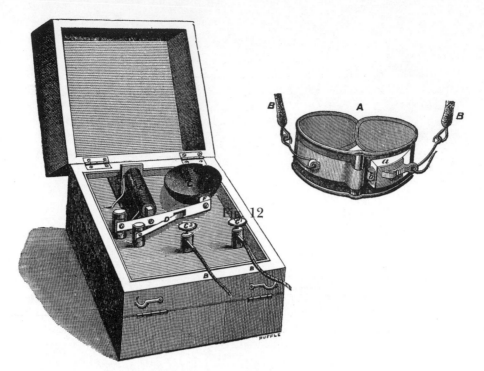

12 and 13 Devices recommended by Milton for the prevention of nocturnal emissions, either by producing painful pressure on the penis, or sounding an alarm to awaken the sleeper (from J. Laws Milton, *On Spermatorrhoea*, 1872).

at a time when doctors were trying to establish that they were the ones who 'knew' about sex, even if very few of them really wanted to have much to do with the subject.[88]

Peterson has argued that Acton, far from being a pillar of the medical profession, was motivated less by idealism than by lust for profit.[89] While this should not be dismissed, Acton appears to have managed to become an authority on sexual matters in a manner appropriate to a member of a profession ever more on its dignity,[90] gaining approval from his peers, and widely praised in the medical press.[91] Paget's own glowing obituary tribute has been cited (p. 135), in which he marked off Acton from other practitioners in a field 'not usually decent'. Possibly Acton had cunningly perceived which way the wind was blowing, and manoeuvred himself into being the consultant in his specialized area to whom other practitioners referred their tricky cases, instead of advertising himself in the press and on broadsheets. This suggests that there was something in his work which did appeal to the profession: both its manner, which gave assurance that he was a 'real doctor' of

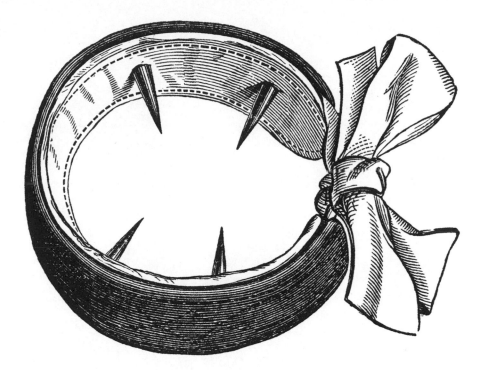

serious intent rather than a mercenary quack, and also the moral and medical acceptability of his messages.

The audience to which even doctors, permitted to discuss sexual matters, might communicate was debatable. Was sexual knowledge to be disseminated, or kept for secluded discussion in medical circles? The complexities of medical ideas on sexuality were illuminated in the mid-1860s by the *cause célèbre* over the clitoridectomies performed by Isaac Baker Brown in his London Surgical Home. Could a serious medical work on the delicate subject of female masturbation resemble 'the class of works which lie upon drawing-room tables', with the author's name in gilt letters? The *British Medical Journal* reviewer of Baker Brown's book *On the Curability of Certain Forms of Insanity, Epilepsy, and Hysteria in Females* thought not.[92] 'Reasonable and thinking men,' editorialized the *Journal,* could only feel disgust at 'public discussion, before mixed audiences, of sexual abuses'. Only duty could possibly 'induce professional men to meddle . . . as far as possible in strictly technical language' with 'such a dirty topic'.[93]

Colleagues (or some of them) perceived Baker Brown as improperly exciting 'the attention of non-medical persons, and especially of women, to the subject of Self-Abuse in the Female Sex'. He was attacked

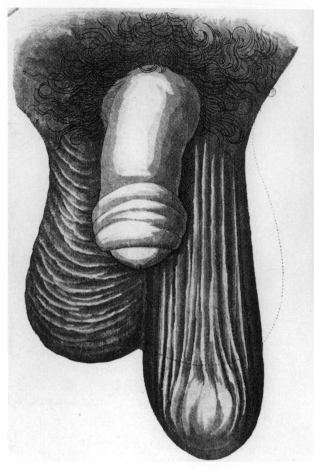

14 and 15 Male sexual organs suffering from varicocele, 'generally attributable to masturbation and excessive venereal indulgence' (from Samuel La'mert, *Self-Preservation*, c. 1850s–60s).

for addressing audiences of clergymen, and disseminating rather too freely circulars advertising the London Surgical Home. This debate certainly reveals no universal acceptance of notions of female sexlessness, and the significance of the clitoris was central to it.[94]

Writing about sex was problematic even for a doctor: George Drysdale, the Malthusian writer of *Elements of Social Science: or Physical, Sexual, and Natural Religion*, a doctor and a radical, cautiously issued early editions anonymously. Appearing in 1854 and constantly reissued at least until the First World War, *Elements of Social Science* promoted a Malthusian gospel of 'preventive intercourse', early marriage with the use of contraceptive measures. Drysdale's views on sexuality were antithetical to the notion that it was a dangerous force requiring constant vigilance to keep in check. For him, sexual problems resulted from the unnatural restraints placed on indulgence of natural urges, and

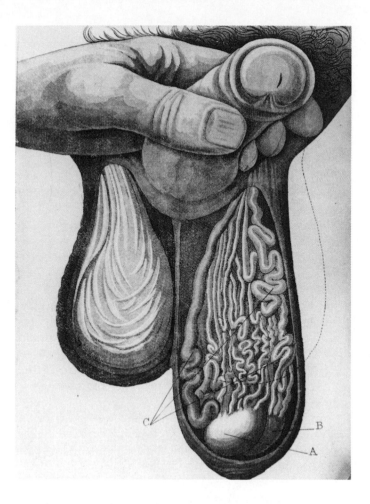

celibacy was blamed for ailments attributed by other authorities to indulgence.[95] Prolonged continence during the years of youthful vitality, Drysdale contended, could not fail to result in 'injurious habits of self-pollution' which, he believed, laid the foundations of lingering disease.[96] Nor was he of the opinion that nocturnal emissions were Nature's way of relief: his predictions of spermatorrhoea as their sequel seriously alarmed the youthful Havelock Ellis.[97] The healthful course was for the generative organs to experience 'due exercise from the time of their maturity', that is, from puberty.[98]

Drysdale joined both Samuel La'mert and the reviewers and leader-writers of the *Lancet* in deploring the neglect of sexual problems by the medical profession.[99] 'Pernicious feelings of delicacy' commonly led physicians to neglect inquiry 'into the history, past and present, of the genital organs in each patient', so that the sexual disorders 'at the root of all the symptoms' were never discovered.[100] Drysdale's views were predicated upon an assumption of female desire equal to that of the male. Under the existing social dispensation, he claimed, most women suffered from sexual starvation, while an unhappy few suffered the effects of a prostitute's life.[101] Though accused of intending to reduce all women to the state of prostitutes, Drysdale believed that his prescriptions would eradicate prostitution and its consequences.[102]

Elements of Social Science enjoyed considerable circulation. Havelock Ellis suggested that although 'by no means in every respect a scientific or sound work . . . it certainly had great influence, and it came into the hands of many who never saw any other work on sexual topics'.[103] Its status was ambiguous: produced primarily for a lay audience, kept in print at low price at some personal cost, it was nothing like the cheap or gratuitous volumes or pamphlets issued by La'mert and his ilk. Although Drysdale offered a panacea, this was not obtainable exclusively from himself but was a practice – contraception – which anyone could pursue. His message was taken badly enough by fellow secularists, some of whom claimed that Malthusianism aimed at a society in which 'all women would be virtually prostitutes',[104] and his sincere idealism was not directed towards issues of a kind likely to endear him to the medical profession. On its publication, *Elements* seems to have been ignored by the medical press.[105]

However, it did avoid legal proceedings, unlike other works advocating contraception. Knowlton's *Fruits of Philosophy*, reprinted by Drysdale's fellow-Malthusians Charles Bradlaugh and Annie Besant,[106] with his own editorial emendations, and H. A. Allbutt's *Wife's Handbook* were the subject of legal prosecution.[107] *Elements of Social Science* may have escaped as chiefly a philosophical, medical and political justification for the artificial limitation of families rather than a birth-control tract as such.

Perhaps the climate of opinion was becoming stricter, with the rise of a self-conscious movement for social purity connected with the agitation against the Contagious Diseases Acts, and anxieties about increased literacy among the lower classes.[108] Couples seem to have successfully limited family size by diverse means from about the 1870s,[109] largely without assistance from the medical profession, who regarded the entire subject as thoroughly reprehensible.

C. H. F. Routh, condemning contraception in his 1879 paper, 'On the Moral and Physical Evils likely to follow if practices intended to act as Checks to Population be not strongly discouraged and condemned', was extremely careful to point out that only the desire of 'distinguished members of the profession' induced him to open such discussion. Aware of 'the responsibility of having one's notions misconstrued', nevertheless he was 'ready to fulfil a manly and generous part'. During his diatribe he declared that though it was 'almost defilement even thus cursorily to allude to these vile practices . . . sexual fraudulency, conjugal onanism', it was the medical man's duty to point out the dangers. It seems clear that the very mention of the subject, even in outright condemnation, was regarded with suspicion.[110] While Allbutt 'might have ventilated his views without let or hindrance from professional authority had he been contented to address them to medical men instead of to the public',[111] it seems improbable that he would have met a favourable reception had he done so. However, he might have avoided deletion from the Medical Register for the professional crime of publishing *The Wife's Handbook* at a price placing it within the reach of all except the very poorest.

Sermons on 'impurity' from the 1850s treated fornication – either with prostitutes or intended brides – as the major and real danger.[112] It seems to be only by the 1880s, emerging from the movement to repeal the Contagious Diseases Acts, that there was more general vocal anxiety about masturbation. The *British Medical Journal*'s 1881 editorial, 'A Grave Social Problem', summarized existing debates and made various suggestions, extending the problem beyond the purely medical. Both 'the exaggerations of some of the earlier medical authors' and denial of 'the frequency of the evil and the permanently bad effects which it produced' had to be avoided. 'Certain forms of vice', never explicitly named, were 'a parasite' which had 'deeply eaten its insidious way' into the heart of the public school system. For an attempt at opening up discussion of a taboo subject, very little was actually being said, and the explicit warnings of Acton and others were deprecated. It was very hard to warn 'without entering into repulsive and suggestive detail', though 'vague and mysterious warnings' might suggest 'evils which might otherwise have remained unknown'. Tension existed between the urgent need to warn of impending dangers and the fear of putting undesirable ideas into formerly untouched minds.[113]

Masturbation was regarded as disgusting and sinful, deleterious to health, and also as the first step towards debauchery, disease and death through eroding self-discipline and self-control. Edward Lyttelton in *The Causes and Prevention of Immorality in Schools* alleged that 'The least defilement by hand enormously increases the difficulties of continence in manhood.'[114] 'The precocious indulgence of boyhood' might as 'the ungovernable passion of manhood . . . become responsible for the support of prostitution'[115] but masturbation might itself become 'the one absorbing and uncontrollable passion of life'.[116] Far more readily pursued to 'excess' than fornication, it dangerously depleted the vital forces, especially in adolescents, who needed these for the maturing process.

Although masturbation was supposedly so much more harmful than fornication that copulation was often advocated as the remedy, it is hard to find doctors actually recommending this (though see the case reported to Marie Stopes, above, p. 135); purity literature reiterated warnings against unprincipled medical men advocating fornication as essential for male health. Drysdale and the Malthusians could be regarded as doing this by implication, though Drysdale's belief in the medically deleterious effects of the existing sexual system hardly had the corollary that young men should resort to prostitutes, with the associated risk of disease.

Although masturbation (and indeed all sexual arousal in any connection except procreation within marriage) was so universally reprobated, there was a flourishing trade in pornography. Several historians who have analysed Victorian pornographic themes suggest that there was no escape; 'pornotopia', as Marcus called it, held up a mirror to Victorian sexual anxieties.[117] Earlier associations of pornographic publishers with radicalism and free thought had faded by the mid-century, as radicalism itself became respectable, and ideological libertinism or politically seditious obscenity were subsumed by commercial considerations.[118] Donald Thomas has suggested that erotic writing's exile in a pornographic ghetto of dubious legality led to 'greater psychological and physiological unreality' (and increasingly sadistic leitmotifs) in a genre always prone to be 'the fairy tales of adult society'.[119]

Questions need to be asked about the circulation of pornographic literature, much of which was highly priced 'masturbatory fantasies for frustrated upper-class males', in limited editions for a restricted market.[120] What exactly was being hawked by 'the filthy traders of Holywell Street' (the thoroughfare off the Strand in London notorious for the sale of obscene publications) and the itinerant vendors who visited markets and fairs up and down the country?[121] 'Feelthy pictures' seem to have figured more than letterpress, according to figures accumulated by the Society for the Suppression of Vice. In 1845 (prior to Lord Campbell's Obscene Publications Act), there were confiscated from two dealers alone 27,646 prints, 555 books, 447 copper-plates, 109 lithographic stones, $34\frac{1}{2}$ cuts of letterpress and 114 pounds of stereotype.[122] Obscene stereoscopic slides and 'indecent pipe heads' also figured.[123]

It is questionable how pornographic much literature sold as pornographic was; Mayhew described the 'Sham Indecent Street-Trade' in

spuriously obscene 'sealed packets'.[124] The unfulfilled lubricious prom-
ise of banal feuilletons like *The Confessions of a Lady's Maid or Boudoir
Intrigue, disclosing many Startling Scenes and Voloptuous [sic] Incidents, The
Confessions of a Footman or The Secrets of High Life Exposed, containing the
History of the 'Young Man' of Great Parts founded on Such Facts as are Rarely
Revealed to the Public, The Fortunes and Misfortunes of a Balletgirl. A Peep
Behind the Scenes* presumably justified the price of a shilling apiece.
However, *London by Night; or Gay Life in London* (extensively cribbed
from Mayhew), and the equivalent volume for Paris (though including
a good deal of comment on French life probably not of interest to
purchasers) were a slightly better bargain. Nuns, convents and the
confessional also seem to have been capable of generating erotic *frissons*
in a Protestant nation.[125]

It has been suggested that literature overtly aimed at suppressing
sexual vice itself has a pornographic function, and that works condemning masturbation may in fact lead to it. 'A certain unsavoury
suggestiveness' was found in Acton himself[126] – while he condemned
the salaciousness lurking in Lemprière's *Classical Dictionary*.[127]

Far from being an area of silence, a matter swept beneath the carpet
under the probably apocryphal pantalooned piano legs, sex was a recurrent topic of debate during the Victorian era. What were the messages,
and the tones of voice, of this debate? The dangerousness of sex was the
unavoidable theme, though differences might appear concerning
where, precisely, the danger lay. If sex was not concealed, there were
strong feelings that its manifestations ought to be, if they could not be
eradicated.

Contradictions were rife: how should we relate Acton's pronounce-
ments on female coldness to Baker Brown's fervid (and widely
condemned) excision of clitorises? How calibrate Drysdale's plea for
healthy contracepted sexual indulgence against his dire warnings of
the perils of spermatorrhoea? Syphilis was rife, but quacks and doctors
alike preached on male debility and the deleteriousness of masturbation. Media salaciousness lubriciously condemned the vices of
'debauched aristocrats' and 'French harlots', presumably remote from
their readers.[128] Mayhew classified women living with men in unmarried
fidelity as prostitutes.[129] Preachers condemned premarital fornication as
just as sinful as promiscuity.[130] In his famous articles on 'The Maiden
Tribute of Modern Babylon', W. T. Stead turned to the service of the
purity cause, as Walkowitz has so incisively demonstrated, themes and
motifs connected not merely with sensationalism and melodrama but
with outright pornography.[131]

By the 1880s new ways of thinking about sexuality were beginning to emerge, which endeavoured to escape or avoid association with pathology, individual or social. These will be discussed in the following chapters.

CHAPTER SEVEN

From the Primeval Protozoa to the Laboratory: the Evolution of Sexual Science from 1889 to the 1930s

In *The Descent of Man and Selection in Relation to Sex* (1871) Darwin argued the importance of sexual reproduction to the evolutionary process. This created the possibility of sex becoming a subject of scientific study distinct from the purely medical – no longer a question of pathology or disease, but a 'natural' phenomenon – though few took up this challenging task. The initial influence of these ideas of Darwin's seems to have been on 'The Woman Question'.[1] It was some time before the wider implications of treating sexuality as a proper field for scientific rationality were engaged with. So marginalized, indeed eccentric, was this development that it cannot be discussed without some consideration of the individuals engaging in it.

In 1889 a broader approach was adumbrated in *The Evolution of Sex* by Patrick Geddes and J. Arthur Thomson, the first volume in Havelock Ellis's Contemporary Science Series, small volumes presenting contemporary scientific developments for the average intelligent reader.[2] Although 'to place such a subject at the forefront of the scheme seemed daring to many people', Ellis found 'the book was well received and soon acquired high reputation and many readers'.[3] As a cheap volume of popular science, *The Evolution of Sex* doubtless circulated far more widely than Ellis's own subsequent massive, hard to obtain project, *Studies in the Psychology of Sex* (1899–1910, 1928).

Geddes, Professor of Biology at University College, Dundee, was a polymath whose holistic views, diverging from current trends in biological science, militated against the success many thought he deserved, although his personal influence was considerable. A major synthesist creating a 'bridge between biology and social science', his career was filled with potentially vast exciting projects, few of which came to full fruition.[4] A pupil of T. H. Huxley, he had worked with leaders of contemporary physiology such as Schäfer and Burdon Sanderson, but *The Evolution of Sex*, he alleged, was 'practically boycotted by the physiologists, zoologists, and botanists' because he had deserted ' "the Pack" ' by dropping his early connections with the Sanderson-Schäfer connection. This, though his best-known work, failed to reach the scientists, and was also neglected, he claimed, by 'the advanced people – from Shaw, etc. etc.', who might have 'written plays, novels, etc., not to speak of reviews, on these lines' had they not believed it to be 'technical – (or reactionary, as many advanced women did)'.[5]

J. Arthur Thomson, his friend and disciple, was allegedly the only person able to 'screw real collaboration' out of Geddes (which 'bled him of the last ounce of moral and intellectual energy!'). He brought to the partnership the 'stability, clarity and continuity needed for the production of popular scientific works', and a 'romantic brand of moral earnestness', in tune with the feelings of the period. Initially a theology student intending to become a missionary, Thomson studied natural science with Geddes, who was anxious not to lose this brilliant student. During the 1880s (prior to the writing of *The Evolution of Sex*), Thomson studied in France and Germany and is recorded as sending 'sex papers' from Berlin to Geddes in 1886 and talking about some kind of collaboration, although he was still contemplating the mission field.[6]

Geddes and Thomson viewed human sexuality as a 'fundamental unity underlying the Protean phenomena of sex and reproduction', and claimed to take 'an altered and unconventional view upon the general questions of biology'.[7] Their arguments were based on the theory of 'the divergent evolution of the sexes', expressed in terms of the 'anabolic' or constructive and conservative energies of the female, and the 'katabolic' or disruptive and destructive energies of the male. The 'average truth throughout the world of animals', in their view, was 'the preponderating passivity of the females, the predominant activity of the males' (a conclusion supported by an account of the cochineal insect, further illustrated by the threadworm).[8] Illustrations from all of organic creation proved that 'what was decided among the prehistoric protozoa cannot be annulled by Act of Parliament'.[9] Study of the lower forms of creation demonstrated for humanity 'the temporarily exhausting effect of even moderate sexual indulgence'; given their katabolic nature males were 'especially liable to exhaustion'.[10] However, Geddes and Thomson, while seeing the sexes as essentially distinct, emphasized that they were 'complementary and mutually dependent ... each is higher in its own way. ... Man thinks more, woman feels more.'[11] It seems that Geddes, in particular, came to feel that there was a necessity for the female principle to figure more largely in public life, and for increased co-operation between the sexes.[12]

Geddes and Thomson had some sympathy with neo-Malthusian arguments: 'the survival of a species or family depends not primarily upon quantity, but upon quality',[13] a view which also appealed to them on humanitarian grounds. However, their attitude to the employment of artificial birth control was, like that of many contemporaries, ambivalent; by admitting 'egoistic sexual pleasures' separate from reproductive responsibility it could 'multiply temptations', but conversely, 'the very transition from unconscious animalism to deliberate prevention' might 'decrease rather than increase sexual appetite'.[14] They advocated temperance and 'a new ethic of the sexes',[15] and social, rather than individual, approaches to the problem.

While the 'biological factors of the case' asserted with 'all scientific relativity' do not appear to lead to very different conclusions to the teachings of the 'dogmatic authority' they claimed to supersede,[16] it was nonetheless radical to put sex on the scientific agenda in this way. Edward Carpenter, much further to the left of the reform spectrum, read the work with interest and pronounced it 'first-rate'.[17] It could certainly be perceived as subversive: an early reader wrote: 'your book which my husband offered to our new public library here was courteously rejected under the plea that it was quite impossible to have such books in a library where unmarried or young people might find them!'[18] Mingling biology with 'social and ethical problems' disturbed the reviewer in *Nature*: praising its 'wealth of knowledge . . . lucid and attractive method of treatment . . . rich vein of picturesque language', he nonetheless felt that though useful for biologists to grapple with the work was not suitable for public consumption.[19]

The book's influence on the common reader was suggested by a contemporary's comment that 'multitudes of young men in Scotland and in England owed their souls to the teachings of Patrick Geddes', and found his idealism and optimism, his emphasis on the co-operative rather than the competitive aspects of Darwinism, an inspiration.[20] But it did not do much professionally for its writers. A colleague of Geddes's at Dundee reportedly remarked: 'I always stood up for you old chap. . . . you know, the book on Sex. But I always told them you'd given up that sort of thing long ago.'[21] It did not, immediately, appear to influence other scientists or the course of research, although Alfred Russel Wallace wrote thanking them for his copy, raising some queries concerning their discussion of evolution. He praised their 'labour and care' in 'summarising and coordinating . . . facts on one of the most interesting and most important branches of biological study'.[22] Geddes and Thomson's emphasis on the biological norm also set them outside the mainstream of the emerging new sexology of the 1890s which was concentrating on the pathological and the deviant rather than the 'normal'. While biological, *The Evolution of Sex* was in no way 'medicalizing', nor was it clinical in its approach, which may explain why it was not reviewed by the major medical journals.

A further reason for its neglect within the mainstream of British physiology may relate to the internal dynamic of research in the field, following Schäfer's influential early work on the importance of internal secretions: a certain puritanism among physiologists of the Schäfer school should not be excluded. During the 1890s Brown-Sequard's work in France on 'rejuvenation' using testicular and ovarian extracts stimulated study of the secretions of the sexual organs. His results were scantily and rather critically reported in Britain, and ignored by endocrinologists. This neglect of the potential of treating the gonads as endocrine glands was to some extent due to available methods for assessing endocrine action, more suited to adrenaline or the thyroid. Schäfer's extremely late conversion to the internal secretions hypothesis *vis-à-vis* the sexual organs, however, does suggest typical British puritanism, and a strong desire not to be associated with the fashionable clinical use of 'glandular extracts'. The association with sexual rejuvenation was particularly abhorrent to British scientists.[23]

The new sexology and its categorization of the deviant appeared to many yet another dubious continental import. The *British Medical Journal* reviewer in 1893 admitted to having taken some time to consider whether to notice the English translation of Krafft-Ebing's *Psychopathia Sexualis*. Conceding that 'many morally disgusting subjects . . . have to be studied by the doctor and by the jurist', the reviewer felt that 'the less such subjects are brought before the public, the better'. The book, potentially 'valuable as a book of reference', was 'altogether one not to be left about for general reading'.[24]

Edward Carpenter (1844–1929) was writing at this time on issues of sexuality from a mystical-reformist rather than medico-scientific approach. Himself a member of 'The Intermediate Sex', Carpenter had initially trained for the Church before resigning his curacy and becoming involved in socialism, anti-imperialism, Indian mysticism and allied issues such as vegetarianism, 'the simple life' and anti-vivisection. Though opposed to what he perceived as increasing scientific materialism, he was happy to adduce scientific evidence (including that of Geddes and Thomson) in support of his arguments, while his synthesis of the available evidence gained credence among many committed to the scientific materialist outlook. His vision of transformed human relationships was previewed in the long Whitmanesque poem *Towards Democracy*, written in 1881–2, published in 1883, and much reprinted, depicting a celebratory attitude towards the body and a comradely relationship between the sexes. In 1894 he produced a series of small pamphlets on sex reform questions: *Woman and her/, Sex Love and its/, Marriage and its/, Homogenic Love and its/Place in a Free Society*, published by the Manchester Labour Press. These pamphlets formed the basis for the book *Love's Coming of Age* (1896), although due to hesitation by the publisher T. Fisher Unwin in the aftermath of the Oscar Wilde case the section on 'The Intermediate Sex' was not included until 1906.[25]

Love's Coming of Age was highly influential, and often reprinted during the following forty years. While Carpenter believed in essential biological differences between the sexes, he regarded the existing excessive social differentiation as highly deleterious; the sexes ought not to be 'two groups hopelessly isolated in habit and feeling from each other'. Given that 'the extreme specimens at either pole are vastly divergent', those of a middle range in spite of physical differentiation were 'by emotion and temperament very near to each other'. He argued for the symbolic function of sex as union, not just for reproduction. The 'immense diversity of human temperament and character in matters relating to sex and love'[26] meant that there were

> no limits of grace or comeliness, or of character and accomplish-
> ment, or even of infirmity or age, within which love is obliged to
> move . . . no defect, of body or mind, which is of necessity a bar –
> which may not even (to some special other person) become an object
> of attraction.[27]

Men and male predominance bore much responsibility for the trouble civilization was in; the significant regenerative role that Carpenter assigned to women was surely flattering to female readers, despite the very traditional nature of some of his assumptions. He believed in improved sexual education, opposed the double standard, and held to an ideal of a central, but not necessarily exclusive, monogamous relation between individuals. His ideas enjoyed a wide influence well beyond the specifically 'Uranian' constituency, and his books were read and admired in moderately progressive circles by both sexes.

This is not to ignore his highly influential treatment of the problems of 'The Intermediate Sex'. The discussion of these in *Love's Coming of Age* may have reached a broader audience than his books addressed more specifically to the topic.[28] Those of the 'Uranian type' were not 'necessarily morbid' but often 'fine, healthy specimens of their sex, muscular and well-developed in body, of powerful brain, high standard of conduct'. Carpenter was definite that the intermediate's 'special affectional temperament' was inborn, and he believed it possible that they might 'have an important part to play in the evolution of the race'.

Far from being 'libertines having no law but curiosity in self-indul-
gence', their attachments were 'often purely emotional in character'.
He saw the intermediate as possessing in some degree the characteristics of the opposite sex, in the ideal type being more or less the perfect
balance of the best qualities of both sexes.[29]

It was in this milieu of increasing debate on problems of sex, in the
face of considerable ambivalence, if not deliberate evasion, among the
medical profession over the subject, that Havelock Ellis (1859–1939) set
out to write his enormous work *Studies in the Psychology of Sex*. A proem,
the volume *Man and Woman* (1894), published in the Contemporary
Science Series, synthesized existing data on secondary sexual differences.[30] Ellis, after a mystic revelation while teaching in Australia had
directed him to the study of sex, had acquired the licentiate of the
Society of Apothecaries, the minimum qualification necessary for medical practice, so had the not inconsiderable advantage of being a medical
man. Nevertheless he encountered enormous problems in the early
stages of his project.

His collaborative first volume, *Sexual Inversion*, was undertaken with
J. Addington Symonds, himself an 'invert', who died while the volume
was in preparation. Symonds had already privately printed and circulated to possible sympathizers two short tracts on homosexuality, *A
Problem in Greek Ethics* (1883), and *A Problem in Modern Ethics* (1891),
probably the first British statements on the subject, although there had
been debates on the continent for some decades.[31] Ellis's choice of this
introduction to the project appears partly to have been motivated by
the approach from Symonds, but he claimed to Edward Carpenter, 'I
have been independently attracted to it',[32] possibly by the revelation
that his wife Edith was a lesbian. The volume appeared with disastrous
timing shortly after the Oscar Wilde trial, under Ellis's name alone,
after a first edition under both names had been bought up and
destroyed by Symonds's literary executor in order to spare the feelings
of the family.[33]

There had been problems in finding a publisher for a volume on
such a controversial topic and it eventually appeared under the dubious
imprint of the Watford University Press, which was run by an equivocal
character of obscure antecedents. This firm also published the *Adult*,
the journal of the small but vigorous Legitimation League, which combined the practical object of improving the legal status of illegitimate
children with a wider critique of contemporary marriage and sexual
mores. Meetings of the League attracted anarchists, and had brought
the organization to the attention of the police, who assumed the strongest connections between free love, anarchism, and 'books of the "Psychology" type'. The secretary of the League, George Bedborough, sold
a copy of *Sexual Inversion* to a police detective in May 1898, and was

arrested: the police hoped, while suppressing 'a certain lewd, wicked, bawdy, scandalous libel' (namely, *Sexual Inversion*), to kill two birds with one stone by also destroying the Legitimation League with its politically subversive associates. A Free Press Defence Committee was set up, but after six months of waiting Bedborough was brought to trial and pleaded guilty. Ellis was not accused, but nor was he allowed any opportunity to defend his work, which was labelled scandalous and obscene uncontested.[34] The whole episode was extremely traumatic for a shy and highminded man like Ellis and led to his increasing shrinking from public life.

The seizure and prosecution of *Sexual Inversion* was the subject of comment in medical journals. The *Lancet* was prepared to admit that the subject had 'proper claims for discussion', and though 'odious in itself', ought to be faced. A 'book written solely in a spirit of scientific enquiry' could not be 'indecent literature', but discussion of the subject had very definitely to be restricted 'to persons of particular attainments'. It was not a matter for 'the man in the street', or even worse 'the boy and girl in the street', and the work might become indecent 'if offered to the general public with a wrong motive'.[35] The *British Medical Journal* conceded that no attempt had been made 'to advertise the book in any general way or to expose it for sale otherwise than in a technical sense', and that it in no way pandered 'to the prurient mind'. Members of the medical profession indeed ought to have some acquaintance with this 'extremely disagreeable' topic.[36] No British physician, however, was prepared to join those supplying testimonials to the Free Press Defence Committee as to Ellis's scientific respectability and serious motives.[37]

Meanwhile, a number of issues specifically relating to female sexuality were being debated by women themselves, perhaps given confidence by their participation in the campaign to repeal the Contagious Diseases Acts. Science seemed at least a potential ally in clarifying what were perceived as murky distortions of truth imposed by a male-dominated social order. This sexual theorizing usually took place in the context of a wider and immediate concern with reform, and is also discussed in Chapter 8, and in Chapters 9 and 10 in the context of changing discourses on conjugal sex and on sex education.

Feminist thoughts on sex appeared in such forums as Margaret Shurmer Sibthorp's short-lived feminist journal of the 1890s, *Shafts: A Paper for Women and the Working Classes*, and in publications of various kinds by women. Questions were raised about, for example, the alleged greater degree of chastity manifested by women: was it an innate trait, thus nothing to be boasted about, or a real, therefore meritorious struggle?[38] 'Ellis Ethelmer' (pseudonym of Elizabeth Wolstenholme Elmy) elaborated in her poem 'Woman Free' (1893) upon the theory of T. L. Nichols (in his widely circulated *Esoteric Anthropology*) that sexual indulgence excited the ovaries and caused menstruation to degenerate into a 'real hemorrhage . . . depraved in its character'.[39] Where Nichols had seen this as a personal pathological consequence of overindulgence, Elmy attributed the 'unhealed . . . scars of man's distempered greed', 'the heritage of woe', 'spurious function' (etc.) to primeval rape. She hoped that a 'purer phase of life' would release women from the 'burden of wasting weariness', as women once more took control of their sexual lives.[40] This interpretation of menstruation as 'indiscriminate violation of . . . sacred laws' establishing as ' "habit" a morbid malady, unquestionably due to primeval man's uncontrollable depravity', was also argued in correspondence in *Shafts*.[41]

Shafts also paid attention to writings such as Carpenter's. About *Sex-Love*, the reviewer had 'a fault to urge . . . he writes with a masculine pen, he reasons with the masculine bias, he sees with the masculine dimness of vision'. The writings of 'a masculine pen on such subjects as these should be taken up and threshed out by women'; Carpenter was, however, conceded to be, in his dim masculine way, on the right track, and worth reading as a stimulus to further thought.[42]

As a new century dawned the medical profession continued to contend that medical men had some need to know about disgusting subjects such as sexual perversion. However, Carpenter's *The Intermediate Sex* was subjected to a scathing four-column review in the *British Medical Journal* in 1909. This animadverted against the 'many publications of this character since *Psychopathia Sexualis* and *Sexual Inversion*', and concluded by suggesting that 'Urnings' ought to emigrate to

> some land where their presence might be welcome, and thus serious people in England might be spared the waste of time reading a low-priced book of no scientific or literary merit, advocating the culture of unnatural and criminal practices.

The reviewer was positively obsessed with the cheapness of the work, referring to it once as 'low-priced' and twice reiterating that it cost 3s. 6d. (18p): perhaps the worst offence, since it placed it within reach of that 'man in the street' who was to be protected from such knowledge.[43] Ellis commented to Carpenter that although the book was 'more needed in England than in Germany' (where it was initially published) 'England is scarcely yet ripe for it.'[44]

This attack on Carpenter contrasts with growing respect accorded Havelock Ellis by his professional peers. His subject-matter might be 'disgusting and nauseous', but his 'honesty of purpose' was commendable, in spite of 'regret that it is not turned to better account'.[45] In 1910, the *Lancet*'s reviewer recommended *Sex in Relation to Society* (giving 'the dignity of scholarship to a very delicate and difficult subject') 'to the medical world and to serious students of social problems'.[46] *Studies in the Psychology of Sex* was the result of serious scholarly labours, available only in limited, expensive and hard to obtain editions, even if Ellis also wrote works of a more popular nature. It also helped to be both a doctor and British: Arthur Cooper's little textbook *The Sexual Disabilities of Man and Their Treatment* (1908) was favourably contrasted by the *Lancet* with 'certain turbid continental outpourings'.[47]

Turbid continental outpourings gained little sympathy in England, particularly among the medical profession. In the same year as Cooper was praised the *British Medical Journal* published a leader, 'Professor Freud and Hysteria', on the 'particularly interesting and lively controversy' over Freud's theories of the aetiology of hysteria and the value of psychoanalysis: of which it was not at all in favour.[48] Dean Rapp has ably demonstrated that, prior to W. H. R. Rivers's article in the *Lancet* of 1917, most discussion of Freud and psychoanalysis was to be found in lay periodicals and among intellectually progressive groups of lay people (and even they preferred Carl Jung who placed less emphasis upon sexual aetiology).[49] It is far from clear whether Freud and his teachings were much known beyond a rather limited circle: in 1912 J. A. Campbell deemed it necessary to explain to Patrick Geddes (apparently in response to a query), 'Freud is an Austrian Dr... his effort is to break up morbid psychological conditions by tracing them to their sources generally to the inhibition of emotional expression in childhood.'[50] By 1914, in their Home University Library volume, *Sex*, Geddes and Thomson alluded to 'the remarkable work of Freud' and his 'most important recent contributions to the pathology of sex'.[51] Rivers, however, in his ground-breaking *Lancet* article of 1917 on psychoanalysis, explicitly deplored overemphasis (attributed to over-enthusiastic disciples rather than Freud himself) on the role of sex in the aetiology of neurosis.[52]

In spite of the *British Medical Journal*'s somewhat constrained imprimatur of 1893, less than ten years later the 1902 translation of the tenth edition of Krafft-Ebing's *Psychopathia Sexualis* was savaged as 'the most repulsive of a group of books of which it is the type', not sparing 'the minutest and the most nauseous detail'. The *British Medical Journal* reviewer preferred 'that the book should convey solace by being put to the most ignominious use to which paper can be applied'.[53] It seems probable that even while Krafft-Ebing himself was still alive, *Psychopathia Sexualis* had already gained, through pirated and unauthorized editions, its scabrous British reputation as little more than a work of scientific pornography.

'Turbid continental outpourings' may also have included Otto Weininger's notorious *Sex and Character*, of which an English translation (from the original German) was published in 1906, to what appears to have been at least a *succès de scandale*. Weininger had killed himself in 1903, at the age of twenty-three; the book had been written when he was twenty-one. He claimed to be investigating principles rather than details; not despising the investigations of the laboratory while finding these limited in scope compared to 'introspective analysis'. In the first section Weininger collated evidence supporting the thesis that no human being is ever entirely male or entirely female. Sexual attraction, in his view, most strongly existed between beings having complementary proportions of male and female, thus making up a complete one of each. In the second part he elaborated the view that far from being separate but equal, or having different but equally valuable functions, the sexes (in ideal and unmixed form) were totally different, the male positive, the female negative. Woman was 'nothing but sexuality, she is sexuality itself', and fell into two classes, the maternal type and the prostitute.[54]

The book certainly seems to have gained notoriety, being mentioned noticeably more often in surviving correspondence of both Geddes and Edward Carpenter than anything by Freud or even Krafft-Ebing, and in the case of Geddes more often than Havelock Ellis. Requesting a review from Geddes, the editor of the *Saturday Review* remarked

> I have a very shrewd suspicion that the work is more than one half the work of a quack, and I want a really first-rate man to deal with it. . . . The English translation . . . is put forward with a considerable flourish of trumpets.

An annotation on this letter by Geddes reads 'Morbid in tendency. Sophistical in treatment.'[55] The (anonymous) review in the *Saturday Review* pointed out that Weininger's main thesis had already been adumbrated by Geddes and Thomson. Criticism of the work was however 'no mere reclamation of priority': major objections were registered as to its adolescent and narcissistic misogyny.[56]

Carpenter's friend Grace French called it a 'terrible book', urging him to 'publish a counter-blast – and demolish his anathemas!'[57] Carpenter wrote to Ellis in October 1906 that he was reading the book 'with great interest' and although 'a very unequal book, juvenile in parts, rash and dogmatic in conclusions, often illogical' it was 'quite a work of genius'. While agreeing with Weininger's 'general estimate of woman . . . provided of course you apply it as representing the extreme type' Carpenter considered it 'a pity he did not balance the book by shewing the absurdities of the Absolute Male'.[58] Ellis's own view was presumably encapsulated in his dry 1916 comment 'I should not myself have been inclined to *recommend* Weininger's book, a brilliant piece of fireworks which is already being taken seriously by many.'[59] Carpenter in later editions of *Love's Coming of Age* mentioned the 'true German manner' of Weininger's 'algebraic formula for the different types of men and women'. 'Though we may mock a little at these fanciful divisions and dissections,' he added, they did 'help us to realize the enormous, the astounding number of varieties' to which human nature was susceptible.[60] Carpenter's extensive account of *Sex and Character* to Ellis contrasts, perhaps significantly, with his brief and rather dismissive sentence on returning 'Über den Traum' in 1914: 'I can't say that I find it very interesting – rather *forced* I think.' While he thought he would like to look at Freud's book on the subject he did not want to do so immediately.[61]

The extreme feminist and theosophist Frances Swiney referred to *Sex and Character* as 'this remarkable book', with its 'cry from the abyss of human suffering, misery, and despair' as man was 'confronted by the perverted sex-principle in human depravity'. Her views almost exactly inverted Weininger's: she too believed the sexes to be antithetical, but conceived that the corrupt male was hindering the higher evolution of the superior woman.[62] Although of a theosophical bent, she allowed that scientists were 'doing the grandest, the most indispensable, work for the reformer, the metaphysician, and the philosopher'. Among those 'laying bare the foundations of the eternal temple' Ellis and Geddes and Thomson had 'in a measure elucidated the mystery of sex'.[63] She cited Geddes and Thomson in confirmation of her argument that 'the male element is invariably associated in all ages with destruction, disintegration, force, impurity, and evil'; contact with it rendered the female – the true source of creative energy – impure.[64]

A continental author less favoured than Weininger was Iwan Bloch, whose *Sexual Life of Our Time* was condemned to be destroyed at Bow Street early in 1907. Eden Paul, the translator and a member of sexual reform circles, was prepared to take the case to the 'House of Fossils' (i.e. the House of Lords), but Havelock Ellis expected, rather cynically, that 'a compromise will be arranged and that the publisher will agree to limit the sale to doctors, etc.'.[65] The edition which appeared in 1909 did indeed have just such a limitation. The 'Publisher's Note to the English Edition' conceded that the subject was 'no doubt one which appeals to and affects the interests of all adult persons'. However 'after very serious and careful consideration' the sale was to be 'limited to members of the legal and medical professions'.[66]

Although sex might be a subject which ought to be discussed (if only with all due precaution among the medical profession), Continentals were suspect, even when medical men themselves. Lay persons were not supposed to tamper with it. Within the British medical profession Havelock Ellis therefore had almost a clear field, although there were a few writers – such as Arthur Cooper – writing approved textbooks on the clinical manifestations of sexual disorders which might appear in the consulting room. Ernest Jones, Freud's British disciple, addressing Ellis in 1910 as a 'fellow worker in the field of sexology' remarked on his 'relatively lonely path'.[67] There was no one approaching the subject with anything like Havelock Ellis's grandeur of vision, which was allied to a particularly elegant style. It cannot have hurt his critical reception that he wrote pellucid prose in the tones of the Victorian gentleman scholar, described by the writer Rebecca West as 'delicate, grave, rectory English', in which she averred Ellis sustained 'in the most difficult circumstances' the 'inveterate appearance . . . of being a character out of *Cranford*'.[68]

The monumental *Studies in the Psychology of Sex*[69] drew upon an enormous variety of sources, from medical writings, the researches of anthropologists, the work of biologists, literature from many countries, and the self-disclosures of individuals about their own sexual experiences. His research was conducted under conditions not always favourable: he wrote to the anthropologist Edvard Westermarck in 1902, 'I have to buy so many books that are not accessible in English libraries that I am obliged to refrain from buying books that are accessible.'[70] The *Studies* form among other things a valuable archive for what was being said and thought about sex at the time. If they could be said to have one underlying theme it was that all sexual behaviour lay somewhere upon a continuum, that the 'perverse' often merely exaggerated 'normal tendencies', and that liberal toleration for difference was a high virtue. Ellis was an old-fashioned liberal with a strong belief in the power of education: although he sympathized with the contemporary eugenics movement his emphasis was placed on its educative role, and he was extremely chary of anything smacking of compulsion. His name became a metonym for the sexology of liberal celebration of diversity, as the name Krafft-Ebing became for the cataloguing of pathology.

Ellis is perhaps mainly remembered for his contribution to studies of the sexually anomalous and his depiction of the vast range of sexual behaviour. His sober non-judgemental treatment of *Sexual Inversion* has been often commented upon – 'the voice of common sense and compassion' as his biographer Phyllis Grosskurth describes it.[71] His somewhat unsatisfactory formulation of female sexuality as essentially responsive to the male and founded on her reproductive function has also been discussed.[72] However, he wrote essays and pamphlets on marriage, eugenics and motherhood in the context of his philosophy of a changed and more egalitarian relationship between the sexes: he was a passionate advocate of the 'erotic rights of woman' and within the context of his time the importance he gave to 'the play-function of sex' must surely have struck readers far more than the biologistic assumptions they as much as he must have taken for granted. His approach by its very openness, its reluctance to force conclusions, provided a potent model for further explorations.[73]

Ellis's method of approaching subjects normally treated in pejorative and pathologizing terms can be seen in the essay on 'Auto-Erotism', in Volume I of *Studies in the Psychology of Sex*, first published in 1899 as Volume II. In this he turned a radically critical gaze onto received wisdom. Auto-erotism, formulated as extending far beyond deliberate masturbatory practice, had 'rarely been viewed in a scientifically sound and morally sane light'; attention had been concentrated upon masturbation 'in insanity and allied conditions'. In fact, masturbation was 'a specialized form of a tendency' affecting 'all the higher animals'.[74] Ellis exploded contemporary myths that masturbation was inevitably physically, mentally, or morally debilitating, a uniquely human trait, or a sad side-effect of civilization. It was 'found among the people of nearly every race of which we have any intimate knowledge, however natural the conditions under which men and women may live'.[75]

His mild caution that deliberate masturbatory practices might divorce 'the physical sensuous impulse and the ideal emotions',[76] was a long way from the awful warnings of most writers, although Ellis did suggest that the persistent and habitual masturbator might suffer from traditional 'morbid heightening of self-consciousness' and lowering of self-esteem – still a long way from insanity, consumption and death.[77] 'Auto-Erotism' was much more likely to alleviate than create anxiety, since Ellis foresaw undesirable results only in specified circumstances.

While the *Studies* were not easy to obtain, the name of Havelock Ellis became associated with sexual enlightenment and people did manage to get access to his works. He commented in a long letter to Carpenter in 1910 on the completion of the *Studies*, that 'the work is becoming known as rapidly as I care for, and I shall not publish in England,' and some years later that 'intermediates' wrote or called 'at almost regular intervals' having come across *Sexual Inversion*.[78] Many of the ideas discussed at length in the *Studies* were presented more simply and accessibly in his essays, for example, those collected in *Essays in War-Time* or *Little Essays of Love and Virtue*.[79]

He had enormous influence on other writers. Some acknowledged this, including the anthropologist Radcliffe-Brown, who described his works as 'one of the most potent influences that have shaped my life

. . . a lasting inspiration'.[80] However, the 'spate of books on the sexual question' appearing after the war were, according to C. P. Blacker, largely 'secondhand versions of Ellis's ideas presented with little of his literary distinction and none of his philosophical detachment', whose authors nonetheless received 'nothing but sympathy and encouragement' from a pioneer 'completely devoid of petty jealousies'.[81] When Marie Stopes protested to Ellis about the virtual plagiarism of her *Married Love* by another writer,[82] he replied that

> (though I do not feel any admiration for the people who do this sort of thing) I am pleased to see ideas to which I attach value put into circulation, whether or not they are labelled with my name.[83]

The new sexology was widely regarded as, and in many cases even intended to be, dangerously radical. This was certainly so in Britain, where the leading figures in the field were also involved with politically radical movements. However, although talking about sex and arguing for its investigation was initially a subversive and progressive project, it was by no means uncomplicated in its implications. Ellis and Carpenter, like Geddes and Thomson, believed that difference did not imply hierarchy, that society grossly exaggerated adventitious characteristics of gender, and that because of their very difference women should be given a greater voice in the ordering of society; nevertheless, many of their arguments were founded on the assumption that profound differences between the sexes existed.

Their work could be – and was – turned against their own aims, by succeeding writers with very different, indeed antithetical agendas. The reforming sexology of Ellis and Carpenter was to some extent overtaken, if not entirely superseded, during the second decade of the twentieth century. There arose a new, laboratory and experiment-based scientific study of sex and reproduction, drawing upon animal studies and the gradually increasing knowledge about the gonadal hormones and their action, with considerable input from clinical observations by gynaecologists. The study of sexual phenomena was increasingly abstracted from the realm of human behaviour and social influence, and (apparently) depoliticized.

However, because of the stigma hindering investigation, against which the reformist figures had been struggling, little was known about reproductive biology. In most textbooks of physiology the subject was either 'restricted to a few final pages seldom free from error, or else . . . entirely omitted'.[84] Studies appearing from 1910 onwards did not scorn the information or hypotheses of writers such as Geddes and Thomson, Havelock Ellis, Otto Weininger, Krafft-Ebing, Edvard Westermarck, Auguste Forel and Iwan Bloch, in attempts to establish some kind of basis for research.[85] The influence of these writers on sex with their social and psychological orientation on sexual problems, and often radical political agendas, on the laboratory-centred study of reproductive biology has yet to be fully elucidated.[86]

In 1910 F. H. A. Marshall set out to supply the want of a comprehensive treatise pertaining to the reproductive processes.[87] 'A milestone in the history of biological literature',[88] his book, *The Physiology of Reproduction*, aimed to 'give a connected account of various groups of ascertained facts' not hitherto placed in relation to one another. 'Addressed primarily to the trained biologist', its subject would also interest the medical man.[89] Though Marshall failed to make outstanding discoveries, he was 'an invaluable guide and stimulus', whose synthesis of available evidence 'cleared the ground for others',[90] without ignoring the controversies and uncertainties within the field.[91]

Marshall's synthesis demonstrated that knowledge of all aspects of the reproductive processes was both scanty and in a state of flux. Marshall enumerated the varied conjectures about the relationship between the menstrual period and ovulation, a question not to be resolved conclusively for nearly another twenty years. Though obstetricians had concluded from empirical observation that 'women menstruate because they do not conceive', Marshall, whose own experimental work had been on animals with a marked oestrous cycle, was inclined to be more cautious.[92] It was still an open question at what point in development sexual differentiation took place, whether at conception or at some stage of foetal development.[93] But what seemed incontrovertible was the existence of latent characters of one sex in the other so that no individual was entirely male or entirely female; indeed it was arguable that everyone was 'potentially hermaphrodite'.[94]

By 1910 the influence of the sexual glands on general metabolism had been much discussed, but conclusions were far from definite and often contradictory. Though removing testicles and ovaries, transplanting them, or injecting extracts had proved their influence to be chemical rather than nervous, results were far from conclusive.[95] The relationship of secondary sexual characteristics to 'the essential organs of reproduction' was not clear-cut,[96] and the role of the other ductless glands (thymus, thyroid, pituitary) had already become apparent.[97] Marshall expressed characteristic British scepticism towards Brown-Sequard's views on the 'invigorating properties' of testicular extracts; he thought it 'not unlikely that some of the effects . . . attributed to the use of the extract were in reality due to suggestion'.[98] His own tests of commercially produced ovarian extracts revealed their inefficacy.[99]

Buried within Marshall's text were a number of sexual facts which might seem obvious and hardly needing to be said, but which a perusal of the revelations of sexual ignorance received during the 1920s by the advice-writer Marie Stopes suggest were not entirely self-evident, even among biological scientists.[100] Not everyone seems to have been aware that the penis was 'the intromittent organ of copulation', with the 'function of conveying the semen into the genital passages of the female . . . dependent upon its power of erection under the influence of sexual excitement'.[101] Similarly, it was not necessarily a matter of general knowledge that 'the clitoris in the female . . . undergoes erection during coitus', leading to 'a reflex discharge of motor impulses in both the female and the male'.[102] (Marshall gives no indication that this latter effect might not be the automatic outcome of intromission, though he had surmised that 'higher nerve centres exercise an inhibitory influence over the sexual processes'.)[103] He granted that it was 'conceivable . . . that the process of erection is after all a more complex phenomenon than is generally believed', but was unable to cite experimental evidence illuminating this issue.[104]

The task of isolating the hypothetical gonadal hormones gave investigators of sexual physiology a clear-cut goal. Research had proceeded with some vigour since Schäfer, the doyen of British physiology, had declared his very belated conversion to the view that 'internal secretions containing special hormones' from the testicles and ovaries exerted significant influence on secondary sexual characteristics. Monitoring and measuring actual changes posed technical difficulties in the absence of data on all aspects of the reproductive process as the baseline for monitoring the effects of hormones. In spite of the vast gaps in knowledge and the need for further experimental work, however, the nervous energy theory of sexuality was already losing predominance to the glandular theory.[105]

Around 1912, investigators in three different countries discovered 'the secret of the ovarian hormone' ('extraction with lipid solvents) but for another ten years ovarian endocrinology remained in confusion.[106] This was presumably at least in part due to the disruption of war, which affected biological research within the countries involved as well as communication between researchers of different nationalities, given the enormous advances that were made during the 1920s.

Several works influenced by the current investigations into and debates about sexual physiology appeared in Britain during this confused period. Among them were *Sex Antagonism* (1913), a polemic statement by Walter Heape, a zoologist who had worked closely with Marshall and to whom *The Physiology of Reproduction* was dedicated, and *The Sex Complex* (1916), by the gynaecologist and obstetrician William

Blair Bell. They indicate the kinds of idea 'in the air' about sex at the time. Something of a reaction against the ideas of Carpenter and Ellis, they give the impression of having been negatively affected by the militant suffrage movement, and possibly the emancipatory upheaval of the war.

Eschewing Marshall's caution in the face of equivocal evidence about sex differences, Heape argued that the sexes were not merely innately different, but that antagonism between their aims in life had existed since the earliest epochs of human existence. Contemporary social unrest resulted from neglect of the natural laws ruling the relations of the sexes. The male was 'active and roaming, he hunts for his partner and is an expender of energy', passionate, promiscuous and polygamous.[107] Suppression of the powerful male 'generative impulse' was penalized by 'derangement throughout the body'.[108] The female, 'passive, sedentary, one who waits for her partner and is a conserver of energy', was predominantly interested in motherhood and preventing her mate from straying.[109] The sexual requirements of the two sexes were thus vastly at odds, and the imposition of monogamy generated sex antagonism.[110]

Though complementary, the sexes in primitive society (and implicitly though less obviously in contemporary civilized life) were engaged in constant struggle for supremacy.[111] Rigid societal laws of sexual conduct favoured 'the growth of drastic sex antagonism', as society became 'more and more complicated and the life led by its members more purely artificial'.[112] But although Heape considered that, by their pernicious constraint upon natural tendencies, 'the present sex laws weigh as heavily, if not much more heavily on men', he found a remarkable 'complacency of the dissatisfied man'.[113] 'Sex antagonism' due to 'Neglect of Nature's laws', led some women, 'undoubtedly spinsters', exhibiting 'mental derangement . . . associated with degeneration of the functional capacity of the generative organs', into vociferous opposition to the existing state of affairs. Their interests were, Heape contended, antagonistic to those of women concerned with the production of children.[114] Woman would be better advised in his view to cultivate 'dominant female qualities, by increasing their value, she will gain power which no man can usurp'.[115]

Blair Bell too was well aware of participating in a 'controversy concerning the differences between Man and Woman' with social and legal implications, rarely conducted 'on unbiased and scientific lines'. His project seems to have caused him some ambivalence, given his allusions to tearing aside 'the veil overhanging the mystery of sex', and the 'ravages of science'. Nonetheless he suggested that dissecting the complexity of sex would 'not disturb the sex instincts of a single normal individual'. Unlike Heape, and although believing humanity was evolving towards yet greater differentiation,[116] Blair Bell considered that whatever the predominant sexual identity of the individual, 'latent traits of the opposite sex' in various degrees of development were always present.[117]

His particular revelation, however, was that '*femininity itself is dependent on all the internal secretions*': the gonads did not act alone to influence female characteristics and genital functions.[118] Woman's mental characteristics came under 'the dominating influence of her special functions'.[119] Although 'individuation' might not negatively affect fertility, the discharge of female functions might not be compatible with the degree of individuation normal in males.[120] The human female's highly developed mental processes were to assist with sexual selection and the care and upbringing of offspring, keeping pace with the general mental evolution of the race.[121] Males had evolved intelligence 'to sustain their mates and offspring in an environment compatible with advanced civilisation' and to deal with the 'intricate processes' of modern life.[122] Reproduction made fewer demands on the male metabolism, therefore men's 'nerves [were] steady, the mind stable and the physical strength great'.[123] Men's 'more diverse and intellectual secondary reproductive functions', however, were in no way superior to woman's 'patient and absorbing work': in modern conditions this was 'a far greater self-sacrifice'.[124]

A normal woman's mental processes depended upon her metabolism, which in turn was controlled by her internal secretions ('Women with very active ovaries' being 'usually energetic and lively').[125] The functioning of a woman's organs of internal secretion varied during her life-cycle, though further work was urgently required on 'normal periodic variations'.[126] Female characteristics included dependence on the male, 'associated with an ardent desire to be loved'.[127] 'Sexual and maternal capacity' depended upon the 'proportion of femininity' in the individual woman's make-up. 'The normal woman' found 'pleasure in sexual intercourse', desired children, and the 'truly feminine' woman 'menstruates freely, her breasts are well formed and her mind is feminine', with all natural functions 'perfectly coordinated and correlated'. The higher type of woman, with a more developed 'reasoning faculty' had 'less need for the lure of sexual gratification to ensure the perpetuation of the race'.[128] Civilization, however, had produced women who wanted children but not sex, and vice versa. There were even those who shunned both, their femininity 'almost neutralised' by physically apparent 'masculinity'.[129]

Ovarian insufficiency in women was at least capable of treatment by 'what is known as organotherapy'.[130] Excessive ovarian secretion, however, manifested in women 'extremely feminine in appearance and character',[131] produced 'excessive sexuality, amounting perhaps to sexual insanity', leading to masturbation or even 'inversion'.[132] Women thus either had healthily functioning ovaries and were adapted to their prime function, or malfunctioning ovaries and manifest pathology. While it was not the scientist's business to suggest remedies for social conditions forcing 'women out of their natural sphere', women's demands for remedies were 'a tacit admission of abnormal circum-stances'.[133] But modern woman's rejection of maternity was possibly 'Nature's plan for securing the disappearance of Man to ensure further evolution'.[134]

The conservatism of these writers, their relative disinclination to problematize the male, an attitude to social conditions heavily reliant upon opposing 'the natural' to 'abnormal modern conditions', assumed and stated rather than described, underlines the radical-ism of predecessors like Ellis and Carpenter, and even Geddes and Thomson. Thomson indeed criticized Heape's biological determinism in a review of *Sex Antagonism*, although conceding that emphasizing that women's usefulness lay in her dissimilarity to man was 'good biology'.[135] Comparison with Marshall also calls into question how far Heape or Bell could truly be described as 'scientific'. Rather than endeavouring, in however compromised or naive a fashion, to maintain an open mind in the face of contradictory evidence, they both employed 'scientific' arguments to shore up existing prejudices. Merriley Borell has shown how little scientists actively engaged in studying reproductive endocrinology contributed to debates of the 1920s on issues such as birth control.[136] They were fully aware of the complexities of existing knowledge and the gaps in it, though they may also have thought their work was regarded quite dubiously enough without entering the realm of social controversy.

Research into less socially immediate questions in the field of repro-ductive biology continued, although Swale Vincent remarked in 1922 the temptations besetting physicians and physiologists to imagine an 'easy solution of sexual abnormalities by their reduction to mechanical failure of the gonad'.[137] This work took place in an international con-text, in Germany, the Netherlands and the USA as well as in the United Kingdom, while Voronoff, one of the pioneers, notorious for his 'monkey-gland operations', ran a rejuvenation clinic in Algiers. British representatives on the international delegation to this clinic in 1927 returned a 'very cautious' report to the Ministry of Agriculture.[138] Allan and Doisy in the USA produced purified follicular hormone in 1923;

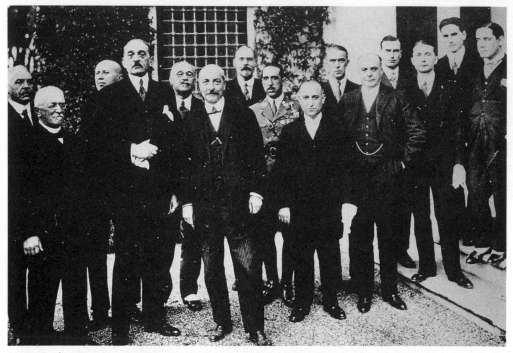

16 and 17 The respectable face of sex research: the European delegation to Voronoff's establishment in Algiers, 1927 (above); members of the First International Conference on the Standardisation of Sex Hormones, London, 1932 (below).

1. E. A. Doisy   2. F. H. A. Marshall   3. H. H. Dale   4. E. Laqueur   5. J. B. Collip
6. A. S. Parkes   7. G. P. Marrian   8. A. Butendandt   9. E. C. Dodds   10. A. Girard

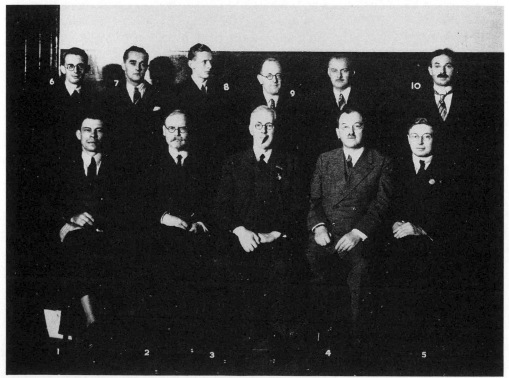

shortly afterwards the young Alan Parkes at the National Institute for Medical Research irradiated some female mice by mistake and discovered that even though their ovarian follicles had been destroyed they were still producing ovarian hormones.

The assumption of the early 1920s was that the female sex hormone had to be exclusive to the female, found only in her sexual organs: 'the chemical messenger of femininity', it was antagonistic to masculine form, function and behaviour. And similarly for the more elusive male sex hormone. Yet once the sex hormones had actually been isolated and were available for study, they tended to produce results which did not straightforwardly underwrite this simplistic, 'commonsense' biological paradigm.[139] In 1928, for example, testicular extract was discovered to produce the vaginal cornification used as a biological assay for ovarian hormones.[140] So when Marie Stopes wrote in *Enduring Passion*, 1928, that 'what is good in restoring normal virility to a man is also good in restoring her vitality to a woman'[141] she was up to the minute in assuming that male and female sex hormones were not necessarily the antagonists authorities such as Steinach had claimed them to be.[142] However, it is to be doubted that scientists who spent their days assaying the minute effects of hormones on the vaginal tracts of mice would altogether have concurred with Stopes's conclusions on the health benefits of generous doses of 'freshly prepared' glandular extracts in gelatine capsules.[143]

The subject was moving out of the hands of the gynaecologists, embryologists and physiologists who had engaged in the pioneering work and into those of chemists, and at this stage of transition from physiology to chemistry British scientists assumed major significance in the field.[144] It seems improbable that levels of competence varied greatly between British scientists pursuing different scientific disciplines; but as research into the problems of sexuality became to an ever-increasing extent a matter of chemical compounds tested on small laboratory animals it must also have become an acceptable field of study to career-minded individuals and, at least as important, to funding bodies such as the Medical Research Council. It could be presented as 'scientifically interesting' without any necessary reference to the messy problems of human sexuality.[145]

Conversely, R. A. McCance's detailed study with colleagues at King's College, London of the effects of female periodicity in a sample of 200 women in 1929–30 had great difficulty even in getting published; it finally appeared in the *Journal of Hygiene* in 1937. 'Somewhat before its time', according to McCance, it was twice rejected by the Royal Society, the first time apparently without even being sent to referees, and the second time, in 1936, after being sent to a highly unusual five for comment before being withdrawn. Numerous papers were being accepted at the same period on the sexual and seasonal cycles of ferrets, hedgehogs, monkeys and other 'lower animals'.[146]

The experiences of scientists working towards practical developments in contraception were somewhat similar. F. A. E. Crew in Edinburgh obtained funding from the Rockefeller Foundation in New York, as birth control research within the USA faced legal problems, whereas in Britain it could be undertaken 'by scientists of the highest standard and the results of their work made available without serious governmental interference'. The Birth Control Investigation Committee (BCIC), funded by the Eugenics Society, supported the not very scientifically challenging testing of existing spermicides.[147] J. R. Baker and Solly Zuckerman received some American funding for work on spermicides and the menstrual cycle (and the lifespan of sperm and ovum) respectively, but when this expired they sought assistance from the Eugenics Society; this was granted on the grounds that their research promised methods suitable for the most 'dysgenic' groups in the population (those which were the reverse of eugenically desirable on physical or mental grounds). Baker derived additional support from the pharmaceutical company, British Drug Houses Ltd.[148] Even with funding guaranteed, Baker had difficulties. Some tests required human semen, supplies of which were difficult to obtain. The Oxford Professor of Zoology was uncomfortable with birth control research in his department though the Pathology Department then provided facilities. Baker found research for the BCIC 'rather prejudicial' to his career, losing him at least one professorship and having to be kept quiet when he applied for another. However, he also claimed to 'care little for traditional morality', which was possibly a contributory factor, and one that aligns him with an earlier generation of sexologists.[149]

Other developments in the making of sexual knowledge from the 1890s exist in a definite if not necessarily definable relationship to the increasing 'scientific' discourse of sex. It is by no means apparent that the theories of deviancy, for example, mooted by sexologists ever achieved hegemonic status in medical thinking; it certainly took decades for them to have any practical effect on the administration of the law as it stood or legislation to amend it, although the insights of sexology were increasingly from the 1910s adopted and co-opted by sex educators of a predominantly social purity bent. The rise of sexology provided a corpus of evidence and theory that could provide a basis for very different agendas, and it was raided by both feminists and anti-feminists, social reformers and social purists. It could be liberatory or it could be oppressive. But by, at least in intention and however compromised, setting out to apply the rigours of scientific rationality to a highly emotive area, it provided a radically new way to make, unmake and remake sexual knowledge.

CHAPTER EIGHT

The Authority of Individual Experience and the Opinions of Experts: Sex as a Social Science

As scientists and thinkers began tentative endeavours to make sexual phenomena a field for scientific investigation, attempts emerged among the relatively educated and articulate to discuss questions of sex, in order to make some kind of sense of this ferment of new ideas in the light of their own experiences and emotions, which had been stimulated by such public manifestations as Stead's 'Maiden Tribute of Modern Babylon' and the subsequent passing of the 1885 Criminal Law Amendment Act. A few small, relatively informal groups drawn from among networks of existing friends and acquaintances engaged in this project of basing a new knowledge about sex on the experience of the individual. Wider progressive agendas of socialism and feminism (as well as eugenics) were of considerable influence, but these explorations were perceived as essential groundwork for tasks of reform.

Perhaps the most well known, and most extensively written about, is the Men and Women's Club of which Karl Pearson and Olive Schreiner were members. It is clear that Pearson hoped to elicit from the female members privileged insights into female nature and sexuality. Olive Schreiner's criticism about his 'omission of "*Man*"' from his opening paper to the club does not seem to have been seriously registered, and the club continued on the line laid down by Pearson, which was that its object was 'to discuss woman, her needs, her mental and physical nature, and man only in as far as he throws light upon her question'.[1] (Schreiner's objection was one to which efforts at studying sexuality continued to be open to over a long period of time.) Pearson's aim was not fully achieved, as he seems to have been more successful in inspiring the female members of the club to undertake massive tasks of historical research in the British Museum Reading Room, than in encouraging them to reveal the inmost secrets of female nature.

The women were, as Lucy Bland has pointed out, painfully aware that the men regarded them less as equals in the endeavour to advance knowledge than as interesting specimens for study. Furthermore, uneasy with the male debating society style of the club, the women experienced difficulty in finding a language in which to articulate questions of sexuality; the ones available for them were drawn largely from the debates on prostitution generated by the campaigns for the Contagious Diseases Acts. It also seems probable that the somewhat tense interpersonal dynamics of the group, added to Pearson's personality and style – 'impersonal, cold and rationalist', as Walkowitz sums it up – on top of the offence caused by both his views on 'The Woman Question' and his condescending manner, militated against the creation of a safe space in which the women might have felt capable of arguing more openly from their own experiences. The other groups mentioned by Carol Dyhouse in *Feminism and the Family* such as the Legitimation League and the Fellowship of the New Life may have operated very differently, but in the absence of a copious archive such as that of the Men and Women's Club (retained along with a great deal of other material relating to his career and associations by Karl Pearson) it is impossible to say.[2]

That speaking their own experiences was not wholly impossible for respectable middle-class women of the period – for indeed, some of the very women associated with the Men and Women's Club – is demonstrated by Havelock Ellis's ability to elicit comments and full case histories from his women friends and associates over the period when he was accumulating the material for, and writing up, *Studies in the Psychology of Sex*. Ellis laid down the rationale for eliciting these case histories in his appendix on 'The Development of the Sexual Instinct' (*Analysis of the Sexual Impulse; Love and Pain; The Sexual Impulse in Women*, 1903). Normal sexual phenomena were the key to abnormal phenomena, which were 'exaggerations of instincts and emotions . . . germinal in normal human beings', but it was impossible even to know what was normal without being 'acquainted with the sexual life of a large number of healthy individuals'. Only then would it be possible to lay down 'reasonable rules of sexual hygiene'.

Ellis made particular efforts to obtain sexual histories of men and women 'by themselves and others considered, ordinarily healthy and normal'. The difficulties of this, he remarked, were 'sufficiently obvious'. There was 'natural reticence to reveal facts of so intimately personal a character', while 'prevailing ignorance and unintelligence' meant that the phenomena were 'obscure to the subject himself'. There was little motivation to produce such records, and no realization of their value. However, he did manage to obtain a large number, 'for the most part offered spontaneously', along with offers to answer further inquiries. Unlike, for example, the cases presented by Krafft-Ebing on

the various manifestations of 'Psychopathia Sexualis', these accounts
were self-observations, and their subjects did not present themselves
'as patients desiring treatment'; their stories were not aimed at the
illumination of pathology. Even when the histories revealed subjects 'on
the borderland of the abnormal', they were playing 'active, sometimes
even distinguished, part[s] in the world'.[3]

The idea, naive though it might seem, that honest accounts by ordinary persons of their ideas and feelings about sex might contribute to
discovering 'the truth' about the subject surely represented a democra-
tization of knowledge, and a move away from religious or medical
prescription. Few people, however, took the subject with the seriousness
of F. H. Perrycoste, who solemnly noted his own nocturnal emissions
over a period of years in search of the pattern of male periodicity.[4]
Foucault's theory of the 'confessional' in the making of late nineteenth-
century discourses on sexuality[5] is somewhat problematic when applied
to a Protestant country with a tradition of reticence; indeed, an almost
hysteric loathing of Roman Catholicism and its appurtenances is
demonstrated by the recurrence of scandals and the persistence of a
prurient genre of revelations about nunneries, the confessional and
so on.[6]

The meaning of confessional accounts of sexuality is bound to be
different in certain respects in societies where it is not a standard
practice, imposed from above, regularly to examine conduct and even
thoughts for evidence of sins against purity. (British educators were apt
to decry continental or Roman Catholic practices of surveillance and
warnings as likely to excite immorality rather than contain it.)[7] The
making of sexual knowledge in Britain has largely been characterized by
attempts to get away from human confessions and into hormones,
hamsters or dry statistics.

Ellis's case studies aimed to establish a new narrative form for sexual
histories, even if these could not altogether escape from earlier models
of the recital of sin or the recounting of pathology to a doctor. There is
a very different tone to Ellis's writings and the 'confessions' received by
him than that of the arguments of, for example, Samuel Solomon in
support of the need to 'confess' onanism.[8] Marion Shaw contrasts,
without fully exploring the difference, the 'pathogenic memories . . .
pressed out' of his patients by Freud to create a 'confessional narrative . . .
of the truth of sex' with Ellis's more fragmentary, less theorized case
histories.[9] While the voluntaristic nature of the stories elicited by Ellis
could be subsumed to a confessional model, perhaps analogous with
the compulsive confession of uncommitted crimes, they were voluntarily submitted, and Ellis does not seem to have been concerned to
know better than his informants the 'truth' of their narrations or of sex.

Inconclusive, unshaped, these 'mythlike . . . Gothic fragments' stand alone.[10]

Ellis can also be, and has been, indicted on the count of giving far more attention to women, problematizing the female in ways not extended to the male. In *The Sexual Impulse*, he declared 'special and detailed study of the normal character of the sexual impulse in men' to be unnecessary. He defined it, surely in contradiction to his personal experience, as 'predominantly open and aggressive', expressed in the 'written and unwritten codes of social law'. Ellis was neither the first nor the last to sigh over the 'elusiveness', the 'mocking mystery' of the female sexual impulse,[11] while that of the male continued to be the object of implicit assumptions never perceived as in need of either defining or investigating.[12]

Other groups besides the Men and Women's Club were engaged in similar explorations, stimulated by the writings of Pearson as well as Edward Carpenter and, slightly later, Havelock Ellis. The Fellowship of the New Life in which Ellis was a leading figure was presumably discussing the same issues. Young provincial Fabians in the circle of John Bruce Glasier and Katherine Conway engaged in similar discussions, circulating a notebook of their thoughts on 'free love, sexual emancipation, and the possibility of socialist revolution'. Carolyn Steedman, discussing the child-educator Margaret McMillan's involvement with this group, points out the 'many heterodox sources' in the 1890s, including theosophy, that provided ways of articulating sexual and emotional ideas and the discussion of women's issues in the context of social reform.[13]

Evidence from periodicals such as *Shafts* and the *Adult* (and in the new century, the *Freewoman*) and correspondence received by figures such as Edward Carpenter suggests that both individuals and groups were engaging in such explorations, on a perhaps less formalized basis. The *Freewoman* Discussion Circle considered, among other issues, such questions as 'Sex Oppression', 'The Problems of Celibacy', 'Neo-Malthusianism', 'Prostitution', and divorce law reform.[14] If, unlike contemporary social purity organizations, they did not aim at activism on the basis of implicit ideas about sexuality and society, instead querying such ideas, it was within a context in which the potential for deriving from their study a sound basis for social action was implicit. More work certainly needs to be done on the investigation of these activities, and the ties between members of such discussion groups and bodies with a more activist agenda.

If the evidence provided by the British Society for the Study of Sex Psychology, founded in 1914 after preliminary meetings in 1913, can be generalized, the existence of such links between investigation and activism seem entirely probable: its members though largely 'keen propagandists on various subjects' nonetheless supported the Society's 'advocacy of that attitude of mind . . . which makes investigation possible', that is, detached and non-judgmental.[15] The founding members of this Society generally had a special interest in the improvement of the legal position of, and a lessening of the social stigma against, homosexuals, but the Society's aims were much broader; so broad, in fact, as seriously to hinder its effectiveness in action. The founders perceived a pressing need for 'discussion from the point of view of the ordinary thoughtful person as well as from that of the doctor and scientist' of 'problems and questions connected with sexual psychology from their medical, juridical, and sociological aspects'.[16]

The Society attracted a cross-section of individuals interested in the open study of sexual phenomena: as well as those who desired greater understanding of the problems of the homosexual, there were a number of early adherents of the British psychoanalytic movement, divorce law reformers, sex educators, those more generally interested in education, Malthusians, nudists, feminists, social hygienists, a few doctors, several clergymen and a handful of anthropologists.[17] They were perceived, even to some degree by themselves, as eccentrics. According to Lytton Strachey they were 'a third variety of human being', who were 'surprisingly frank'; the American educational psychologist Homer Lane described them as 'hairless perverts with twitching lips'.[18] There was a certain anxiety about the public face of the group: they did not want to become a 'happy hunting ground for Mayfair in search of "thrills"', or the prey of gutter journalists.[19]

Over approximately thirty years the Society held regular meetings, built up a library of rare volumes on sexology for reference and loan to members, and early in the 1920s established a headquarters office in – perhaps naturally – Bloomsbury. It published a series of pamphlets, some of which are now recognized as classic works: for example Havelock Ellis's *The Play-Function of Sex* (1921) and Stella Browne's *Sexual Variety and Variability among Women* (1917, based on a lecture of 1915). These works sold well and had considerable circulation among the general public.

Lectures were given on a wide variety of topics, drawing average audiences of between thirty and fifty, including non-members attending as guests. Subjects presented and discussed at meetings included obscenity, coeducation, repression of the erotic impulse, sexual crime, sex ethics, the sex lives or views on sex of various historical figures, divorce, birth control, homosexuality, children, eugenics, intersexuality, psychoanalysis, adolescence, anthropological approaches, the art of love and sex in art.[20]

Study groups intermittently investigated specific aspects of sexual problems: at various times Sex Education, Inversion, Heterosexuality and Psychoanalysis. Little record survives of the groups' activities. Occasionally they were mentioned in minutes of the Society at large, but of their own records only some accounts (mostly rather scanty) survive of meetings of the Heterosexuality Group and the joint meeting of the Education, Heterosexuality and Psychoanalysis Groups on 16 March 1921.[21] There were occasional flurries of interest in undertaking systematic collection of information from members and other interested individuals about their own sex life, or aspects of it, but these remain tantalizing hints among the records.[22] A questionnaire was produced by the Sex Education Group of the Society – which may or may not be the same as a questionnaire produced by the Heterosexuality Group, as these two groups amalgamated – but not a single example appears to survive.[23]

As sexology as a science was being increasingly co-opted into the more scientifically neutral field of reproductive biology, and investigation focused on non-human animals (as discussed in Chapter 7), the approach to problems of sexuality by appealing to the authority of individual experience continued in parallel. Individual experience itself gradually came to be evidence for experts, though methodological problems and a continuing sense of taboo hindered the development, at least in Britain, of extensive sex surveys. This was related to the 'enduring amateur tradition of social investigation' in Britain well into the twentieth century, which continued to be 'untouched by what then passed for academic sociology'. Empirical social research consisted largely of ad hoc local surveys: by 1939 'little progress had been made in . . . making sociological surveys more analytically sophisticated [by] . . . linking them with . . . sociological theory'.[24]

Early in the twentieth century some tentative endeavours were made to assess the prevalence of the use of birth control by married couples. In 1905 the Fabian Society set up a sub-committee to consider the birth rate and infantile mortality. Given proven decline of the birth rate since the mid-1870s, of a differential nature, which suggested that national degeneration was an unlikely cause, and 'common report that . . . deliberate regulation of the married state' was widely prevalent, 'direct individual evidence that volitional regulation exists' was sought. In order 'to obtain a voluntary census from a sufficiently large number of married people who could be relied upon to give frank and truthful answers to a detailed interrogatory' some 600 to 700 persons (members of the Fabian Society, or recommended by them)[25] were approached, drawn from 'a most varied selection of occupations, extending from the skilled artisan to the professional man and the small property owner'. Information was supplied anonymously, 'the form being so arranged as to enable it to be filled up by nothing more easily recognizable than crosses and figures'. Six hundred and thirty-four forms were sent out, but after a number of returns had been deducted from the total for various reasons, 'significant replies were received from 302 persons'.[26] This mode of selection was criticized by Karl Pearson as statistically inadequate and biased in favour of intellectuals.[27]

The majority of these marriages were 'limited', and this limitation appears to have succeeded in reducing the number of children born to the couples concerned. 'Voluntary regulation of the marriage state among this tiny sample of (presumably) very deliberate and foreseeing citizens' had brought about a reduction in the birth rate greater than that for the country as a whole. The deduction could be made that 'volitional regulation of the married state' was 'at work in many different parts of Great Britain, among all social grades except probably the very poorest'.[28] No indication of methods employed were sought by this survey.

A survey of the birth rate in the northern counties of England undertaken by Ethel Elderton of the Galton Laboratory (headed by Karl Pearson) in 1911, published in 1914, gave more details. However, information on the prevalence in particular districts of coitus interruptus, the use of sheaths, douching or pessaries, or abortion, was supplied by 'correspondents' whose precise status was not defined. On internal evidence, many seem to have been asked for birth control or abortion advice in some professional capacity. The survey's interest in 'propagandism by way of advertisement' for family limitation may explain the emphasis on appliances, although correspondents indicated that withdrawal and even some form of safe period were in use, or that desire for limitation outran actual knowledge.[29]

Investigations emerging from and influenced by Victorian traditions of delving into the pathology of social problems – and even Royal Commissions, such as the one on venereal disease – continued to feature as one mode of exploring the realm of the sexual, well past the Second World War. These included a Royal Commission on Population in the 1940s, the Home Office Departmental Committee on Homosexuality and Prostitution (the Wolfenden Committee) in 1954, and the Lane Committee, which investigated the working of the 1967 Abortion Act in the early 1970s.

The National Council of Public Morals, under Sir James Marchant, established a National Birth-Rate Commission in 1913. Over the next

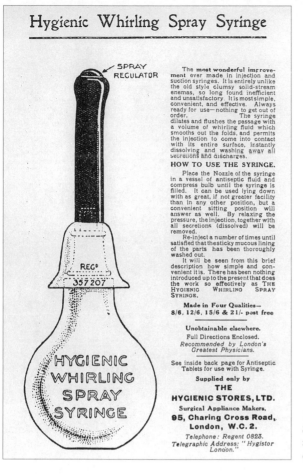

Hygienic Whirling Spray Syringe

SPRAY REGULATOR

The most wonderful improvement ever made in injection and suction syringes. It is entirely unlike the old style clumsy solid-stream enemas, so long found inefficient and unsatisfactory. It is most simple, convenient, and effective. Always ready for use—nothing to get out of order. The syringe dilates and flushes the passage with a volume of whirling fluid which smooths out the folds, and permits the injection to come into contact with its entire surface, instantly dissolving and washing away all secretions and discharges.

HOW TO USE THE SYRINGE.

Place the Nozzle of the syringe in a vessel of antiseptic fluid and compress bulb until the syringe is filled. It can be used lying down with as great, if not greater facility than in any other position, but a convenient sitting position will answer as well. By relaxing the pressure, the injection, together with all secretions (dissolved) will be removed.

Re-inject a number of times until satisfied that the sticky mucous lining of the parts has been thoroughly washed out.

It will be seen from this brief description how simple and convenient it is. There has been nothing introduced up to the present that does the work so effectively as THE HYGIENIC WHIRLING SPRAY SYRINGE.

Made in Four Qualities— 8/6, 12/6, 15/6 & 21/- post free

Unobtainable elsewhere.
Full Directions Enclosed.
Recommended by London's Greatest Physicians.

See inside back page for Antiseptic Tablets for use with Syringe.

Supplied only by
THE HYGIENIC STORES, LTD.
Surgical Appliance Makers,
95, Charing Cross Road,
London, W.C. 2.
Telephone: Regent 0823.
Telegraphic Address: "Hygistor London."

REG⁰ 357207

HYGIENIC WHIRLING SPRAY SYRINGE

18 'Hygienic Whirling Spray Syringe': 'washes away all secretions and discharges', i.e., a contraceptive douche.

ten years this investigated the declining birth rate and its causes, and associated problems of population; it also explored the problem of the 'Development and Education of Young People for Worthy Parenthood', taking on the vexed question of sex education. (There was also an inquiry into the effects on morality of the cinema.) While the Commission seems to have enjoyed a certain official friendliness – for example the presence on it of Dr T. H. C. Stevenson of the General Register Office and Dr Arthur Newsholme of the Local Government Board, with the consent of the Registrar-General and the President of the Board – it had no official status in spite of the announcement in Parliament that the government would await its report with interest. (Such sympathy, costing nothing, was a not uncommon response of governments to initiatives of this kind: see Chapter 10.) The Commission might not be able to accomplish as much as a Royal Commission, but there was no

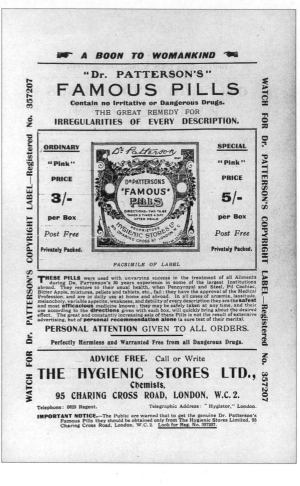

19 'Dr Patterson's Famous Pills': a widely distributed abortifacient. Testimonials included the euphemistic but suggestive comments: 'had the desired effect', 'everything was as wished', 'acted like magic'.

prospect of one on the birth rate for some considerable time. Furthermore, it might accomplish things an official inquiry would miss, as 'witnesses will feel more free to speak'.[30]

There is no indication of how the witnesses to this first investigation were selected; they included a wide range of individuals with opinions across the entire spectrum of views on population decline and birth control. The second report, however, commented that

> We have been fortunate in securing witnesses of competence and authority, most of whom voluntarily offered their services, and all of whom were eager to assist in the enquiry. Indeed, their numbers could have been multiplied many times.[31]

A very similar statement was made in respect of the inquiry into 'Youth and the Race'; the Commission had secured 'witnesses of competence and authority, representing Psychology, Education, and Medicine', the majority of whom had voluntarily offered their services, all manifesting 'keen anxiety to assist the enquiry in every way'.[32] Witnesses produced statements as to their views and recommendations, and underwent questioning by the members of the Commission.

This system, though it might have some virtues, had the disadvantage of privileging those who had an existing agenda on the subject. It relied on, and presumably valued, the opinions of experts more than inquiry into the actual views and practices of specific couples, though there were undoubtedly strong feelings against any such inquiry. The strong and well-formulated opinions held by these expert witnesses militated against a disinterested consideration of the subject: Enid Charles suggested in 1932 that evidence given to the Commission that contraceptives caused sterility was 'based on personal observation and embodies a type of fallacy which vitiates much current discussion on contraception'.[33]

In 1918, just before the end of the war, the Association of Moral and Social Hygiene (AMSH) initiated a Committee of Enquiry into Sexual Morality, whose findings were summarized in *The State and Sexual Morality*, published a few years later.[34] A strong moral agenda underlay this investigation. The qualifications for membership of the committee were

1. A real desire for Social Reform.   2. Acceptance of the equal standard as a basis (but not necessarily acceptance of what seem to us the implications).   3. Knowledge and experience of some aspect of the subject matter; or alternatively, a definite contribution of something the Commission otherwise lacks, eg legal training, or knowledge about reformatory institutions, etc.[35]

The inquiry seems to have emerged from the widespread objections to the Defence of the Realm Act (DORA) Regulation 40d, which penalized communication of venereal diseases by women while ignoring men. Heads of inquiry were organized around existing laws regarding public (sexual) morality, suggestions for alterations to existing law or for new legislation, and the question of the provision of prophylactics for venereal disease.[36]

Twenty-two organizations co-operated with the AMSH, but the members of the committee sat on it as individuals, not as representatives of particular bodies. 'The advisability of obtaining evidence from representatives of all possible sections of the community as to the current standards of sex morality' was discussed. It would be helpful 'to receive evidence . . . as to the special dangers and difficulties and viewpoint of various sections of people'. Suggestions were made as to groups which might be canvassed, such as women workers, workers in factories, working men, domestic servants (with special emphasis on dangers from employers). However, the employment of a special worker to undertake such inquiries (as was already being done in America) was vetoed as being outside the scope of the investigation.[37]

Efforts were made to gain a wide spread of expert opinion: Havelock Ellis, as usual shrinking from the public domain, declined to give evidence, while the offer by George Ives, founder member of the British Society for the Study of Sex Psychology (BSSSP) and a member of the Howard League for Penal Reform, was taken into consideration.[38] Those who gave evidence were almost entirely those who had some professional involvement with the problems of sexual morality: an army chaplain, a magistrate, doctors with a specific interest in venereal disease (including Robert Lyster, secretary of the Society for the Prevention of Venereal Disease), women police, social workers, social purity workers, women prison doctors, and so forth. Some attempt seems to have been made to include modern sexological opinion: besides Ellis, suggested witnesses were Dr Jessie Murray, a very early British convert to psychoanalysis, and Norah March, editor of *National Health*, both of them active in the British Society for the Study of Sex Psychology. There was a considerable bias towards women among witnesses suggested and called, but this perhaps reflects the role of women in social purity organizations and the belief that women had particular insights to offer in the area.[39]

The evidence recorded illuminates, among other things, the operation of prostitution during the period, from a viewpoint characterized by sympathy for the prostitute, possibly to be expected given the Josephine Butler tradition upheld by the AMSH. A police magistrate declared of the offence of solicitation that 'men are not all annoyed. It is the fate of every man to be spoken to. One's feeling is sorrow, not annoyance', and claimed that he invariably penalized 'a man insulting a respectable girl' more severely than a girl speaking to a man.[40] Several witnesses reported that professional prostitutes conducted themselves with quiet discretion, seldom verbally soliciting customers. Men persistently annoying women in the streets usually got away scot free (even when complained of to the police) while young girls 'larking' might be arrested.[41]

The sympathy extended to those upon whom the laws bore so unequally (a point made by several witnesses) was not extended to the male prostitute. W. J. H. Brodrick declared that

The professional boys are about the most degraded being you could find. They have no talk except obscenity; no ideas except unnatural vice; they are usually diseased and a pest and a nuisance to everybody with whom they come in contact. Personally I should be glad to see them put in a lethal chamber and have done with it.

Even slighter evidence than with female prostitution was accepted by the police: 'as a rule the evidence consists of rouge and powder puffs and things of that kind. It is quite easy to get.' It was alleged that cases were seldom pursued 'unless there is active solicitation'; police were anxious lest 'advertising does . . . more harm than good'. Brodrick seemed dubious about prosecuting in 'individual cases, such as often occur in the country, people who are not professional'.[42] The Reverend A. Herbert Gray, formerly an army chaplain, mentioned counselling a man 'guilty of . . . an offence with boys', which 'to his horror' he had 'only just realised to be illegal'; he noted the salutary effect on the man's mind and the 'benefit to his character', when he was led to seek help to 'chuck it'.[43]

It is far from clear that psychoanalysis made much real contribution to the elucidation of sexual matters in Britain, outside strictly psychoanalytical circles; however, the close involvement of several early British Freudians in the BSSSP should be noted, and Ernest Jones's greeting of Havelock Ellis as a 'fellow worker in the field of sexology'.[44] But as Jeff Weeks has pointed out, it was 'in a fairly bowdlerised form that Freudianism made its main penetration into Britain'. British sexology was strongly influenced through Ellis by a biologistic tradition, leading to dilution of Freudianism as it was popularized.[45] The desire of psychoanalysis for wider acceptance may also have led to a playing down of the sexual elements, as in W. H. R. Rivers's 1917 defence of its value.[46] Terms such as 'complex', 'repression', 'fixation' or 'sublimation' were loosely tossed around with purely cosmetic effect, providing a language and to some extent an explanatory model for fashioning sexual histories, but not necessarily any deeper rethinking of sexual categories. The fascinating unpublished autobiography of physiologist V. H. Mottram (who underwent 'the proddings . . . of psychoanalysis' with a Jungian), attributed his own homosexual 'phase' to a 'deep-seated Oedipus complex', and remarked that 'people, psychologically, are bisexual'; but Mottram described a difficult colleague as 'a feminine soul in a masculine body'.[47]

By the late 1920s surveys of actual sexual behaviour were being published in the USA,[48] but this was not imitated in Britain. Although the Social Survey in Britain had its roots in concerns about population, studies of sexual conduct, if they occurred at all, continued to focus rather narrowly on specific problems around fertility, with some interest in social deviancy. Sex as an index heading barely figures in historical accounts of the Social Survey in Britain, although demography was a continuing area of interest; this may be due to the fact that surveys relating to sex were, even more than most, eccentric amateur efforts shaky in their methodology.[49]

Havelock Ellis had not been very systematic about acquiring the case studies published in *Studies in the Psychology of Sex*, nor had he engaged in any kind of statistical enumeration, although such accounts continued to be sent to him as his fame grew. Leonora Eyles's conclusions about the sex lives of the working classes, in *The Woman in the Little House* (1922), seem to have been based largely on five separate women telling her 'I shouldn't mind married life so much if it wasn't for bedtime',[50] a somewhat impressionistic mode of data collection. Marie Stopes had not initially set out to undertake the role of adviser when soliciting correspondence from the readers of *Married Love* for the purposes of scientific research, in particular further data on female curves of desire. However, while she found that she was appealed to more in the capacity of an agony aunt than a scientist, her readers did provide her with (unsystematically gleaned) data about their sex lives. In *Enduring Passion* she wrote that correspondence received after writing *Married Love* had made her aware of 'the wide prevalence of premature ejaculation' among the British middle classes (and therefore encouraged her to deal with the subject in more detail).[51]

Her more systematic attempts to obtain information focused on contraception rather than wider aspects of sexual behaviour. In 1922 she circularized medical schools about their teaching of birth control (almost universally non-existent),[52] and sent out a questionnaire to members of the medical profession on their personal contraceptive practices. One hundred and twenty-eight completed forms survive, and a few torn up or otherwise defaced by indignant recipients. The returns from this statistically unsatisfactory sample provide some suggestive impressions. Several respondents claimed that abstention for greater or lesser periods, amounting to years, was the only method of deliberate limitation employed.[53] Members of the clergy were also circulated about birth control practices.[54] Stopes additionally compiled studies from the case records of her Mothers' Clinic – *The First 5000* (1925). From the rather different angle of appeal to women's own experiences, she published selections from her letters from working-class women, in *Mother England: A Contemporary History self-written by those who have no historian* (1929), taking up a genre pioneered by the Women's Cooperative Guild in *Maternity: Letters from Working Women* and *Life as We Have Known It*.[55]

Stopes occasionally received charts from readers illustrating her own theories of female periodicity. The question was subjected to a rather more thorough investigation when the biologist R. A. McCance (best known for his studies in nutrition) and colleagues at King's College, London undertook a survey of periodic variations among women in 1929–30. The forms included space for subjective comment as well as daily squares for marking off with data on physiological, emotional and mental phenomena. Of their sample, 167 women kept charts complete enough to be of use to the investigation, if not for as long as the full six months envisaged. These women, almost entirely from the educated middle classes, manifested great 'willingness and co-operation' with the project. There were 100 single and 51 married, with 5 women recording sexual relationships treated as married. Problems were encountered in obtaining even so restricted a sample of 'women of a certain degree of intelligence' capable of carrying the survey through. Institutional sources such as women's colleges and medical schools 'took exception to the forms on the grounds that sexual feeling was abnormal in unmarried women students' (among the data to be recorded were sexual feelings as well as actual intercourse). However, 'few women once approached on the matter objected' although some married women abandoned their record-keeping because of objections by their husbands.

An interesting discrepancy was noted between data recorded in the preliminary sheets filled in by the subjects and their more detailed day-to-day records, for example between women's perception of whether their periods were painful and actual episodes of pain recorded. Additionally women's interpretations of the term 'regular' were seen to bear no particular relationship to actual regularity of cycle. This led the researchers to query the usefulness of questionnaire surveys asking for such general comments. The day-by-day records revealed rhythmic periodicity of both physical and mental symptoms (not all anticipated), but in certain individuals the periodicity, though marked, differed from the combined results. Enough questions remained, or had been generated by this preliminary study, for McCance and colleagues to hope for 'repetition of the work by more experienced and competent investigators'.[56]

Such an investigation seems to have baffled and bewildered the referees to whom it was sent in 1936 by the Royal Society; there were five in all – two eminent figures in reproductive physiology, a psychologist, a physician and a surgeon. While there was general consensus that the paper was a good and worthwhile study, there was hesitancy about giving a definite opinion as to whether 'papers of this kind should be published by the Society'. The only referee explicitly opposing publication argued that 'it would seem to be undesirable to put all such details of human clinical affairs in publications that are read chiefly by men who are not concerned with clinical work', even though reproductive biology (admittedly in non-human mammals) was currently an area in which large numbers of papers were being published in the *Proceedings* or *Memoirs* of the Society.[57] 'Somewhat before its time,' McCance thought subsequently.[58]

Another survey about the same time, similarly reliant upon the testimony of 'women of at least average intelligence in comfortable economic circumstances', was Enid Charles's analysis published in *The Practice of Birth Control* in 1932. The 900 women claimed by the subtitle appears misleading. Of 874 women, only 432 returned questionnaires deemed suitable for analysis, though these were said to cover '966 separate experiences' of contraceptive methods.[59] Additional sections were based on data (pertaining largely to the Dutch cap) gathered by Nurse E. S. Daniels, and at the Birmingham Women's Welfare Centre.[60] Charles found it necessary to emphasize that 'it should now be possible to discuss contraceptive methods without reference to moral issues'. 'Applied science' could 'legitimately enquire . . . [into] different types of contraceptive method without concern for the ethics of their use in any particular cases'. Charles discussed the problems of acquiring information: existing clinics often relied on one specific method, rendering them unrepresentative; furthermore, clients lost touch and continuous histories of contraceptive practice were seldom maintained.[61]

On behalf of the Birth Control Investigation Committee (BCIC) an attempt was made to collect information from a random sample of the population by means of a questionnaire, with the inherent defect that most answers returned might be from women 'more intelligent than the average of their social group', and 'possibly more than usually interested in the subject of birth control'.[62] Given the difficulty of extracting 'statements with reference to . . . sexual life corresponding at all accurately with behaviour', the virtue of the questionnaire was its assurance of anonymity, combined with the absence of a reporter. However, it was recognized that the survey involved 'matters of behaviour about which human beings rarely if ever tell the truth'. 'Enquiry into intimate details of sexual habit limits the number of replies which can be obtained', or so it was generally believed. To avoid offending sensibilities and to maximize the number of replies, data on frequency of sexual intercourse was not sought, even though recent research indicated that this had an important effect on frequency of conception.[63]

McCance and his colleagues had specifically included spaces for the recording of both feelings of sexual desire and occasions of intercourse

in their data-sheets, and their respondents do not seem to have hesitated to fill these in. One woman even helpfully differentiated episodes
of sexual desire arising from what she defined as 'original sin' and those
in response to outside stimulus, and others indicated whether sexual
intercourse included orgasm.[64] It seems odd that individuals who had
already undertaken to answer questions about the still highly sensitive
matter of birth control, which was only gradually winning acceptance
and far from a subject of common conversation, would be deterred by
questions on frequency of intercourse. Three respondents to the BCIC
questionnaire did after all frankly admit to practising 'sexual variations'
in which 'the form of intimacy adopted was not normal copulation
nor coitus interruptus' (unspecified by Charles, except in the single
case of 'karezza' – prolonged intercourse without ejaculation; recommended by Stopes and other writers for its spiritual and emotional, as
well as contraceptive, benefits).[65] Or was it precisely because they were
being asked about such a touchy subject that it was decided not to risk
increasing the touchiness factor?

   Although the two main methods in use were employed by men, it was
still women who were being asked about birth control. The survey
indeed indicated that there were significantly different outcomes in the
practice of contraception by the man rather than the woman; or at least
'methods used by the female partner'. In cases where comments were
made on the unsatisfactoriness of the sheath, 'dislike on the part of the
husband' was mentioned: and some answers had even been written by
husbands.[66] Charles did not intimate whether, as with McCance's survey,
objections by husbands led to failure to complete questionnaires. It
seems probable that there was a persistent, never explicitly stated or
examined, belief that men would not or could not respond to these
investigative projects in the way women did. Given how explicit many
men were in their letters to Marie Stopes about their problems and
their sex lives generally,[67] the assumption may have been wrong.

The British Sexology Society (as the British Society for the Study of Sex
Psychology was renamed in the 1930s) claimed to have a less narrowly
focused investigative agenda. In spite of the persistent 'impression that
it concerned itself almost exclusively with the homosexual question',[68]
the Society's revised 'Aims and Policy' of 1932 emphasized the development and maintenance of 'a suitable machinery for the scientific
investigation of sexual phenomena' as its prime aim, as well as promotion of 'a more rational attitude towards sexual conduct'. 'All subjects
coming within the scope of the Society' were 'frankly discussed, thus

providing for the systematic investigation of special problems, exchange of views' and accumulation of material as a basis for the reform of sexual ethics; a claim which does not seem altogether capable of substantiation from the records which survive.[69] One member wondered cynically in the 1930s if the Society's chief purpose were not

> to supply us elderly people . . . with an opportunity, denied us in our younger days, for the occasional enjoyment of the thrill – sometimes, I should suspect, slightly exhibitionistic in quality – of discussing intimate and unsavoury sex matters before a public audience of both sexes.[70]

There were other, even smaller, more localized societies with similar or possibly even more radical aims, besides such covert organizations such as the homophile Order of Chaeronea founded by George Ives, also of the British Sexology Society (BSS).[71] Dora Forster Kerr (also involved with the Malthusian League and the Fabian Society) mentioned in correspondence with the BSS a Sex Study Circle of which she was part, based in Croydon. This group produced a newsletter, *More Light Letters*, contributions to which were apparently concealed by pseudonyms.[72] A local group which may have been similar existed in the Welwyn area (Welwyn Garden City had roots in the Fellowship of the New Life),[73] where Aldous Huxley spent a weekend, during which he had 'taken off his clothes among the cabbages, & read Waste Land. Necessary to say penis and fuck.'[74] Provincial members of the BSS occasionally wrote to headquarters in hopes of setting up, if not a local branch, at least occasional meetings with other members in their vicinity (there is some evidence that a branch did exist in Brighton).[75]

The Mass Observation organization was established in 1937 by the anthropologist Tom Harrisson in order to produce 'an anthropology of ourselves', that is, the people of Britain; Martin Bulmer suggests that ornithology provides a better model for what they actually did. Besides accumulating diaries and reports by volunteer observers of contemporary social phenomena, it undertook investigations into particular topics using full-time observers and canvassing the opinions of 'the man in the street'.[76] Generally 'unsystematic and magpie-like',[77] Mass Observation did not at first make any concerted investigation into sexual mores or attitudes; however, Mass Observers endeavoured to scrutinize alfresco courtship as part of a wider survey in the seaside resort of Blackpool one summer. In such surroundings the observation of embracing couples was so common (especially, according to the report, by 'older men of scoptophilic tendencies') that the attendant risk of voyeurism was less than might normally have been the case. While a wide range of sexual behaviour was observed, the investigators

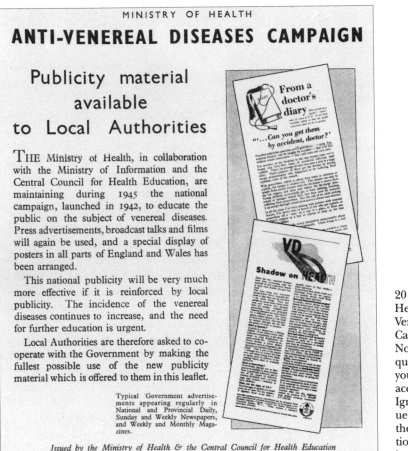

20 Ministry of Health: Anti-Venereal Diseases Campaign, 1945. Note the headlined query ' . . . Can you get them by accident, doctor?'. Ignorance contin-ued to flourish as the Mass Observa-tion investigations indicated.

concluded that very little actual copulation was taking place.[78] A few reports dealt with sexual issues; the subject also occurred in observers' diaries, and reports of pub conversations.[79]

In 1942–3 the organization was commissioned by the government to undertake an investigation of the efficacy of the anti-VD press cam-paign. Men observers were to approach men, and women women, and ask a series of questions, starting by ascertaining if the respondent had seen the adverts. They were then to find out what the respondents felt about them, whether they were getting too much, too little or about enough information about VD, if there was anything special they wanted to know, whether they had any views about the dissemination of the necessary information, if there were any words they felt should not be used, and their own views on prevention. Indirect comments were also to be recorded, as were all refusals, and an estimate of the degree of embarrassment.[80]

The 'great willingness, and often active desire' among the public to know more about the subject and to have it brought into the open was striking,[81] though it was sometimes described as 'dirty', 'nasty', even 'horrible'. Views on control were frequently heavily authoritarian, advocating supervision of prostitutes, establishment of properly run licensed houses, regular compulsory medical examinations, and punitive measures for the infected who avoided treatment. One man claimed that there was 'No way other than sterilisation.'[82] Others believed education and dissemination of information were needed, rather than driving the subject underground, while some recommended old-fashioned moral discipline. One lady of 73 advised: 'Keep clean.'[83] Among groups blamed were 'Little cheap loose-living girls', soldiers and the women's services, Americans and foreigners generally. 'Any woman who's had four men is bound to either have it or be a carrier,' alleged one man.[84] One 30-year-old woman 'didn't like that word intercourse I don't think any woman would.'[85]

A very different approach was taken by the Royal College of Obstetricians and Gynaecologists' 'Enquiry into Family Limitation and its Influence on Human Fertility during the past fifty years' for the Royal Commission on Population in 1944. There was much agonizing over the methods of acquiring both sample and interviewers, given anticipated difficulties. Questioning members of the normal married female population on such a supposedly sensitive subject was believed to require great tact. The Committee was convinced that 'only qualified members of the medical profession who stood to the women in the relation of doctor to patient' were suitable interviewers. Doctors specially hired to conduct the interviews (paid 5 shillings [25p] apiece per interview) approached married women in general hospital wards. The importance of random selection and not just picking out women who looked likely to respond favourably was emphasized but it is not clear how this ideal worked in practice. Objections and refusals by women approached were said to have been rare, and it was a 'pleasure to be able to record the friendly co-operation given . . . at all levels, and including the thousands of women who voluntarily provided the essential information', although problems arose in obtaining a sample population of the more well-to-do classes, since private hospitals and nursing homes were reluctant 'to risk incurring unpopularity among their clientele'.[86]

In 1951 *Patterns of Marriage: A Study of Marriage Relationships in the Urban Working Classes* reported on an investigation of 200 families carried out over 30 months between October 1943 and April 1946 by the psychiatrist Eliot Slater and psychiatric social worker and researcher Moya Woodside. The survey was based on two groups: soldiers who succumbed to neurotic illness while in army service; and soldiers hospitalized for non-neurotic ailments. While aware of possible objections to this apparent over-representation of neurotic subjects, Slater and Woodside suggested that 'neurotic individuals compose a respectable fraction of our total population'. Although it was not 'a truly random selection of the population', the sample was 'fairly representative . . . of Londoners of working and lower middle-class, married, and between the ages of twenty-two and forty-seven'.[87] Some bias was also introduced by the tendency of men whose marriages were breaking down to refuse collaboration.

The survey was conducted by means of interviews initiated by a questionnaire. Being questioned about matters of sex was 'provocative of emotion'. This may have owed something to the semi-official status of the interrogators, who were connected in their subjects' minds with 'the Government', which at that time was engaged in debating Family Allowances and setting up a Royal Commission on Population. There was recurrent prejudice against 'social workers', associated with the prying investigations of charity and Public Assistance, among the wives, while 'strange rumours' about the project circulated among the soldiers in the hospital wards. Even with subjects willing to co-operate there were practical problems in organizing times and places for the interviews. In spite of initial reluctance and suspicion, this 'opportunity for people to talk in confidence about marital and personal problems' was appreciated. 'Getting things off their chest' was found, even within the restricted parameters of short, research-orientated interviews, to have benefited the subjects. Simple advice on various topics was requested and gratefully received.[88]

As Eustace Chesser (see below, pp. 199–201 and Chapter 9) was similarly to find, premarital sex was already increasing among younger age cohorts, with a continuing predominance of men over women. However, the authors found some uncertainty over the definition of 'sex relations'; in some cases this might not have gone as far as full intercourse.[89] Among reasons for marrying, the purely sexual was regarded ambiguously. Sexual desires were 'thought of as being natural and inevitable, but at the same time not quite respectable, and are usually referred to with evidence of shame', while among women respondents there was 'a good deal of self-righteous complacency about frigidity'.[90] Sexual factors were found to play a by no means straightforward role in individuals' assessment of married happiness.[91] Frequency of marital intercourse varied very widely – with 1 per cent never having intercourse at all – and the figures were noticeably lower than those recorded by Kinsey in his American sample, *Sexual Behaviour in the Human Male* (1948). There was a prevalent notion that there must be some standard to which most people conformed, along with the assumption that everyone was much the same.

Women were more forthcoming than men, perhaps because of the sex of the interviewer. The men seemed to be less troubled on the subject, or at least time and again things were said to be 'all right', blocking further inquiry. There was a distinct pattern of male dominance, with sexual responsiveness in wives hardly expected and in some cases disapproved, and even feared. Women, though more articulate than the men, manifested a widespread puritanism and a high degree of sex antagonism. The attitude to conjugal relations was compliance with the husband's demands and a pride in passive endurance, shading towards boredom and dislike. Husbands were valued in an inverse relation to sexuality, 'he doesn't bother me much' and 'he's not lustful' being terms of praise. Perceptions of discord in the sexual relationship were found to correlate with wider conflicts in the marriage.

Reliable information about orgasm and sexual satisfaction in women was difficult to obtain. The question was hard to word and it was unclear 'how far there was sufficient self-knowledge of the physiological event', given that 'Many who said "yes" sounded unconvinced.'[92] Women's expectations were low and fears of pregnancy were an inhibiting factor. Ignorance was rife: in spite of the increasing acceptability of, debate about and accessibility of birth control, Slater and Woodside found that coitus interruptus (withdrawal) was not considered to be birth control, which was defined as 'something chemical or mechanical', while others confused contraception and abortion. A 'Mrs D' was reported to have said: 'they don't use birth control as "there's no need" but also says her husband is "careful"'.[93]

Shortly after the war, Mass Observation (MO), inspired by the Kinsey survey in the USA, undertook a 'Sex Survey' in the United Kingdom, though with aims and methods somewhat different to those of Kinsey. It was hoped to discover 'what people's feelings really are towards sex morality in this country' (rather than to conduct Kinsey-style investigations into sexual behaviour, although a small sample was asked to complete a more detailed questionnaire on this). The teams of investigators worked on the basis of a questionnaire, rather than the famed interviews of Kinsey and his colleagues.[94] It is notable among British sex surveys for not being rooted in either pathology or hygienic or moral problems. Even surveys not specifically concerning 'pathology' – those carried out by the Royal College of Obstetricians and Gynaecologists,

Slater and Woodside, and Eustace Chesser – drew their material from individuals who had in some way come to medical attention, and MO's own VD survey had of course been undertaken for public health reasons.

The results of the survey were written up but never published *in extenso*.[95] The typescript 'Report on Sex' is held in the Mass Observation Archives. It includes around 3,000 completed questionnaires, a total not including pilot surveys and the survey of 'Leaders of Opinion' (clergymen, doctors and teachers), but incorporating replies by members of the Mass Observation 'Panel' (individuals who undertook to record their own views and to observe public opinion for the work of Mass Observation) who were perhaps more middle class in general social standing and more unorthodox in attitudes than average. An outstanding discovery was 'the contrast between our own initial expectation of inhibition, embarrassment and rebuff – and the friendly and cooperative manner with which our questions were answered'. Only 1 per cent of the street sample refused to continue responding once they had learnt of the survey's emphasis, though one woman was reported to have terminated the interview claiming, 'We never mention the word sex in the class of society I belonged [*sic*] to.' One problem was the tendency of respondents to try and give a 'correct' reply; but preconceptions to do with the reticence of the British were certainly not fulfilled. Respondents regarded the subject as important – with 'the constant insistence that "sex is natural"' – though there was an apparent tension between this view of sex as natural and healthy and fears of 'uncontrolled' sex.[96] In relation to gender differences, the survey concluded: 'Men appear to have experienced fewer troubles, on the surface at least', and that men seemed

> to be more complacent about their lack of sex instruction; perhaps in any case street-corner bandying of sex facts is more open and casual amongst boys – or perhaps men are less willing to admit to sex doubts and difficulties.[97]

However willing respondents were to discuss general attitudes, the face-to-face questionnaire method of the survey probably deterred discussion of personal fears and problems.

In the early 1950s Eustace Chesser undertook a massive study of *The Sexual, Marital and Family Relationships of the English Woman*, with the assistance of three collaborators and an advisory committee including F. A. E. Crew, Kenneth Walker, a psychiatrist, a woman doctor, and a canon. He was also assisted by 1,498 doctors in obtaining his research material, a total of returns relating to 6,500 women.[98] The study was based on various presuppositions, such as Chesser's belief that the

background was 'one of progressively weakening taboos, and of continuous change in feelings and attitude on the subject of sex, marriage
and family problems'. Given this assumption, he aimed to discover
the present experiences of and attitudes towards marriage among a
sample of Englishwomen, the association between certain childhood
experiences and these experiences and attitudes, and to assess the
factors linked with feelings of happiness or unhappiness in marriage.
It was not, as he explicitly pointed out, merely a fact-finding inquiry
but was designed to test 'certain hypotheses suggested by sociological
and clinical findings'.

Chesser was influenced in organizing the data he had gleaned by
'clinical observation and theoretical considerations' by both psychoanalytical ideas and previous sociological investigations in the field. His
belief that family background and early upbringing would be influential
in later development, embodied in the design of the study, indicates the
way in which psychoanalytical ideas had managed to infiltrate the discourse of sexual knowledge in Britain. This bias differentiated Chesser
from Kinsey, another important influence, but one who concentrated
on the taxonomy rather than the aetiology of sexual development. Also
implicit was Chesser's own view that the changes that had occurred and
the weakening of taboos were beneficial.[99]

Chesser was aware of social survey methods, but for reasons which
appear principally to have related to practicality, he invited a large
number of GPs to distribute the questionnaire to a cross-section of their
female patients. The survey thus depended on voluntary co-operation
rather than random sampling. Chesser admitted that such an approach
might introduce bias, but since the establishment of the National
Health Service, a high proportion of the population visited their doctors at least occasionally during the year, and were known to them, while
women might consult on behalf of their children. He hypothesized (but
had no means of testing) that a widely representative sample of woman
patients would not differ substantially in most respects from the general
female population. The doctors distributing the questionnaires employed various criteria for selection liable to create bias. In some cases
these criteria were self-cancelling – specific choice of patients in marital
difficulty or without problems – and sometimes the doctors selected on
grounds of 'intelligence', social status and age, tending to favour the
educated, literate and articulate middle class. An additional biasing
factor was the non-response level, but although some doctors were
reluctant to distribute questionnaires to single women (McCance had
had similar difficulties), single women were over-represented. The age
group between 21 and 40 was also over-represented in relation to its
percentage in the general population.[100]

The survey, not surprisingly, tends to bear out Chesser's preconceptions. In spite of the supposed tendency of sexual advice in the 1950s to stress the importance of complementary and differentiated sex roles, Chesser found significant correlation between perceptions of parental happy marriage (and a happy childhood) and a fairly egalitarian relationship in which neither father nor mother appeared to be 'boss'; where there was a boss, those families in which this was mother seemed less happy than those in which it was father.[101] A most significant finding was the noticeable difference between older and younger age groups in openness of discussion of sexual matters. Forty per cent of the women born before 1904 had discussed sex with other women, and around 14 per cent with boyfriends. Sixty per cent of those born after 1914 had discussed sex with other women, and over 20 per cent of those born after 1924 with boyfriends. By the 1950s more sex education literature was available and perused, and the subject was discussed more readily and in ways distinct from 'street-corner smut', within marriage and between friends. Fewer women had 'picked up' sexual information from no one in particular.[102]

Nearly all these later investigative initiatives had a somewhat Whiggish bias. Although the paradigm shift away from pathology was by no means complete, in many cases the feeling that things were already improving ('new outlook . . . new conception') was combined with a sense that it was now possible to 'bring about constructive reform along rational lines'. The aim was to discover what was 'needed for the elaboration of a more enlightened, juster and more satisfactory sexual ethic':[103] not merely to add to the sum of human knowledge, but through that knowledge to increase human happiness.[104] There was rather a serious blind spot to much of this investigation: a lop-sided focus on women, and for various methodological reasons, intelligent, educated and articulate middle-class women at that. Furthermore, just as scientific research into sexual questions had become dissociated from the wider context of human sexuality, the progress of social investigation into sexuality had narrowed down to specific topics and statistical tables, from Ellis's extended case studies to Chesser's numbered paragraphs, and the graphs, pie-charts, Venn diagrams and percentages in the 1994 publications of the British National Survey of Sexual Attitudes and Life Styles,[105] in a (not altogether successful) attempt to contain and make respectable an innately messy and problematic subject.

CHAPTER NINE

'Good Sex': the New Rhetoric of Conjugal Relations

The idea of sex as licit conjugal pleasure did not completely vanish during the nineteenth century. Even William Acton had decreed that moderate exercise of conjugal rights was beneficial to health. Malthusian writers stressed the healthy pleasures of a conjugality relieved from the economic strains of too frequent pregnancy. Writers from alternative health perspectives, such as prolific phrenological writer O. S. Fowler, and hydropathist T. L. Nichols, often consulted 'as a desirable source of information' on 'these secret subjects',[1] discussed sex and conjugality among more general problems relating to health care.

The 1873 and subsequent British editions of Nichols's *Esoteric Anthropology* omitted the free-love rhetoric of earlier American editions,[2] and Nichols was cautious about allowing too much sexual indulgence. He believed that healthy women desired sexual union for a period of several days monthly, when 'full of ardour' they had 'a great capacity for enjoyment' and were 'seldom satisfied with a single sexual act'. However, once conception had taken place, intercourse was taboo, and remained taboo until the cessation of nursing and the inception once more of menstruation. Men, though not subject to female periodicity of the reproductive function, ought to abide by these 'requirements of natural law'. While emphasizing that (though necessarily infrequent) sexual intercourse should be mutually pleasurable, Nichols was more concerned to give hints for the maintenance of continence. He described the factors stimulating to the organs of generation, but so that amative excitement could be avoided: his list included the usual targets of Victorian moral diatribes such as immodest dress and dancing, but he also cautioned against the arousing effects of lip-kissing and caressing of the bosom.[3] Furthermore he considered that in the corrupt state of modern life many women were not only incapable of sexual enjoyment, but could be 'deeply injured in their nervous systems by the efforts of their husbands to make them participate in, and so heighten, their enjoyments'.[4] Men were cautioned that 'after fifty, sexual pleasures are very exhausting', liable to produce paralysis or apoplexy.[5]

During the latter decades of the nineteenth century, and also originating from the other side of the Atlantic, there appeared the new literary genre of the marriage manual, an entire volume devoted to questions of conjugality. Two popular examples were *Sexual Physiology and Hygiene* by R. T. Trall, MD,[6] and *Confidential Talks with Husband and Wife* by L. B. Sperry, AM, MD,[7] both of which achieved numerous UK editions well into the twentieth century. In their emphasis on the marriage relationship and its right conduct, some themes were already emerging which laid foundations for the efflorescence of the genre in the 1920s. One was the importance of the wedding night, and the dangers that lay in wait there: according to Sperry it was 'one of the most delicate and important events' in a man's life, when he had to 'show himself a man, instead of a selfish sensualist or a careless and ungovernable brute'.[8] Another was that sexual intercourse was important to the married relationship itself as well as to its generative function: abstinence, however much praised by 'theorists', was likely to cause 'indifference and formality, not to say actual coldness and irritation', whereas 'occasional sexual connection . . . unquestionably cultivates affectionate mutual regard and unselfish devotion'.[9] Trall concurred with Sperry that 'normally exercised, no act of an intelligent being is more holy, more humanising, more ennobling'.[10]

The problem of how much was permissible continued to tax these writers: although sexual indulgence in moderation was not perceptibly injurious to the normal husband or wife, moderation was hard to define with exactitude.[11] Distinguishing love from lust was not always easy, since the appetites of most people were 'to a great extent morbid'.[12] Husbands in particular were exhorted to cultivate restraint,[13] given their tendency to let sexual intercourse become a habit, indulged 'reckless and thoughtless of its consequences to themselves or to their wives'.[14] Conjugal relations 'should be as agreeable as possible to both parties',[15] but these writers did not find it necessary 'to describe in detail the proper position for copulation, or the exact methods of procedure in exercising the sexual function'.[16] While adumbrating a new ideology of marriage relations, these works still eschewed exact physiological instructions for rendering the act mutually pleasurable. With a couple in good health, not vitiated by the corruptions of modern life, the act, if not abused or perverted, was assumed to be naturally agreeable to both. Its pleasurable, but ambiguously so, character, was stressed by reiterated warnings against excess and sexual gluttony.[17]

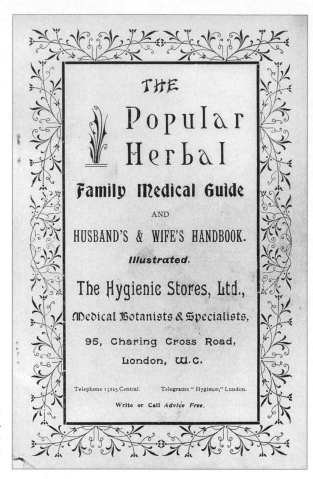

THE

**Popular
Herbal**

Family Medical Guide

AND

HUSBAND'S & WIFE'S HANDBOOK.

Illustrated.

The Hygienic Stores, Ltd.,

Medical Botanists & Specialists,

95, Charing Cross Road,

London, W.C.

Telephone 13215 Central.   Telegrams " Hygistor," London.

Write or Call *Advice Free.*

21   The cover of *The Popular Herbal:* marital handbook in the form of promotional literature for alternative practice, in this example, medical botany.

Such ambivalence about sex even when consecrated in marriage was pervasive. *Nature's Revelations for the Married Only* (*c.* 1904) was produced by the Electric Life Invigorator Company at the price of one shilling (5p), to promote the company's products, and is a rare example of a kind of literature that presumably enjoyed considerable circulation. Although the weakening dangers of sexual excess would respond to remedial application of invigorating electricity, nevertheless the purchasers of the work were given exhortations about the sanctity of marriage. Pleasures were to be mutual, for 'Intercourse which is not reciprocal must in a measure be demoralizing and unhealthy.' No healthy woman would refuse intercourse, with the weasel proviso 'when it is right and proper'. Intercourse could not be agreeable if the husband's premature emissions prevented 'the orgasm of the woman and the ejaculation of semen of the man in the same instant'. There was an assumption that so long as the wife had not been traumatized by having 'tired body and lacerated person' subjected to a 'mistaken sense of manliness' on the wedding night, and was not the victim of selfish husbandly excess, mutual pleasure was a matter which needed no instructions.[18] The work reiterated the theme that, provided it was not abused, sex within marriage was a natural and unproblematic pleasure.

The possibility that female sexual desire might not be a simple response, even when not turned to disgust by male brutality, was not an issue. It appears to have been thought of as an innate potentiality (capable indeed of corruption through seduction) which would blossom in the wake of considerate male conduct. Information on the clitoris as 'the seat of venereal pleasure', homologous to the penis, was to be found in the much reprinted, clandestinely circulated, *Aristotle's Master-piece*. However, though emphasizing the necessity of 'equal ardour', editions of the later nineteenth century somewhat coyly advised couples 'to excite their desires mutually, before they begin their conjugal intercourse', without further details.[19] (While the circulation of *The Master-piece* was obviously wide, given its continued reprinting, it is far from clear who bought it where and for what purpose, and how it might have been read.)

Edward Carpenter advanced a critique of marriage as it existed and recommendations for what it could be. The 'special property-relation between the two sexes' – man 'only half-grown' and woman 'a serf or a parasite' – led to 'sex-starvation and sex-ignorance' wedding 'mere licentiousness'; not, in his view, conducive to a successful, living relationship. Ignorance was most acute in women, who were 'led to the "altar" often in uttermost ignorance and misunderstanding as to the nature of the sacrificial rites about to be consummated'. Husbands were commonly 'unaware that love in the female is . . . more diffused than in the male'. Injured and horrified through male ignorance, many women found 'the thought of Sex brings but little sense of pleasure': fulfilment of conjugal duty constituted 'a real, even though a willing, sacrifice'. A factitious and dangerous 'glamor' about the opposite sex coexisted with nearly total ignorance of thier real nature. The lack of true companionship between the sexes meant that even when there was initial sexual satisfaction, the sequel was frequently 'mere vacuity of affection, then . . . boredom, and even nausea'.[20]

'Mere pleasure-seeking', however, was not the end of marriage and Carpenter was convinced that permanent and life-long unions existed. In those men who had attained 'a certain grade of evolution' (and almost all women) 'deep rousing of the sexual nature' led to 'romance and tender and emotional yearning towards the object of affection', which endured beyond the waning of sexual attraction. Though he gave some credence to the perception that the human male was by nature and needs polygamous, the development of the race was leading towards 'deeper alliances [becoming] more unitary'. He inclined towards relaxation of formal barriers and legal forms, in spite of common assumptions that this would lead to 'an utter dissolution of all ties, and the reign of mere licentiousness'. Essential reforms were the emancipation of women, rational sex-teaching in youth, 'freer, more companionable, and less pettily exclusive' marriages, and modification of the artificial binding of couples on a lifetime basis. Legal changes alone would effect limited improvement in a commercial society whose idea of marriage was based on property relations: real change would only accompany major societal change, though widespread premarital sexual activity would largely be 'foreign to the temper of a northern nation'. In a utopian flight Carpenter wondered if 'triune and other such relations' might (albeit rarely) be permanently maintained. Altering society was necessary but not sufficient 'so long as the human heart is what it is', and short of the millennium natural tragedies would always occur.[21]

In Carpenter's radical agenda marriage was a central but non-exclusive sustaining relationship, which the social changes he advocated would make more attainable, though changes of heart and racial evolution also had parts to play. Although he deplored the widespread ignorance consequent upon inequitable gender and social relations, his work did little on a practical level to lift it, never setting out those facts he felt were being withheld from the young, to their detriment. The emphasis in his works was on the emotional and spiritual, physical acts standing almost metaphorically for human union on these other planes, rather than as a positive good in themselves. Though Carpenter decried the contemporary suppression of the body, his tentative recommendations in connection with intercourse (against artificial contraception, for sex in the open air among the beauties of nature rather than in stuffy dark rooms) savour of the mystical.[22]

Feminist writings on marriage began to take on the specifically sexual aspects of the relationship with a greater explicitness towards the end of the century. Certain gains had already been made: since 1857 a circumscribed right of divorce, some child-custody rights in the case of marital separation, broader grounds of judicial separation, the passing of the Married Women's Property Act.[23] Women writers tended to pick up, and give additional emphasis to, themes already present in the literature of marriage, such as male brutality, and the notion (adumbrated by, for example, Nichols) that sex was only permissible at intervals of several years for the purpose of procreation.

The role of women in marriage and the place of restraint in conjugal life were debated in, for example, Margaret Shurmer Sibthorp's *Shafts: A Paper for Women and the Working Classes*. While the tenor of editorial policy was anti-Malthusian, one female correspondent pointed out that motherhood was not the sole sanctifying end of marriage and that some women were refusing to bring children (or too many of them) into the world as it existed at present. Articles advocating 'the use of scientific checks to undue and immoral reproduction' appeared,[24] generating correspondence for and against. One article decried the employment of 'scientific checks' by the wife as enabling the husband to indulge himself without restraint; and Sibthorp concurred in an editorial that 'Women must themselves be the controlling power, the arbiter and the authority on this point.'[25] Though continuing to give space to advocates of Malthusianism such as Jane Clapperton, Sibthorp 'earnestly believ[ed] . . . that there is no justifiable remedy for overpopulation but self-restraint'.[26]

Havelock Ellis was perhaps the first British writer explicitly both to advocate and describe a combination of 'the art of love' with the 'science of procreation' as essential to marriage.[27] This problematization of the conjugal relation is perhaps the flip-side of Ellis's agenda, rendering 'natural' practices popularly supposed to be 'unnatural', by demonstrating how for many people they were indeed felt to be 'natural', and to show furthermore that they were continuous with more apparently orthodox leanings. Deconstructing assumptions that 'natural' 'normal' sex was unproblematic and needed no discussion, Ellis pointed out that in the state of sexual ignorance commented upon by such austere high Victorian figures as Sir James Paget, 'even the elementary fact of coitus needs to be taught'.[28] Sex-love in contemporary Western society was sternly repressed if physical, laughed at if emotional,[29] and both sexes married in sexual ignorance or misapprehension.[30] But although the basic facts could be taught, love as an art was 'far too subtle, too complex, too personal, to be formulated in lectures and manuals'.

Ellis did, however, make some essay towards indicating in what the art of love might consist. Too much written about marriage had been 'framed to suit the supposed physiological needs of the husband', neglecting those of the wife.[31] In spite of his powerful advocacy of the sexual rights of women, Ellis claimed that 'in the art of love the man must necessarily take the initiative'. Sexual intercourse was not 'a mere physical act to be executed by force of muscles'; the man, aware of the signs of sexual desire in woman and capable of evoking them, was to woo and court the woman herself into reciprocal desire.[32] Though a woman might be capable of revealing the secrets of love, she would only dare to do so with a man who had already 'shown himself to be an initiate'.[33] Ellis's very modest allusion, accompanied by citations from various authorities, to the necessity of foreplay, drew criticism from the otherwise laudatory reviewer of the volume in the *Lancet* in 1910. Ardent young husbands might be 'apt to be too hasty and too clumsy in the introduction of their wives to the mysteries of the marriage bed', but it was nonetheless dubious whether 'the refinements in the *ars amandi* detailed in this chapter' should be generally adopted.[34] This may however refer to the mentions of variant positions for intercourse and the use of oral stimulation.[35]

It was some years before such idealism about the potential of mono-gamous marriage coupled with recognition of the need for erotic instruction reached a wider audience, though changing attitudes towards marriage as a relationship were implicit in demands for change in the divorce law, which was finally achieved in 1923.[36] While the war appeared, through the flood of divorce and illegitimacy, to be undermining the institution of marriage, after 1918 there was a sudden efflorescence of a new form of marriage manual. This provided the kind of detail that Ellis had mentioned in his chapter on 'The Art of Love', while the idea that sex within marriage had functions besides the purely reproductive gained much wider currency. In order that it might fulfil its other potential function of consolidating the married couple's relationship, physically, emotionally and spiritually, new guide-lines were needed, for a mutually satisfying (and non-procreative) physical relationship between husband and wife did not necessarily come naturally.

The book which breached the dam of reticence was *Married Love: A New Contribution to the Solution of Sex Difficulties*, published by Marie Stopes early in 1918. Stopes has been the subject of several biographies and studies,[37] and Laurie Taylor has pointed out her affinities with such apparently different contemporary figures as D. H. Lawrence and Wilhelm Reich, sexual radicals whose visions centred upon a profound, multilayered union of transformed monogamy.[38] The emphasis in her works was on the normal, the natural, the healthy, the clean: *Married Love* aimed to give 'average, healthy, mating creatures . . . the key to happiness' and to save 'years of heartache and blind questioning in the dark'.[39] *Married Love* went through five editions, selling 17,000 copies in the first year alone, and outsold bestselling fiction of the era.[40]

By 1925 sales had passed the half-million mark. The reasons for this success are not hard to find. Readers' responses demonstrate that Stopes was writing in the right place at the right time, attuned to the spirit of the age in her descriptions of what many couples sought in marriage and were failing to find. *Married Love* was also short, something that could be read in one evening, and got straight to the problems of human marital sexuality in contemporary British society without climbing the evolutionary ladder and covering the globe first: 'two thirds of every book seems to be directed to primitive customs which have no bearing on our needs,' Stopes observed.[41]

It also advocated the use of artificial birth control, though without giving details (Stopes's *Wise Parenthood*, published later the same year, dealt more explicitly with the matter), a radical departure in books of this kind. Earlier works – apart from those of the Malthusians – when making a token gesture to the need of some couples to restrict their families had usually recommended the safe period, calculated from biblical formulae and even less reliable than the present-day rhythm method ('Vatican roulette'). But Stopes's message that sexual fulfilment for both partners was necessary to marriage, independently of reproduction, struck a profound chord in her readers, as she combined the practical prescriptions of the Malthusians with a poetic idealism. Above all, *Married Love* was technically helpful in explaining what to do to obtain pleasure in the sexual act: the writer Naomi Mitchison remarked in her autobiography: 'It seems incredible now that this book was such an eye-opener. Why had none of these elementary techniques occurred to either or us before?' and attributed to it 'a marked increase of happiness'.[42]

Stopes's work revealed the deficiencies of the medical profession as advisers on marital sexuality. The *Lancet* called *Married Love* 'an extremely sensible little book . . . really needed as a public adviser', containing things 'which thousands of people would be happier for knowing',[43] while the *British Medical Journal* paid tribute to Stopes's 'literary skill, sympathetic insight, idealism, and more than common courage'. Her volume could be given to 'the married and those about to marry, provided they are normal in body and not afraid of facing facts',[44] thus sparing doctors the excruciating task of actually having to discuss such things with patients themselves: the response to *Married Love* uncovered a mass of sexual ignorance and suffering which doctors had ignored or believed negligible.[45] Stopes retained few illusions about the state of sexual ignorance prevailing among the medical profession; in 1920 she wrote to Havelock Ellis that she seriously contemplated 'publishing "Letters to Marie Stopes", every one containing a pretty revelation of doctors' incompetence!'.[46]

3 TEA TIME TALKS

AT

CLARIDGES (BROOK STREET)

BY

Marie C. Stopes, D.Sc., Ph.D., F.L.S., etc.

(Author of *Married Love, Enduring Passion*, etc.)

ON

DIFFICULT PROBLEMS IN MODERN MARRIAGE

To LADIES ONLY

Questions on relevant personal sex problems from any of the audience will be answered as fully as time permits, and may be asked at the time or sent in in writing

on 3 Thursdays

February 28th. Chair: Dr. Evelyn Fisher, M.D., D.P.H.
March   7th. Chair: Mrs. Laura Henderson
March   14th. Chair: Mrs. Stanley Wrench

Lecture and Questions 5—6.30   Tea served at 4.45

TICKETS :—For the Course of 3 Lectures . £5 5 0
Single tickets for any one Lecture £2 2 0

To be obtained only from the Lecture Secretary,
108, Whitfield Street, W.1

22 'Tea Time Talks': Marie Stopes getting sexual matters discussed in polite society, while raising money for her Mothers' Clinic.

Norman Haire, a Harley Street specialist and member of the British Sexology Society, had the utopian vision that 'the doctor of the future will have a greater knowledge of sex-matters than has the doctor of today', with chairs of sexual science at every medical school, an 'Institute of Sexual Science' in every large city, medical students trained in sexology and contraception.[47] A doctor who had attended a birth control demonstration at Stopes's Mothers' Clinic concurred: 'presumably in the future doctors will not be so apathetic and ignorant';[48] numerous doctors wrote to Stopes deploring the current state of medical education.[49] The British Social Hygiene Council's proposal to set up an advisory bureau on preparation for marriage in 1932 engendered heated correspondence in the *British Medical Journal*:[50] doctors continued to claim the right to speak on and deal with sex, while simultaneously manifesting powerful reluctance actually to do so.[51]

Stopes's name became almost synonymous with the new rhetoric of marriage, but she was not the only successful writer of sexual advice during this period. Many books on the subject were published, some of them exceedingly ephemeral, but several, if not serious contenders for Stopes's crown, had a considerable following, went into several editions, and continued to be reissued over a period of many years.

Published very shortly after *Married Love*, *Wise Wedlock* by Dr G. Courtenay Beale[59] was alleged by Stopes to be more or less a plagiarism of her own work, and 'G. Courtenay Beale' the pseudonym of a syndicate.[53] Certainly no doctor of that name appears in the *Medical Register*; and passages in *Wise Wedlock* echoed the phraseology and general tenor of Stopes's work suspiciously closely. 'Beale' asserted the existence of a fortnightly rhythm of sexual desire in women, an idea particularly associated with Stopes: Havelock Ellis's discussion of the question, in Volume VII of the *Studies*, paid tribute to her formulation of this idea,[54] and it was also recognized by the reviewers in the medical press as one of her most distinctive contributions.[55] It is hard to imagine where else 'Beale' could have found this notion. It is possible that 'Beale' was expressing ideas that were less Stopes's own property than part of the climate of the time; however, although writers on reproductive physiology, such as F. H. A. Marshall, discussed women's rhythmic cycles, this specific fortnightly upsurge of sexual desire does not seem to be mentioned in their writings.

The Reverend A. Herbert Gray's *Men, Women, and God* of 1923 was a more general *Discussion of Sex Questions from the Christian Point of View*, as the subtitle explained. It included chapters on questions of marriage, as well as an appendix on 'Some of the Physiological Facts' by Gray's doctor brother, Charles. This work, typically for the genre, attempted with more or less success to combine the moral agenda of the social purity movement with the 'modern, scientific' insights of psychology and sexology. Charles Gray indeed quoted Havelock Ellis on sexual intercourse as 'an indispensable aid to the best moral development of the individual' even without procreative intent.[56] Published by the Student Christian Movement, *Men, Women, and God* went through many editions and sold hundreds of thousands of copies, having considerable circulation especially in overtly Christian circles.

While the medical status of 'Beale' might be uncertain, Isabel Hutton was a woman doctor who took the daring step in 1923 of publishing a work of marital advice, *The Hygiene of Marriage*,[57] under her own name. Her work, like that of Stopes, stemmed from her 'own past ignorance and difficulties' (she had married relatively late in life after a successful career in psychiatry) though also out of 'the questions patients had asked me throughout the years'. Her aim was a book that would be simple and realistic, containing 'essential information that is not instinctive with the human species'.[58] *The Hygiene of Marriage* certainly achieved this, and, though never one of the most notorious works in this field, enjoyed a modest success, being reprinted several times.

Perhaps Stopes's major competitor in the field was Theo. van de Velde, a Dutch gynaecologist and author of the famous work *Ideal Marriage* (after he had left the Netherlands with a married patient),[59] and other works of less far-reaching popularity. The British doctor Eustace Chesser claimed that *Ideal Marriage* was given to young husbands in the same way as Mrs Beeton on cookery was presented as a vade-mecum to young wives.[60] Influenced by Van de Velde himself, Chesser nevertheless maintained that though 'almost blindly followed by the majority of writers on sexual technique',[61] 'after studying his huge inventory of sexual pleasures, all of them carefully inscribed "normal" . . . nine readers out of ten have felt cheated'.[62] However, the original readers, not to mention its English translator, the feminist Stella Browne, must have found the emphasis on the necessity for mutual sexual pleasure in marriage, and the detailed instructions for achieving it, remarkable and valuable enough for them to ignore, or at least take in their stride, the misogyny and the intrusive 'inter-mezzos' of aphorisms and quotations about love, marriage, manhood, womanhood and so on.

These works shared a major shift in conceptualization of the sexual natures of men and women. Women were not seen as innately frigid, but had lying 'dormant the capacity to become vibrantly alive in response' to their lovers.[63] Initially they were unlikely to be spon-taneously sexually desirous or immediately responsive, although Stopes for one suggested that because of 'concealment of the essential facts of life' women might not recognize the stirrings of desire.[64] As a result of ignorance of what marriage might entail, women approached it with 'a curious feeling of apprehension, and many doubts and fears', exacer-bated by the fact that many of them had never experienced 'any con-scious feeling of sexual desire'.[65] A woman might receive 'physical, mental and moral shocks' sufficient to 'wreck her own and her hus-band's life' on the wedding night.[66] Even if not thus traumatized, she might take quite some time to achieve adaptation and arrive at 'com-plete physical sympathy' with her husband.[67] However, the 'normal' woman was 'capable of intense sexual desire and its intense satisfaction' and could even 'suffer severely from the effects of the non-satisfaction of her wants', though her more diffuse and less readily aroused desire was 'less clamant' than that of the male. Nonetheless she was capable of sharing a 'glorious communion of sense and soul with the man'.[68] Exhortations to wives laid more stress on attitude than activity: they should be 'at least willing to be awakened and made responsive'.[69]

Men were depicted as ardent but clumsy and impetuous; Balzac's image of the orang-utan trying to play the violin was constantly invoked.[70] The male was supposed to contain his urges for as long as it took to arouse the female with foreplay, and then, following intromission, to continue the act for as long as it took to bring about the elusive female orgasm. One of the few dissenters from this new emphasis on male self-control during the act (rather than from performing it at all) was 'Courtenay Beale', who called it 'a severe and probably injurious strain upon the nerves and the emotions alike'.[71] On the whole, however, the assumption was that a man, once aware of the need to control the insurgent spontaneity of his desires, would be both willing and capable, although it was recognized that 'in early married life, the husband is apt to reach orgasm too quickly'.[72]

Male impetuosity, clumsiness and lack of control could imperil the marriage right from the wedding night. Fearsome tales were recounted of marriages ruined as male insensitivity met female ignorance: brides 'driven to suicide or insanity' by 'the horror of the first night of marriage'.[73] Even if not driven mad, 'many a delicately-organised, highly-strung woman' never recovered from 'her horror of what to her appears the revelation of male brutality'.[74] In somewhat less Gothic mode, the husband was warned to be 'specially gentle and considerate in the early days of marriage' lest he permanently ruin his chances of married happiness.[75] Such wedding-night carelessness was not usually attributed to malice or deliberate brutality. Hutton thought it 'very rare for a man to use force intentionally' rather than being thoughtlessly impetuous,[76] and Stopes believed that only a minority of men were consciously careless about their bride's suffering,[77] while 'Beale' maintained 'the brute who has no consideration for the feelings of a woman – and that woman his new-made wife – is happily very rare'.[78] Only Gray struck a positive note, suggesting that many couples looked back 'upon the first night of marriage as on a sacred occasion which they recall with wonder'.[79]

A husband's own performance anxieties, doubtless exacerbated by such warnings, were less often addressed, perhaps for fear of putting ideas of failure into men's minds. Few writers mentioned, as Isabel Hutton did, that 'temporary inability to obtain erection, and so perform the marital functions, is of fairly frequent occurrence in the early weeks of marriage', and might even be due to the man's fear of inflicting pain upon his bride.[80] Van de Velde was particularly reluctant to reveal the prevalence of male dysfunction admitted by Hutton and remarked on by Stopes in *Enduring Passion*, the sequel to *Married Love*,[81] indeed tending to regard impotence (except from temporary fatigue from excesses) as 'distinctly morbid',[82] and premature ejaculation, 'often found in neurasthenic subjects', as 'on the border-line of *disease*'.[83]

Once the traumatic beginning had been safely passed, the couple had to aim for 'Mutual Adjustment'. The perfect sexual act was envisaged as coitus culminating in mutual orgasm more or less simultaneously. 'Naturally educators and initiators of their wives in sexual matters',[84] men (the female role was still essentially passive) had to learn 'to kindle the spark that will flash an answer to his spark',[85] deploying this knowledge with 'tenderness, tact, gentleness and patience'.[86] Few writers dared mention that male arousal was anything but a given response, not needing any encouragement: again Isabel Hutton was unusual in suggesting that the wife ought to 'be ready to help her husband if his reactions are slow' and even to 'master the subject of love-play, and learn what helps sexual response in him'.[87] Stopes put the problems of 'The Undersexed Husband', about which she had heard so much from correspondents, down to the lingering effects, direct or indirect, of wartime strain. She advised the wife to 'woo and encourage her husband in many ways', while 'smil[ing] failure away'.[88]

Once the delicate period of initiation and adjustment had taken place and provided he had made no irreparable mistakes in the early years of marriage, the man might eventually hope for a little more reciprocity, or at least to have some of the responsibility for managing the couple's sex life taken from him, with his wife not only co-operating but occasionally even playing a dominant part. Van de Velde cautioned husbands against recklessly habituating their wives to 'a degree of sexual frequency and intensity' which they were unlikely to be able to maintain,[89] but this seems to have been less of a worry among the British writers than boredom and indifference. The general line was that these largely resulted from ignorance and ineptitude. Stopes suggested (followed suspiciously closely by 'Beale') that ideally intercourse should take place at intervals determined by the wife's recurrent curve of desire, and that the concomitant periods of abstinence would be a form of erotic discipline heightening the eventual experience. However, she warned against 'a clockwork regularity', given that there might be times when, even with the woman's physical passion at 'ebb-tide', she might be stirred by 'emotional and spiritual' factors. Besides, at the 'wave-crest' of the woman's desire, several unions might take place over the relevant days.[90] Hutton, in less lyrical strain, thought frequent intercourse not merely 'debilitating' but that it rendered the act 'somewhat commonplace'.[91]

Female frigidity, whether manifested as revulsion or indifferent passivity towards sexual relations, was regarded as highly deleterious to happy marriage. Stopes considered the frigid wife 'an artificial creation of unnatural circumstances' brought about by 'the artificial falsities of society'.[92] Mostly the problem was attributed to male incompetence or ignorance: 'he, and no-one else, is the cause of the non-responsiveness which he deplores'.[93] Modern man, 'lacking the art of stirring a chaste partner to physical love', blamed the woman's coldness instead of his own 'want of art'.[94] Gray, however, warned women against 'deliberately checking all response', and 'a mistakenly spiritual view' of sexual relations.[95] Most cautions to women, however, were directed against letting romance go out of marriage through personal neglect. To 'cease to try to charm, and take no interest in their appearance' was a recipe for marital disaster.[96] Stopes, indeed, advocated maintaining 'the elation, the palpitating thrills and surprises, of the chase' through the woman's own sensitivity to the behests of 'her natural phases . . . at times to retreat'.[97]

There was no great development in the marriage advice genre during the 1930s and 1940s. The titles already mentioned continued to be republished (indeed, some were still being reissued as late as the 1960s and even the 1980s with superficial, if any, alterations). Further works were added to the numbers of volumes available, but on the whole they continued along the lines already laid down in the wake of Stopes. There was, perhaps, a greater explicitness. Edward F. Griffith (a founder of the Marriage Guidance Council), for example, in *Modern Marriage and Birth Control* gave considerable details as to the stimulation of the clitoris for the woman's satisfaction should her husband suffer from premature ejaculation.[98] Eustace Chesser in *Love without Fear* went beyond the usual recommendations to women to keep romance alive, mentioning the provocative effects of 'the partly clad or artfully concealed body', with examples drawn from the practices of 'some continental licensed brothels'.[99]

One issue emerging as a cause for concern during the 1930s was the danger of single women being aroused by men's casual lovemaking: 'it is difficult to imagine a more refined cruelty than to arouse sex passion in a girl for whom the normal satisfaction of the passion is denied', according to Leslie Weatherhead, a Methodist minister and writer of several popular works on psychology. This may reflect the greater freedom of women and the increasing amount of non-coital sexual experimentation taking place. Some of the male behaviour described in Weatherhead's *Mastery of Sex*, however, would now be categorized as 'sexual harassment' rather than mutual acts.[100] E. F. Griffith, apparently warning against premarital 'trials', argued that 'A woman once loved is an awakened women';[101] the male should not thoughtlessly 'arouse the passions of a woman' when she might be 'prevented . . . from obtaining the natural relief'.[102]

Some writers have argued that this new genre of marriage advice was implicitly oppressive to women, turning wives into eroticized sex objects as their husbands, terrorized by the flood of information about the prevalence of venereal disease, eschewed prostitutes.[103] There is strong evidence to indicate that what most British men sought and found in commercial sex was a somewhat perfunctory sexual experience, more readily associated with evacuation than eroticism.[104] Furthermore, the new marital eroticism required considerable effort and a major change of habit in men, and the main tenor of its message was criticism of the selfishness, ignorance and ineptitude that characterized the average male. The Stopes correspondence suggests that far from seeking to import rampant eroticism into their marriages, most men were still endeavouring to find a sexual position that was comfortable for both partners, and wondering if it might possibly be permissible to be naked and keep the light on while performing the act.[105]

This new phase of writing about sex, begun by *Married Love*, might be seen as replacing one set of anxieties with another. There was a new emphasis on getting it right, in the right place: 'normal and perfect coitus' concluded when 'the man's orgasm begins and sets the woman's acme of sensation in train at once'.[106] There was a growing differentiation between the right and wrong kind of female orgasm: 'digital stimulation of the clitoris' was dismissed as a 'rudimentary act . . . far removed from the mutual, synchronised, mature form of sexual intercourse', although it was also perceived as a sometimes necessary expedient.[107] Undoubtedly 'one of the main avenues leading to complete orgasm', the clitoris could induce 'a full and satisfying muscular orgasm', though differing from 'cervical-orgasm' both in 'quality and result'.[108]

Joan Malleson, a woman doctor prominent in the Family Planning Association, who wrote *Any Wife or Any Husband* under the pseudonym 'Medica' in 1950, appears to have been a convinced believer in the vaginal orgasm, although she found the most common sexual disorder of women to be a lack of vaginal sensation. However, many women were in the fortunate situation of 'being able freely to achieve an outside clitoral climax' (with their husband's assistance), which went 'a long way to compensate for having no internal orgasm'. Indeed, those women whose vaginal anaesthesia was easiest to treat were those in whom clitoral orgasm was attainable given adequate technique on their

husbands' part, and Malleson found no evidence to support the contention that 'vaginal feeling will not be established if clitoral stimulation is
permitted'. She gave permission, even encouragement, to explore clitoral sensations, and felt that orgasmic satisfaction, however achieved, was
superior to frustration.[109] Eustace Chesser similarly dismissed arguments about fixation of sensibility in the clitoris; women who failed to
achieve 'the normal transference of sensibility' once married were
largely the victims of faulty male technique and selfishness.[110]

Certainly fresh anxieties might be aroused. Yet this school of writing
did not employ the punitive and guilt-inducing medico-moral
framework characteristic of so much Victorian and immediately
post-Victorian sex advice. Its agenda was to encourage a more positive
approach to sex within marriage, and while no doubt, given the
charged nature of the subject, any prescriptive writings on sex may
have induced anxiety, this was no explicit part of the programme of
these writers. There were perceptible ambiguities in their own thinking, and any radical intentions were hedged around by an acute
perception of how far they might go: in 1924 Stopes informed a
correspondent that to publish more explicit information on clitoral
stimulation would be deleterious for 'the movement as a whole'.[111]
Alec Craig remarked upon Stopes's 'skill and pertinacity' in conveying
'to a wide audience the maximum amount of sex education possible' at
the date of publication, although she had been forced to some degree
of 'reticence and inexplicitness'.[112] By being very careful to state that
they were talking only about sex between persons of the opposite sex
legitimately married to one another, these writers (whose lives were
often considerably at variance with their public rhetoric) were able to
discuss such delicate topics as 'the genital kiss' and to give details for
accomplishing variant sexual positions.

The sex advice genre in Britain had as ancestors both Josephine
Butler and Havelock Ellis, and its strong links to a progressive liberal
agenda of toleration rather than moral policing can be seen in its
discussions of sex which could not by its very nature be marital. Stopes,
it is true, notoriously gave dire warnings to women about the dangers of
lesbian practices ('this unnatural thing'), but in the context of the
problem of sex starvation in women deprived of 'natural' satisfaction by
their husbands. She did concede that 'a very *very* few women have
strong inborn tendencies of this type', but distinguished this from the
'corruption' drifted into through laziness or curiosity.[113] This distinction between innate and acquired was almost universal. Weatherhead
considered that 'congenital abnormality' could not be defined as
vice, but it was nonetheless 'one of the most distressing disharmonies'
a psychologist encountered. Even 'acquired' perversion was not

necessarily due to vice, but could be the tragic by-product of organic disease, or sexual abuse as a child.[114]

Eustace Chesser's views on the subject appear a little ambiguous. No one was '*completely* masculine or entirely feminine'; and homosexuals were not so immediately identifiable as some people believed. While resisting the belief that homosexuality was wholly acquired, and believing in an innate predisposition, Chesser gave some credence to the seduction theory whereby previously 'normal' individuals were 'led along this by-way of sex', though he conceded that many who indulged in homosexual practices at some stage of their lives did not become 'genuine homosexuals'. 'Genuine homosexuals' suffered from 'a definitely pathological state'; however, this was far from being criminal, and many of them had compensating fine qualities.[115] Malleson had similar ideas; she recognized innate bisexuality but differentiated the profoundly and ineradicably inverted from those in whom homosexual bias was 'not deeply ingrained'. Although she viewed homosexuality as largely a condition of 'immaturity', she looked forward optimistically to ever-increasing toleration and removal of the 'uncivilised unjustice [*sic*]' of the law and the unhelpful 'stigma of crime' attached to the subject. Lesbian relationships were often found among 'normal and stable' women, and tended to be 'more satisfactory and enduring' than the homosexual relationships of men.[116]

The marriage manual as engendered by Stopes was about 'good sex': sex both morally and emotionally legitimate, and also erotically satisfying. It was not the sex of seedy and potentially dangerous encounters with prostitutes; it was not the pathologized sex of quacks and anatomical museums. Even so, though desire for 'good sex' was widespread, the concept was not unproblematic, lying constantly open to contamination by association with 'bad sex': anything that savoured of masturbation was dubious or anything that might seem to class the wife with the mistress.[117] Conversely, however, this re-visioning of sex as an idealism focusing on expression rather than restriction could undermine the rhetoric of marriage to which the writers of this advice carefully adhered. It is even possible that these messages about sex as emotional expression may have contributed to its legitimation in (monogamous and quasi-marital) homosexual relationships in which it could be perceived as validating a loving bond.

Jay Mechling has argued, in the case of child-rearing advice, that it constitutes a literary genre whose relation to actual conduct is tenuous.[118] The warning against taking advice works as descriptive of actual contemporary practice is salutary, but Mechling's blanket use of the

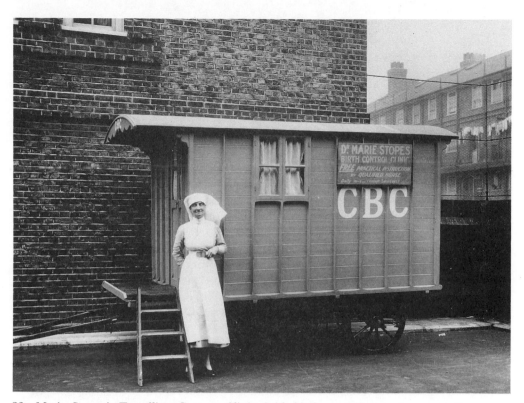

23 Marie Stopes's Travelling Caravan Clinic (with birth control nurse): apparently women preferred to visit this when it was at towns other than their own.

term 'official' advice suggests government propaganda forced on the populace (which may be rather more true when considering child-rearing?), not commercially published volumes written by heterogeneous individuals belonging to varying interest groups, which the public bought on their own initiative, often, as discussed in Chapter 11, with a certain amount of difficulty and effort.[119] Marriage advice-books originated far from the citadels of medical or political power, and were produced predominantly by individuals who themselves were marginalized and who were actuated by the aim of challenging medical monopoly and conspiracy of silence, in order to enlighten the public.

The very production of such works, impinging, as they do, on matters often supposed 'natural' to humanity, certainly raises questions about the kind of society within which such a manifestation takes place and the market for such productions. Nevertheless, it cannot be contended that the writing and reading of such works was merely an intellectual exercise, without any influence on behaviour. The response of a large group of readers to a popular work of sexual advice can be seen in the vast amount of correspondence received by Marie Stopes. (Hutton was also startled by 'how many people wrote to me of their problems . . . many, diverse and unexpected', but the letters do not appear to have survived.)[120]

Although Stopes's publishers had so little confidence in the book's success that she had to pay towards the cost of its printing, and early print runs, due partly to this attitude and partly to war restrictions, were very small, on the first publication of *Married Love* Stopes immediately began to receive letters from readers. Her ideals of marriage found a ready response among members of the respectable working classes, the expected middle-class readers, officers of the armed forces, members of the Indian and other colonial services, and even the aristocracy. The few criticisms focused on Stopes's advocacy of birth control and a philosophy of marriage in which continence and restraint were not the highest conjugal good: 'the true enemy is licence not self-control . . . far from helping mankind you are debauching them'.[121] By far the most common response was outright praise and congratulation, expressed in fulsome phraseology. Correspondents praised the 'cleanness' along with the lucidity and beauty which they found in her works, and the courage needed to publish them. Her works were 'courageous and beautiful',[122] 'sorely needed but . . . which nobody seems to have had either the ability or the courage to publish',[123] and gratitude was expressed for the 'love and courage you have shown', 'your courage and kindness to humanity', 'the fearless spirit in which you have issued your books'.[124] *Married Love* in particular struck her readers with the light of revelation, and many wished it had been available earlier: 'only wish it had been available seven years ago'; '[I] wish I had read it 25 years ago', '[it] might have altered the whole course of my married life'.[125]

Many early readers were anxious to share their experience. *Married Love* was said to 'adorn our bookshelves'; it 'will occupy an honoured place in our home'[126] (so was not hidden in corset-drawers, like *Aristotle's Master-piece* or *Esoteric Anthropology*). It was handed about among friends: 'we have already ordered half a dozen copies for presentation to suitable friends'; 'I intend to help in future by sending a copy of your book to any of our acquaintances about to marry'; 'we shall take pleasure in spreading the good news'.[127] It was given openly as a wedding present by close relatives, even from parent to child: 'we have decided to present a copy to each of our children as they marry',[128] in one case by a father-in-law described as 'a particularly clean-minded parson'.[129] A not uncommon comment was: 'if these books were read by all who are about to be married and those that are already there would be many more happy unions'.[130]

Stopes's books broke through taboos on open discussion of sex matters and, above all, they opened up a channel of communication
between married (and engaged) couples.[131] Michael Gordon, in a paper
on changing trends in marital advice literature in the USA between
1830 and 1940, has suggested that the growing concern with technique
and foreplay during the 1920s and 1930s was 'a form of ritual magic', as
sex became a more anxiety-laden area for men in the face of increasing
emphasis on the sexual rights of women.[132] Evidence indicates, however,
that such works aided marriages not by providing husbands with a
compendium of erotic skills but by their power to 'open up communication between spouses and lovers' about 'the sensations, perceptions,
and emotions arising before, during, and after coitus'.[133] E. L. Packer, in
a 1947 article on working-class marriage, quoted the cautionary tale of
a husband who, realizing 'that his part in copulation was deficient in
skill . . . bought a number of manuals on sex education for marriage'.
But he failed to 'impart any of his newly acquired knowledge to his wife
before coition', so she 'maintained the reserve which was customary,
and the maladjustment persisted'.[134]

Randolph Trumbach has suggested that 'middle class companionship and intimacy . . . was brought into existence by the words that
passed between husbands and wives as much as by anything else'.[135]
Works of marriage advice extended the boundaries of subjects upon
which couples could talk, if only by supplying concepts and vocabulary.
They provided women with a language for matters previously shrouded
in euphemism – if spoken of at all – and gave men a mode of verbalizing
sexual and conjugal matters distinct from the smutty male subcultural
discourses from which so many men picked up such sexual knowledge
as they had, as well as from the guilt-inducing pathologizing of social
purity sermons. The talking itself was doubtless beneficial and conducive to conjugal intimacy, and would also, it seems reasonable to
suppose, improve non-verbal communications in the marital bed.
Marriage advice books worked, if and when they worked, less by informing men of the right buttons to push than by encouraging them to
communicate.

Presumably many of the readers who did not write found Stopes's
books sufficiently clear and helpful to work matters out for themselves;
comments and reminiscences by contemporaries reinforce this
impression.[136] It was those whose problems were not readily solved by
her lucid instructions who wrote. Although some wished simply to
convey appreciation and gratitude, most correspondents had some
further question that they wanted to ask: for elucidation of passages
which seemed unclear to them ('not only her arms should embrace her
husband'), to ask for further advice (her prescription of twenty minutes

for ideal mutually orgasmic intercourse seems to have been beyond many husbands), or about the best methods of birth control (not dealt with in detail in *Married Love*) and where they could be obtained. She may have aroused new anxieties (that twenty minutes) but she also allayed fears which her correspondents had hardly known they had or which had silently tormented them for years.

She was even consulted by the unmarried already having some form of sexual relationship. Sometimes this was a single act, as with the couple, engaged for two years, with marriage delayed for financial reasons, anxious about the result of an unconsidered act of union.[137] Other couples appear to have been having fairly regular intercourse, with some form of birth control, usually the highly unreliable coitus interruptus,[138] or in some cases a sheath.[139] Withdrawal was sometimes practised within more spontaneous acts, not without anxiety, as with the young man who wrote that 'the final act took place outside' but wanted to know when they could be sure that conception had not taken place.[140] Some couples practised some form of 'petting',[141] though this did not obviate fears of unwanted conception,[142] while others were concerned as to how far premarital lovemaking might go.[143] Some wondered whether it would be wrong, for engaged couples unable to marry, 'either from a moral or physical point of view, for two such persons to give each other relief – provided that actual intercourse does not take place?'[144] (Some couples had thus discovered the female orgasm eluding many long-married couples.)[145] Others were concerned about the possible harmfulness of 'embraces short of connection' leading to orgasm.[146] One bluntly asked that as marriage was presently out of the question, would it be all right to sleep with his fiancée?[147]

It seems probable that there was a change, at least in perceptions about the matter, from premarital experience being male encounters with prostitutes, to 'anticipation of marriage'; it was in this latter sense that most 'Leaders of Opinion' took the question on premarital sexual activity in the Mass Observation Survey of 1947–9.[148] This would seem consistent with the development of the notion of 'good sex' as something which occurred within an emotionally meaningful relationship, and which was validated by it.

There are questions to be asked about advice and the relationship of the advised person to the adviser. A book can be gone back to and reread, and discussed with a partner and even, from the evidence of Stopes's correspondents, with family and friends. Furthermore, although its purchase may require a degree of nerve and resistance to embarrassment, 'the reading of a book does not demand an act of courage',[149] which for most people the communication of sexual difficulties does require. From the correspondence Stopes received (and in some cases people did write back reporting on the effect of taking the advice she had given them), it can hardly be doubted that her books did have an effect on readers, did modify both their idea of what the conjugal relationship should be and what they did about it. But people took out only what they were ready for: her books were in the right place at the right time. Feedback from readers influenced her own works: for example, *Enduring Passion* dealt in greater detail with the problem of premature ejaculation revealed to be so prevalent among her correspondents,[150] and the notorious phrase 'not only her arms should embrace her husband' did not appear in the earliest editions of *Married Love*.[151]

In spite of the difficulties and embarrassments of obtaining such works (discussed in Chapter 11) they sold in large quantities. As the author of a humorous work on the sex manual pointed out, though without accounting for it, these works 'enjoyed . . . huge sales and an extraordinary influence'.[152] Though their depiction of the relations between the sexes cannot be taken to reflect actuality, they did indeed influence their readers. This distinctively British tradition of the commonsense marriage manual, pragmatic, empirical and reassuring, not only disseminated, but recreated, sexual knowledge.

CHAPTER TEN

Public Faces in Private Places:
Sex, Law, Politics and Pressure Groups

Although a number of issues concerning sex impinged upon the public interest, at least potentially the province of political action, government policy in Britain on sexual matters was characterized by nervous inertia, vacillation and contradictions. Already the subject of governmental intervention by the mid-nineteenth century were the public health problem of venereal disease, the allied question of prostitution, the publication and dissemination of obscene literature, and the regulation of marriage and divorce. Many of these were in fact dealt with on a case level by the judiciary and the police. By the early twentieth century anxieties over population decline, quantitative or qualitative, joined them.

Such matters in the public domain were widely reported and debated not just by sensationalist journals but in the more respectable press, although the relationship between public policy and the press was deeply ambiguous. Different issues became the focus of anxieties at different periods. Vociferous interest groups advanced demands for either greater activity (sometimes in contradictory directions) or less interference. Britain was in some respects subject to less codified regulation of sexual behaviour than other countries both on the continent of Europe and across the Atlantic, and had an influential civil libertarian lobby, but there was a good deal of informal moral policing, with alliances between groups concerned about public morals and official police forces increasing.[1]

The Contagious Diseases Acts were suspended in 1883 and repealed in 1886. The Criminal Law Amendment Act, 1885, raised the age of female consent, while incorporating the notorious Labouchère Amendment altering existing laws criminalizing buggery. The penalty of imprisonment for ten years to life, reduced from death (never imposed since the 1830s) in 1861, was lowered in 1885 to two years' hard labour, but applied to all consenting homosexual acts between adults in private, creating a 'blackmailer's charter'. This was particularly perverse given that in Britain (unlike many countries) it had never been (and continued not to be) illegal to practise prostitution as such, although the trade was regarded as sinful and immoral. The relevant laws concerned public nuisance, brothel-keeping, the age of consent, and vagrancy, however broadly these were interpreted in practice to harass prostitutes. It might have been assumed that logically a similar line between private sexual conduct, however undesirable, and its public manifestations would have been drawn in respect of homosexuality. The aetiology of the Labouchère amendment is deeply obscure, as Davenport-Hines points out in his account of persistently negative attitudes to homosexuality in *Sex, Death and Punishment: Attitudes to Sexuality in Britain since the Renaissance.*[2] The 1898 Vagrancy Act's extension to male homosexuals of tightened-up laws on immoral importuning perhaps derived from the *fin-de-siècle* anxieties depicted by Elaine Showalter in *Sexual Anarchy.*[3] The effects of the 1885 Act on homosexuals and attempts to reform the law have been extensively discussed by historians.[4]

Even before 1883 organizations opposing the Contagious Diseases Acts had moved on to more general questions of social purity, and after this legislative success they increased their efforts. The means to do this were diverse and debatable: some wanted a campaign of moral policing backed by legislative action; others felt that protecting women was more important than cleaning up the streets; some deplored sin but thought it was not, and should not be, a crime; and civil libertarians objected to extending laws.[5] Within the National Vigilance Association, the alleviation of the dangers of sexual molestation and exploitation faced by women and children – leading, for example, to the Incest Act of 1908[6] – was intertwined with a lust for censorship which led to the imprisonment of Vizetelly, the elderly publisher of English translations of Zola's works.[7]

Following the failure of the Contagious Diseases Acts, governments were nervous to the point of inertia about venereal diseases, still a major public health problem. Traditional British medical squeamishness over venereology persisted;[8] policies of exclusion were maintained by voluntary hospitals, and most Friendly Societies refused sick benefit to sufferers. Many venereal cases went untreated, or were attended by 'chemists, qualified and (more frequently) unqualified, and herbalists', through 'fear of disgrace and the consequent desire for concealment'.[9] Well into the twentieth century, ignorance meant persistence of the 'certain superstition . . . that if a man has contracted venereal disease and he can have connexion with a virgin he will transmit that disease to her'.[10]

There were attempts to generate more active policy. Informal contacts in 1896 between concerned members of the medical profession and philanthropic workers, convinced of existing ignorance of 'how great the evil is', resulted in a memorial the following year recommending a Royal Commission to gather evidence on the prevalence of venereal diseases and existing arrangements for treatment. Representatives of eight rescue associations, 96 women engaged in social work, 72 men of all classes and 52 members of the medical profession, submitted a resolution in support of this memorial to the Prime Minister, Lord Salisbury, in 1899. Salisbury believed 'public opinion was not sufficiently informed and enlightened', and may have feared any hint of a revival of the Contagious Diseases Acts. Influenced also by prevalent notions that the problem was declining, and should be fought on moral and religious grounds, he took no action.[11] This memorial was perhaps mistimed. Considerable furore had arisen over control of venereal disease among troops in India in 1897, with demands for the reinstitution in India of what was effectively a Contagious Diseases Act, and outcries against any such proposal. A memorial signed by a number of socially eminent ladies urged effective protection for the British soldier in India: Florence Nightingale (and Mrs Humphry Ward) added a proviso in favour of an independent inquiry.[12] A counter-memorial by the Ladies' National Association (for the Suppression of the State Regulation of Vice), signed by Josephine Butler, was submitted to Lord Salisbury and his government.[13]

Those seeking investigation expected the inclusion of men in any scheme, for both justice and efficacy, and did not intend the registration or licensing of vice. They emphasized protecting 'the innocent from contagion' and checking the spread of VD.[14] The unjust burden upon the innocent was often cited when pleading for wider consciousness of the ravages of sexually transmitted diseases: 'the innocent' were the wives and children of ('guilty') infected men (infection in children, when not congenital, was usually attributed to poor domestic hygiene), those who had shared a cup or an innocent social kiss, doctors or nurses who treated the diseased. Whether many cases were thus contracted is not clear: this emphasis was perhaps intended to counteract the stigma attached to venereal diseases by dissociating them not only from sexual misconduct but from sex altogether.

From the 1880s arguments were increasingly voiced as to the necessity for warning the young about the sexual dangers assailing them on every side.[15] The *British Medical Journal* spoke against the 'complete ignorance regarding the sexual organs and the sexual functions' permitted, even fostered. Most parents were probably 'not well fitted to undertake such a duty', and its delegation to the family medical practitioner 'would be highly disagreeable'. Universal teaching of elementary anatomy and physiology would 'remove the unwholesome fascination which our present habit of secrecy imparts'.[16] The *Lancet*, conversely, while believing that the law should do 'all that it can do, for the protection of the young', felt that the true remedy was 'cultivation of purity'.[17] Meanwhile bodies such as the White Cross League and the Alliance of Honour took the matter in hand by issuing pamphlets specifically aimed at inculcating a high and single standard of chastity. *The Testimony of Medical Men* declared that continence was conducive to health, although its maintenance might be a struggle, given 'the many banks of festering slime' lying in wait to 'tear and rend the unhappy being who is driven against them'.[18] Such literature was widely disseminated through a variety of religiously orientated youth organizations.[19] In 1894 a *New Review* symposium on 'The Tree of Knowledge' came out 'strongly in favour of knowledge' rather than innocence.[20]

From the 1890s a growing amount of literature was available to assist parents in fortifying their children against the dangers of 'contamination' with pure and healthy knowledge about sex. Botany was a prevalent figure: for example calling children's attention to the relation between 'Nature's infinitely varied and beautiful schemes for the fertilisation of flowers' and 'the future plant'.[21] The works of Mrs Wolstenholme Elmy, the suffragist (under the pseudonym 'Ellis Ethelmer'), *The Human Flower* (1894) and *Baby Buds* (1895),[22] were recommended by the feminist journal *Shafts*.[23] Providing children with clean sexual enlightenment might be acknowledged as of national importance, but was still largely a task parents were exhorted to undertake, though a Mrs Kapteyn of Hampstead was organizing classes early in 1896 'for the instruction of the young'.[24]

Although the dissemination of information to adults about birth control was not illegal, neither was it risk-free. H. A. Allbutt was stricken from the Medical Register for producing his popularly priced *The Wife's Handbook* incorporating information on how to avoid becoming a mother too often. The General Medical Council continued to police the profession against doctors publishing 'obscene literature'.[25] Within the National Vigilance Association some members thought that only medical circulars with 'a vicious object' should be prosecuted, but others totally opposed 'promiscuous circulation of this kind of knowledge'.[26] The Post Office resisted the use of its facilities for transmitting 'indecent and obscene' works like *Some Reasons for Advocating the*

Prudential Limitation of Families: in October 1891 the barrister and Malthusian Henry S. Young, MA was deemed to have disseminated this 'broadcast' through the Royal Mail.[27]

In circles in which the discussion of sexual matters was becoming more common, questions of restraint in marriage were debated, often less with personal interest than with humanitarian concern for the poorer woman blurring into wider eugenic anxieties about the national well-being. The educated and articulate might be able 'to rise above the necessity for any such action', but vast numbers 'really incapable of self-control' were liable to swamp the country with 'children too often physically, mentally and morally "below par"'.[28] A contributor to *Shafts* queried whether all were able to exercise desirable restraint.[29] Jane H. Clapperton (a contributor to *Shafts* herself, and associated with the Men and Women's Club) warned Patrick Geddes that 'for the ignorant, the gross, the degraded' only neo-Malthusianism was appropriate.[30]

As the nineteenth century drew to a close, pervasive anxiety arose over the question of national deterioration. Britain was threatened by competitive foreign powers; even within her own Empire by the Boers. Debates about national fitness were phrased in resonant metaphors of virility and fertility, which fed into debates very much concerned with actual issues of virility and fertility.[31] Although the Eugenics Education Society, founded in 1908, never enjoyed a membership far into four figures at its most successful, anxieties about 'breeding' were extremely pervasive within society as a whole. Questions of national fitness and population in both quantity and quality also perhaps seemed an acceptable approach to problems of sexuality: the Eugenics Society (as the Eugenics Education Society was later renamed) enjoyed much more success and status than the British Society for the Study of Sex Psychology (BSSSP), founded in 1913.[32] The concept of 'racial health' pervaded sex education: Baden-Powell's advice on the hygiene of the 'racial organ' in *Rovering to Success*, and the title of Norah March's guide for parents, *Towards Racial Health*, are but two examples,[33] while Marie Stopes christened her recommended contraceptives 'Pro-Race', later 'Racial'.[34] Sex conduct was not merely about morality or personal well-being but about national virility.

As a new century dawned, the problem of venereal disease was considered by diverse bodies deliberating issues of national well-being. The Inter-departmental Committee on Physical Deterioration in its report of 1904 recommended setting up a Commission of Inquiry into the prevalence and effects of syphilis. The 1911 Royal Commission on the Poor Laws recommended that workhouse authorities' powers of

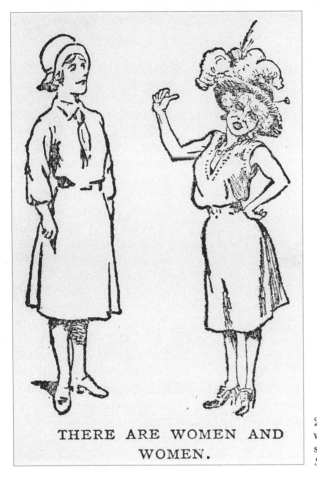

THERE ARE WOMEN AND
WOMEN.

24 'Rocks you may bump on –
women'; the right sort and the wrong
sort from Baden-Powell's *Rovering to
Success.*

detention respecting contagious diseases should be extended to the
venereally infectious.[35] Specialists were beginning to dissociate VD from
professional prostitution, recognizing the implication of 'supposed irre-
proachable women' in its transmission,[36] and the statistically fairly
insignificant role of the 'habitual prostitute':[37] a point of view yet to
enter wider debates on the problem.

Perhaps more positive advance towards a single moral standard
was denoted in the increased agitation for more egalitarian divorce
legislation. The Divorce Law Reform Union was formed in 1906 by
the amalgamation of two recently established societies with that aim.
Questions were asked in Parliament, and in 1909 a Royal Commission
on Marriage and Divorce was appointed. It recommended equalizing
the grounds of divorce to adultery by either party and extending
them to include lengthy desertion, habitual drunkenness, and life

imprisonment. Simplification and decentralization of the judicial procedures were also recommended, to make divorce cheaper and more accessible, as was restricting the publication of reports of cases.[38] Rebecca West prophetically described it as 'A Report that will Not Become Law':[39] over ten years later a very watered-down Act was finally passed.

Prostitution continued to be a matter for public agitation, with new concern over melodramatic tales of young women involuntarily shanghaied into sexual bondage abroad fomenting moral panic about foreign pimps preying upon English girls. The Criminal Law Amendment (White Slave Traffic) Bill introduced in 1909, which permitted arrest of suspected procurers without a warrant, made slow parliamentary progress and was reintroduced in 1912 as a Private Member's Bill, with vague intimations of government support. Much enthusiasm was expressed for its proposals of punishing pimps by flogging (already employed on homosexuals), and it was passed (though in a mutilated form) after a campaign mounted by purity organizations,[40] including further clarification of the law on immoral importuning as related to homosexual offences.[41]

While police action to eradicate 'white slavery' was being urged, prostitutes plying their trade were subject to routine harassment. An 'old sort of tradition' among the police assumed their duty 'to sweep prostitutes off the streets as far as they can'.[42] '6,000 unfortunate women' were 'arrested every year for alleged annoyance of men', but over two or three years a bare 100 or 150 'men annoying women merely by accosting them'.[43] Women were often arrested without any complaint from the man or men allegedly 'annoyed'.[44] A certain level of prostitution took place off the streets through advertisements, heavily coded to evade the Indecent Advertisement Acts. Paul Ferris suggests that the 'prostitute's therapeutic role' was encoded in 'Certified Nurse visits and receives patients for rheumatic complaints', 'Rheumatism Treated with Counter-Irritants', 'Properly qualified and certificated nurse desires Daily Engagements. Therapeutics': ten years previously, however, the code words appear to have been 'chiropody and manicure'. The salacious connotation of 'French' persisted with 'French lady would receive a few paying guests in her well-appointed house' and 'Lessons in French correspondence; also conversation'.[45]

The moral messages of the social purity movement had been supported by argument that following them was also the course leading to good health. As the twentieth century began, the teachings of social purity were also seen to contribute to national fitness and well-being. The dangers of impurity were considered a threat at an ever-early age. It was not only 'children of poor, overcrowded localities' who were at risk of premature sexual initiation ('corruption') but those of 'the more luxuried classes . . . left too much to the care of thoughtlessly chosen servants'.[46] (This apparently paranoid myth-making generated by fantasies about members of lower social classes is to some extent substantiated by the cases of sexual abuse by servants cited in Chapter 11.) The transmission of sexual information or misinformation among young people by (probably) mutual exchange was usually transformed by the proponents of 'clean and healthy' sex instruction into 'the coarser of their companions' disseminating 'degraded ideas on the subject of sex',[47] which were 'generally untrue'.[48] Children who had 'not had all these things properly explained to them' discussed them in a 'wrong and unclean' way.[49] Most deliberate sex education took place in religious settings and through youth organizations such as the Scouts and the Boys' Brigade: there were some experiments in extra-familial sex enlightenment through the educational system, not always success-ful, but this was far from widespread or officially condoned.[50]

With the discovery of the spirochaete in 1905 leading to the Wassermann diagnostic test for syphilis, followed by the 1909 revelation of the arsphenamine drug Salvarsan, which 'stopped the clock' of syph-ilis, a cure for the ravages of an endemic disease appeared to be at hand.[51] The Local Government Board instituted an official inquiry by Dr R. W. Johnstone in 1913, undertaken 'in the midst of other official duties'. The report, though still deploying the emotive terms 'innocent and guilty', advocated improved facilities for early diagnosis and treatment, and ridding the diseases of counterproductive stigma.[52] Nonetheless, approaches to politicians and government departments remained futile. In 1913 Sir Malcolm Morris and others with strong feelings on the problem concluded that

> the only way to get a chance of obtaining a full inquiry was to startle and impress the 'man in the street' in order that public pressure should be brought to bear on the Government.

A 'plain unvarnished statement of the facts' published in the *Morning Post* over many well-known names, including nearly every doctor hold-ing an official position, 'succeeded to perfection': the matter was openly discussed by the press and the agitation for an inquiry spread even to former opponents. The International Medical Congress meet-ing in London that year passed strong resolutions on the subject, and when Parliament next rose the Prime Minister announced the appoint-ment of a Royal Commission.[53] The topic became an increasingly visible public concern; Christabel Pankhurst in articles in the *Suffragette*, subse-quently published as *The Great Scourge and How to End It* (1913), cited the prevalence of the venereal diseases as one of the compelling reasons why women should receive the vote.[54]

The Royal Commission chaired by Lord Sydenham spent several years hearing copious evidence on the prevalence of venereal disease and existing provisions for diagnosis and treatment, as well as recommendations as to what should be done to combat the 'terrible peril to our Imperial race'. The diseases were extremely widespread; though few accurate statistics were available, as many as 10 per cent of the urban population had syphilis and an even greater proportion gonorrhoea.[55] No structures were available to implement recent advances: Wassermann testing was rarely routinely undertaken.[56] British medical practitioners 'failed to appreciate the importance of these diseases' and were 'to a large extent unfamiliar with the newer methods of diagnosis and treatment'.[57] The Commission agreed that only state action could adequately deal with diseases of such national importance. Mindful of the problems involved in venereal diseases, the Commission insisted:

> It is of the utmost importance that this institutional treatment should be available for the whole community and should be so organised that persons affected by the disease should have no hesitation in taking advantage of the facilities for treatment which are offered.[58]

To get away from the old punitive attitudes, and in the interest of public health rather than human rights, the Commission advocated that in provision no distinction should be made between the sexes, between 'good' and 'bad' women, or between the classes. The recommendations, implemented in 1916 in Local Government Board Regulations under existing Public Health legislation, inaugurated a nationwide free, voluntary and confidential system uniting sufferers with adequate expert treatment. The Public Health (Venereal Diseases) Act of 1917 restricted administration of Salvarsan to authorized trained doctors, and criminalized the purveying of purported remedies by any but qualified doctors.[59] Education about the diseases and their prevention was recognized as necessary; the National Council for Combatting Venereal Diseases (composed largely of social purity activists) was subsidized to undertake this.[60]

The subject became even more openly discussible when, somewhat ironically shortly after the Royal Commission had been achieved, the First World War broke out, bringing venereal disease forcibly into prominence as a military problem and a sensitive public issue given the large number of men, including conscripts, exposed to the 'likelihood of permanent damage to the individual, infection to others, and an heritage which might stain an innocent life'.[61] Control presented problems: 'officers and men, knowing how infection is contracted, individually take the risk'.[62] War conditions were considered unusually favourable for encouraging the spread of these diseases: 'The sexual instinct' was 'stimulated in both sexes', and 'gratification of the impulse . . . more easily obtained' in an atmosphere of 'slackening of moral principles'.[63]

There was dissension over the most effective way to reduce the prevalence of venereal diseases among the troops; British forces policies in contrast to those of the US and Dominions appeared *laissez-faire*, even haphazardly *ad hoc*. Lord Kitchener simply exhorted the British Expeditionary Force to resist wine and women.[64] Lectures to the troops were of varying efficacy: men were 'wildly indignant' at some, though 'enthusiastically appreciative of others';[65] one young man found that 'many of the lectures, etc., one ever hears in the service about "dangers" rather pass over my head'.[66] Especially in France reliance was placed on the provision of *maisons tolerées* (regulated brothels); Bridget Towers has suggested that this was approved by a British class leadership convinced that army morale was contingent on sexual activity, although many medical officers by then were committed to a medical rather than a social control approach. Public opinion, in fact, finally forced the closing of these brothels for the troops in 1918.[67]

Early treatment of the potentially infected by establishing facilities for disinfection as soon as possible after exposure was one medical approach; in some units such facilities were provided from early in the war.[68] Some medical officers promulgated the new model of prophylaxis.[69] Dr Lyster of the Society for the Prevention of Venereal Disease claimed that attempts at instituting a 'packet system' were 'thwarted in every possible way by army regulations' – no one was supposed to talk plainly to the men about the existing centres for VD prevention, and official lectures contained no word on prevention.[70] There were vast differences among medical officers: some had 'little faith from lack of experience, others . . . consider the "punishment fits the crime", others . . . have conscientious objections to lecturing on the subject, and still others [are] too tired to do so', though some pursued active policies of ablution or prophylaxis.[71]

A question which came into stark prominence during the war was who was giving disease to these fine fighting men? Soldiers confessed 'they hardly dare venture into the public thoroughfares in certain parts of London because of the temptations with which they are assailed' from the 'vile women who prey upon and poison our soldiers'. The helpless prey of 'harpies', men yielded to the 'depravity' of female solicitation from mere 'human nature',[72] 'persecuted' on the streets by 'girls apparently of only 12 or 13, painted, got up, and with all the manners and phrases of professionals'.[73] It seemed to be not only the prostitute, who might be identifiable and containable, who was the culprit. Over 60 per cent of VD cases among British troops came from women 'not prostitutes in the ordinary sense of the word'.[74] The flappers practically assaulting men in public were not 'vicious or intentionally immoral', but free with their sexual favours in repayment for being taken out and given presents, or simply to 'have fun', not for direct financial reward.[75]

Men preferred women who appeared not to be prostitutes, assuming they would be free from disease (quite apart from the expense aspect: better-paid Dominions troops did contract most of their VD from prostitutes).[76] Lyster claimed that National Campaign for Combatting Venereal Diseases lectures 'frighten people from the professional', convincing 'the average soldier . . . that if he had sexual relations with a woman who was not a professional prostitute, he was safe'.[77] This hindered prophylaxis, which men seem to have felt conveyed unchivalrous 'doubt as to the ladies' chastity or at least immaculateness'.[78] While 'amateurs' were not solely a product of wartime loosening of morals, the problem became prominent and the subject of hysterical outcry during and after the war.

Strategies for prevention in this wartime ambience tended to include the male partner and not just the woman. However, measures were taken early on in some localities to keep 'women of bad character' away from troops and a regulation under the Defence of Realm Act (DORA 40d) provided for the forcible removal for treatment of any woman known to be a source of infection, without including male sources of infection. Soldiers' wives were also intrusively policed for good behaviour.[79] Women were often ignorant of their rights, for example refusal of medical examination when arrested,[80] and in some areas prostitutes still believed that a 'list', something like the CD Acts registration, was in force.[81] Voluntary women police forces set up to 'protect' women seem to have operated often more as snoopers after usually consensual 'indecency', or at least were perceived in this light.[82]

By the end of the war provisions for the treatment of venereal diseases at least in principle aimed to avoid discouraging patients from seeking and continuing treatment.[83] Attempts to make the communication of venereal disease a crime under Criminal Law Amendment and Sexual Offences Bills being debated in Parliament failed.[84] By the mid-1920s the country was covered by a network of nearly 200 publicly provided venereal disease clinics. Despite its continuing low esteem, even stigma, this system was extensively patronized by those suffering from, or fearing that they suffered from, venereal disease. Over a million patients

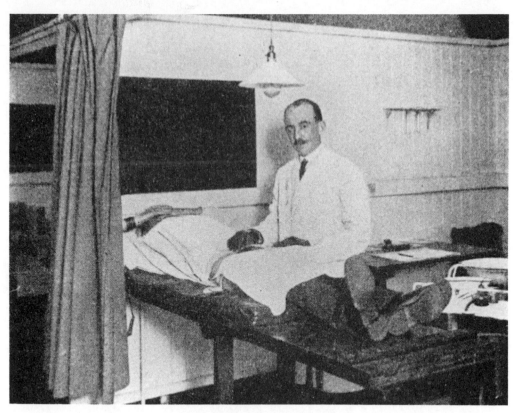

25 Venereal Disease clinic, illustrating post-Royal Commission attempts to combine efficiency of treatment with respect for patient sensitivity.

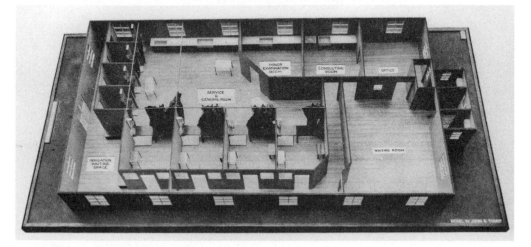

26 Model of a Venereal Disease clinic, Ministry of Health *Memorandum of Organisation of Work at Venereal Disease Treatment Centres* by L. W. Harrison, 1920.

were seen in 1919,[85] and syphilis in particular declined noticeably after the introduction of this system of free, accessible, confidential and expert treatment, though numbers attending actually increased.[86] Attempts to put prevention on the agenda failed. The Society for the Prevention of Venereal Disease (SPVD) seceded from the National Council for Combatting Venereal Diseases (NCCVD) over this issue: they wished information on simple preventive measures to be made more widely available, even over-the-counter self-disinfection kits by chemists. Although an interdepartmental committee (Lord Trevethin's Committee) deliberated this question in the early 1920s, the NCCVD retained its position as favoured body of the Ministry of Health, at least partly because of the reluctance of the Ministry to become embroiled in this politically sensitive matter.[87] There was some anxiety that preventive measures might be confused with self-treatment: the SPVD was promoting calomel ointment, not condoms.[88] The success of the clinic system may bear some relation to the failure of prevention.

Anxiety over the birth rate was extensively documented by the Birth Rate Commission set up by the National Council of Public Morals. Mentioned in Parliament, its report said to be awaited with interest, it was a private inquiry without active governmental support, although the Superintendent of Statistics of the General Register Office and the Medical Officer of the Local Government were included on the Commission, with a remit to provide it with statistical information.[89] In spite of this concern over depopulation, shortly after the war the subject of birth control was openly debated in terms not simply of condemnation. Marie Stopes initially endeavoured to canvass official support for provision of birth control facilities, circulating the Lambeth Conference in 1920 with her *New Gospel: A Revelation of God Uniting Physiology and the Religion of Man*: the bishops were not moved.[90] Advised by Lloyd George 'to make birth control respectable', in 1921 Stopes held a meeting on 'Constructive Birth Control' at the Queen's Hall. Her Mothers' Clinic, opened that year in Holloway, north London, was intended as a model for eventual public health facilities.[91] The Walworth Women's Welfare Centre followed shortly, set up under the auspices of the Malthusian League, though control soon passed to an independent committee.[92] Stopes made birth control widely talked about, if not respectable, in 1923 by suing Halliday Sutherland, a Roman Catholic doctor, for libel over his comments about 'a doctor of German Philosophy (Munich)' who had opened a clinic in the slums to experiment on poor women. The case was extensively reported and gained her enormous publicity.[93]

In 1921 Lord Dawson, the King's personal physician, addressed the Church Congress at Birmingham in favour of birth control: though

James Douglas of the *Sunday Express* (later notorious for his onslaught on Radclyffe Hall's *The Well of Loneliness*) urged 'LORD DAWSON MUST GO', most other press opinion was favourable. Dawson was, however, reluctant to endorse Stopes: 'knowledge as to the applications of birth control should be conveyed by doctors to their patients rather than by books in general circulation'; he aimed 'to make doctors fulfil their proper role'.[94] Although some doctors were willing to work with the clinics, the impetus was largely from lay people, and the general attitude of the profession to the subject remained aloof when not explicitly hostile.[95] Contraception was almost never taught to medical students:[96] large numbers of doctors inquired of Stopes how to advise their patients, and attended her clinic to observe contraceptive methods, as well as seeking information about reliable suppliers;[97] sometimes they commented explicitly on this lacuna in their training.[98] Doctors were not immune to current superstitions about one defective pessary or condom in every packet;[99] one doctor declared this was enforced by Act of Parliament.[100]

In 1922 the Home Secretary was asked in Parliament if the government was likely to make the dissemination of birth control information and contraceptives illegal (as France had just done, and which the Comstock Laws did in the USA). The stonewalling reply, typically reluctant to disturb the status quo, indicated that legislation was not contemplated but that local courts might proceed with prosecutions under obscenity laws.[101] The Minister of Health was 'sympathetic but disconcertingly vague' to a Catholic Women's League anti-birth-control delegation that year, but Dame Janet Campbell, of the Ministry of Health, following the dismissal of Nurse Elizabeth Daniels for giving birth control advice at a maternity centre in Edmonton, stated that this was no part of a welfare centre's function.[102] Early hopes that the Labour government returned in 1924 would promulgate a more liberal line were cast down by the issue of a circular explicitly forbidding birth control advice in welfare centres. It was too sensitive an issue for a government only recently voted into office with a precarious majority, in spite of strong representations from the National Conference of Labour Women. Following this conference a Workers' Birth Control Group was set up.[103]

Anxiety over prostitution, professional and 'amateur', seems to have died down somewhat after the war. The Criminal Law Amendment Act of 1921 is chiefly remembered not for what it did include – tightening up the law on unlawful carnal knowledge of minors, and severer penalties for brothel-keeping[104] – but for what it did not. Attempts to use it to criminalize lesbianism failed (as did attempts to criminalize the transmission of venereal diseases). Purity organizations continued their interest in the subject but not on the legislative level, although in 1925 Lady Astor, a supporter of the Association of Moral and Social Hygiene, introduced a bill to repeal existing laws on solicitation and street offences.[105] The Street Offences Committee of 1928 put forward similar proposals, to include men equally with women under altered laws on importuning and solicitation – there were often more complaints of men accosting respectable women than of men being annoyed by prostitutes – but no measure was passed.[106] Far from promoting moral panic over white slavery purity societies took a rather dim view of the recurrent press scares on the subject.[107] It was widely believed that prostitution as such was on the decline, being replaced by more general, gratuitous, 'promiscuity'.[108]

Though the recommendations of the Royal Commission of 1909 were never implemented, as a result of the upheavals of the First World War an immense increase in divorces occurred. In 1923 a revised Divorce Law put the dissolution of marriage on a gender-equal footing, with a single act of adultery on either part a matrimonial offence deserving of divorce. Divorce was also made easier (and cheaper) by the creation of provincial divorce courts. The inscription of adultery as sole grounds, negated if committed by both parties instead of just one, still left grave objections to the law as it stood. Any hint of collusion between the divorcing couple put the dissolution of their marriage out of court: the law was still bound to concepts of 'innocence' and 'guilt'.[109] The 'spicy reading' provided by publication of evidence from divorce cases in newspapers (not merely the gutter press) was not restricted by law until 1926.[110]

The need for sex education of some kind was becoming easier to acknowledge in public. The National Vigilance Association urged educational authorities 'to provide a comprehensive system which shall secure for future generations a sound and suitable sex instruction, sufficient for self-protection and guidance'.[111] This issue of protection (rather than enlightenment) permeated even women's magazines: the editress of the magazine *Woman's World* in 1925 gave 'A Straight Talk to Mothers' in consequence of a reader's letter:

> my little friend asked her mother to tell her about love and motherhood, the mother was very shocked indeed, and told her that those things were not spoken about, and that she would know all in good time.

Sent out into the world in 'UTTER IGNORANCE', the reader suffered seduction and abandonment as a result of her mother's unwillingness to recognize 'how dangerous life is for young people these days'.[112] Sex was associated with danger: something to know how to handle properly for fear of its effect – rather like electricity.

In some respects sex education was striking a more positive note. The growing eroticization of marriage made it a reward to look forward to for chaste youth.[113] Terrors about masturbation were seen as far more deleterious than the practice itself: modern stress on 'the harmlessness of masturbation' was sometimes declared to be as exaggerated and harmful as the 'distorted fear' and 'exaggerated denouncements' of earlier writers.[114] Most writers trod a very fine line between exploding the old horror-mongering myths, and discouragement of the practice. In spite of self-consciously modern appeals to the science of psychology, with up-to-date parlance of 'repressions' and 'sublimation', these writers were still in the business of issuing warnings against self-abuse and its serious repercussions for normal sex life.[115] The dangers of occasional lapses were minimized, but caution was the keynote: 'once the habit has been begun it is very hard to leave off'.[116]

Birth control as a political issue continued to mutter on without resolution throughout the 1920s, while voluntary bodies, seeing that the government was not immediately going to take action, established clinics across the country.[117] Changes under the Local Government Act of 1929 concerning powers of local authorities could be interpreted to allow birth control in welfare centres, and some authorities took such initiatives. At the Lambeth Conference of 1930 the bishops of the Church of England gave limited approval to the use of artificial contraception within marriage. The Minister of Health of the Labour government in 1930 eventually conceded birth control advice in welfare centres solely on medical grounds, but Memorandum 153/ MCW was sent to local medical officers only in response to specific requests for guidance. Marie Stopes published a leaked copy in *Birth Control News*. The recently formed co-ordinating body, the National Birth Control Council (NBBC), also publicized it, seizing this concession to advance their cause. The British Sexology Society (formerly the British Society for the Study of Sex Psychology) wrote to the Minister (widely disseminating copies of their letter to the press) deploring the restrictive conditions.[118] These were, however, gradually extended by the Ministry under continuing pressure from the NBCC.[119]

The British Social Hygiene Council (formerly the NCCVD) was less positively affected by the 1929 Local Government Act. It promoted sex education beyond its original remit of educational work for VD prevention: instructing teachers, parents and youth leaders, encouraging the teaching of biology in elementary schools, and organizing visiting speakers for schools.[120] Responsibility for its funding was devolved to local authorities and became discretionary; a significant proportion declined to contribute.[121] However, free local authority VD clinics were attracting patients 'who do not properly belong to the hospital class' by the early 1930s: venereologists in private practice complained of 'ruin staring [them] in the face',[122] as the great majority of known syphilis cases were treated in public facilities.[123] The number of cases of early syphilis seen in clinics declined by over 45 per cent between 1931 and 1939, to under 5,000.[124] Nonetheless, continuing stigma located clinics in inconvenient and hard to find areas of hospitals, often with very inadequate privacy for patients. Administrators deemed it 'necessary to close all the doors and windows of the room where a VD patient had been and fumigate it', nursing staff made difficulties,[125] while doctors in the clinics inherited the 'pox doctor's' traditional lowly status.[126] 'It was commonly said that venereology would soon cease to exist as a special subject':[127] in 1937 sulphonamides revolutionized the treatment of gonorrhoea,[128] obviating the instrumental intervention hitherto required for the treatment of this ailment and sending numerous patients back to private practitioners,[129] who were probably willing to treat them once distasteful operations directly involving genitalia were no longer necessary. Emergence of resistant strains soon tempered optimism.[130]

Attempts in the 1930s to legalize voluntary sterilization on eugenic grounds failed: the reasons for this and the anxieties and confusions around the meaning of sterilization have been illuminatingly explored by John Macnicol.[131] Several bodies investigated induced abortion, anxious about its effects on maternal health in a context of growing panic about population decline. In 1936 the Abortion Law Reform Association was founded to seek legalization of a practice which many advocates of birth control shunned. It was available: to the wealthy via the Harley Street racketeer, to the poor from sometimes well-meaning but not always competent or clean backstreet abortionists. A reduced legal risk for doctors performing abortions was established by the Bourne case judgment of 1938. The gynaecologist Aleck Bourne performed a test-case abortion on a 14-year-old girl gang-raped by soldiers, on the grounds that continuation of the pregnancy would cause psychological damage. It is apparent from his comments on this case that he was operating on deeply rooted concepts of 'innocent', 'guilty' and 'deserving', which continued to haunt the provision of abortion.[132]

Such concepts were persistent, heavily weighted for gender. The Association of Moral and Social Hygiene regularly deplored the legal inequity facing under-age girls. Judges tended to encourage the belief that 'decent men are morally defenceless creatures against the wiles of unscrupulous girls under 16', seduced, 'even if they themselves are over 30', mainly through 'the girl's iniquity'.[133] Broad interpretations of 'reasonable cause' led to continued judicial leniency.[134] Innocence and guilt similarly haunted divorce law reform: in 1937 A. P. Herbert's Act

extended the grounds for dissolution of marriage but within the existing adversarial, matrimonial offence framework, although subsequently
90 per cent of divorces, being undefended, presumably involved mutual
consent. New grounds included desertion for three years, cruelty, and
incurable insanity, and, in the male only, rape (though not of his wife),
sodomy or bestiality. (The existence of female homosexuality was not
mentioned, and it did not constitute a matrimonial offence unless it led
to cruelty.) Grounds for annulment were also extended, to include
marrying while suffering from communicable venereal disease, being
of unsound mind, or being pregnant by another man. It was not until
1950, however, that the availability of Legal Aid for divorce finally
implemented equality under the law for rich and poor in escaping
matrimonial misery.[135]

As in 1914, with the outbreak of war there was an almost immediate
upsurge in venereal infections. Within the armed forces mechanisms
allegedly existed to deal with these 'most difficult of all diseases to
control owing to the restrictions imposed on preventive measures by
public opinion'. Information was supposed to be disseminated to all
servicemen about the risks involved and provisions for treatment, but
many patients 'reported never having had a lecture on the subject'.[136]
Nearly all officers and men in the Middle East theatre 'were almost
completely ignorant of the practised methods of prevention of venereal
disease'. There had been inadequate planning for either prevention or
treatment, and facilities for consultant venereologists with the forces
were lacking.[137] Educational films were acquired from the USA, lectures
given, poster campaigns initiated and condoms issued.[138] When peni-
cillin became available in 1944 there was some prejudice against its
use for the treatment of venereal disease;[139] syphilis was sixth on the
priority list.[140]

Anxiety about the incidence of venereal diseases led to a campaign to
increase public awareness of their transmission and the provisions for
treatment, partly breaching the taboo on mentioning venereal diseases
in the press and on the radio.[141] A 'mistaken sense of delicacy' led to
expurgation of advertisements, 'vaguer general statements' replacing
precision; 'a barricade of unfamiliar terms' being used instead of the
demotic 'pox' and 'clap'.[142] The effect of this campaign was investigated
by Mass Observation at government instigation during 1942 and
1943.[143] The 'promiscuous amateur' was made the scapegoat for
venereal infections, although it was also sometimes recognized that
'irresponsible youths',[144] and men engaged in war work who were not
obliged to undergo examination and treatment contributed to the

problem.[145] In 1943 a regulation under the Defence (General) Regulations provided for the notification of carriers reported by more than one contact. Though avoiding obvious gender discrimination, this bore more punitively upon women than upon men.[146] The prejudice against venereal diseases and those who treated them still persisted. A 'sanctimonious attitude of mind' prevailed among the nursing profession and the position of male VD nursing orderlies was 'ill-defined; they were not admitted to the State Register in spite of their skills'.[147]

The popular myth that the prostitute 'knew how to take care of herself' continued, although statistically professionals were far more risky partners.[148] Contact-tracing became more sophisticated, and there was greater interest in the problem of 'the defaulter' who remained infectious.[149] The venereally infected person was coming to be seen, at least in professional journals, as neurotic or inadequate rather than sinful or unfortunate,[150] though some experts continued to claim that 'fighting soldiers of the finest type' contracted these diseases because promiscuity was 'an entirely natural reaction' in such fine specimens, 'subjected to more temptations'.[151] There was an allied perception that the prostitute, once defender of 'the virtue of the middle-class man's sister', drew her clientele from among 'the rejects, the neurotics, the cast-outs' unable to get 'a real woman'.[152]

Though efforts were being made by certain organizations, educational authorities and individuals to bring about more formal sex education, it was only a small minority who encountered this. Very few respondents to the Mass Observation post-war Sex Survey – even among the panel sample, who might have been expected to have been exposed to more progressive styles of education – claimed to have had lessons as part of the school curriculum, or a visiting lecturer on the subject. Any texts used were dependent on non-official initiative. By the late 1940s masturbation was being said to be less dangerous than 'mental conflict which may arise from its condemnation';[153] however, though it had 'no ill-effects, physical or mental', it was still something that efforts should be made to eschew.[154] Young men were warned against 'careless sexual relations' with the 'rather fast girl' who let herself be picked up, rather than prostitutes.[155] Indulging in petting could not only 'play havoc with one's nerves' but 'pervert the ordinary sexual reflexes'.[156]

Perhaps predictably, questions of sexual health remained peripheral under the National Health Service. Venereal disease treatment was consolidated into the comprehensive service under conditions similar to those already described earlier.[157] No provisions for advice and supply of birth control were included, even after the Royal Commission on

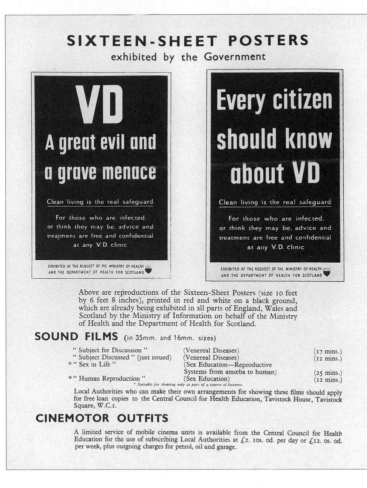

SIXTEEN-SHEET POSTERS
exhibited by the Government

VD

A great evil and a grave menace

Clean living is the real safeguard.

For those who are infected, or think they may be, advice and treatment are free and confidential at any V.D. clinic

EXHIBITED AT THE REQUEST OF THE MINISTRY OF HEALTH AND THE DEPARTMENT OF HEALTH FOR SCOTLAND

Every citizen should know about VD

Clean living is the real safeguard.

For those who are infected, or think they may be, advice and treatment are free and confidential at any V.D. clinic

EXHIBITED AT THE REQUEST OF THE MINISTRY OF HEALTH AND THE DEPARTMENT OF HEALTH FOR SCOTLAND

Above are reproductions of the Sixteen-Sheet Posters (size 10 feet by 6 feet 8 inches), printed in red and white on a black ground, which are already being exhibited in all parts of England, Wales and Scotland by the Ministry of Information on behalf of the Ministry of Health and the Department of Health for Scotland.

SOUND FILMS (in 35mm. and 16mm. sizes)

" Subject for Discussion "	(Venereal Diseases)	(17 mins.)
" Subject Discussed " (just issued)	(Venereal Diseases)	(12 mins.)
* " Sex in Life "	(Sex Education—Reproductive Systems from amœba to human)	(25 mins.)
* " Human Reproduction "	(Sex Education)	(12 mins.)

Suitable for showing only as part of a course of lectures.

Local Authorities who can make their own arrangements for showing these films should apply for free loan copies to the Central Council for Health Education, Tavistock House, Tavistock Square, W.C.1.

CINEMOTOR OUTFITS

A limited service of mobile cinema units is available from the Central Council for Health Education for the use of subscribing Local Authorities at £2. 10s. od. per day or £12. 0s. od. per week, plus outgoing charges for petrol, oil and garage.

27 World War II government anti-VD campaign: posters, films, mobile cinema units were all deployed to this end.

Population, reporting in 1949, strongly commended the Family Planning Association (FPA) and argued that the giving of contraceptive advice should be less subject to restrictions and available within the NHS, though advocating social policies in favour of larger (planned) families. The FPA (and Marie Stopes's Mothers' Clinics) continued to be the only organized providers of these services (and the two most common methods, sheaths and withdrawal, did not require clinic consultation). Marriage guidance, in spite of lip-service to the importance of sustaining the institution, was also marginalized: unlike the FPA the Marriage Guidance Council received Home Office grants in aid of the good work, but no offers to take over the task.[158] Perhaps this freed these bodies to develop in areas such as psychosexual medicine, which government contraceptive clinics might have found more tricky. It was

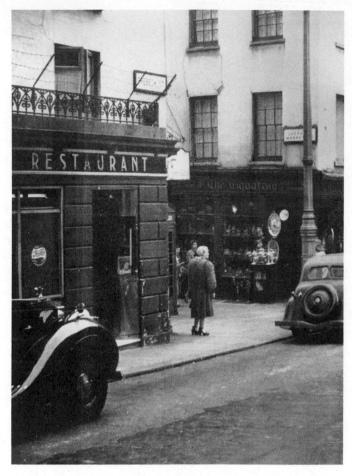

28 and 29 *The Lust Market*: London street prostitution in Shepherd's Market, Mayfair (right) and in Soho (far right) in the early 1950s (H. U. Cross).

not until 1974, a decade after the introduction of the contraceptive pill (requiring medical monitoring but no contact with genitalia) that family planning was incorporated into the NHS.[159]

Thirty years after the collapse of the British Sexology Society during the Blitz nearly all the reforms it had desired had been implemented: easing of obscenity laws, greater availability of birth control and abortion, no-fault divorce, and homosexual law reform. Perhaps it had been in the vanguard of change, or affected public opinion by a process of osmosis, or influenced in their youth individuals who had risen to positions of power and influence by the 1960s, most notably Gerald Gardiner, defence counsel in the *Lady Chatterley* trial and Lord Chancellor of the Wilson government, who was active in the Society during the 1930s.[160] Formerly more successful societies had a less remarkable record: the Association of Moral and Social Hygiene in 1951 obtained a

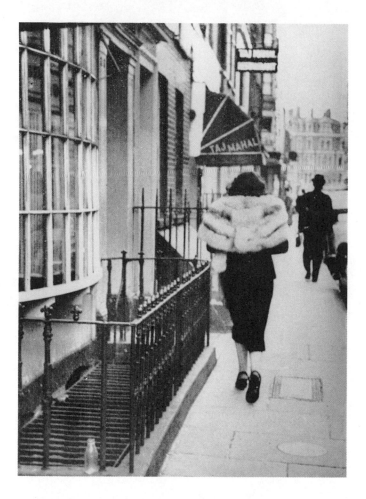

Criminal Law Amendment Act securing prostitutes certain rights against procuration, but the Street Offences Act of 1959 (following the Wolfenden Report) reinscribed the double standard and legalized harassment of prostitutes in the name of cleaning up the streets.[161]

The public arena is often assumed to be a potent force in the making of sexual knowledge – note the fear expressed during debates on the Criminal Law Amendment Act of 1921 that making lesbianism illegal would only bring it to women's attention[162] – but it is open to question how influential it has actually been, particularly as mediated through press report and comment. The relationship between the law of the land and social custom and belief has often been syncopated: divorce in England though lawful from 1857 was widely frowned upon socially for a good hundred years after that (perhaps owing to the centrality of sexual misconduct as matrimonial offence), while although Scottish law was far easier Scots took an even more stringent line on the sanctity of marriage.[163] Much literary censorship was self-censorship by libraries, pusillanimous publishers and even by writers themselves:[164] the British Board of Film Censors, similarly, was a self-policing body set up by the embryonic industry as early as 1912.[165] Prosecutions were most frequently generated by pressure from purity groups, not officially originated.[166]

Folklore about supposed government restrictions and interventions in birth control, such as the statutory dud in every packet of contraceptives, had wide currency, while many women would have been startled at the definition of 'bringing on' menstruation as illegal abortion.[167] In the face of persistent 'establishment' anxiety about the declining population, the population persisted in using contraception. Homosexuals, whom one would suppose must have been aware of their delicate legal position, did not always know the state of the law, or imagined that it affected only those making a public display of themselves.[168] Prostitutes were seldom aware of the dubious legality of their regular arrests and fines for 'annoyance'.[169] The 1994 Wellcome Survey, *Sexual Behaviour in Britain*, suggests that in the 1990s considerable confusion exists over the application of age of consent legislation, with widespread belief that it is illegal for males under 16 to have (heterosexual) sex, and that women under 16 who have sex are themselves guilty of an offence (rather than being victims of one). There is also a widespread supposition that sexual relations between women are illegal.[170]

Such vagueness perhaps reflects governmental reluctance to intervene definitively in sexual behaviour; ostensibly sympathizing with campaigners, it refrains from action, while countenancing social control through the judiciary and police. Policy was little influenced by developments in the field of scientific sexology: some sixty years elapsed between the pleas of Havelock Ellis and Edward Carpenter and the deliberations of the Wolfenden Committee, while the known prevalence of illegal abortion did not result in legislation until 1967. Another notable factor in legislation on sexual matters is that it has nearly always been about someone else, whether altruistic or controlling: birth control was for the poor overburdened working woman, as was abortion; obscenity was something that depraved or corrupted other people; children were to be saved from gutter smut or, conversely, from sex in the classroom. Homosexual law reform was accompanied by a hum of voices proclaiming their own heterosexuality along with their sympathy for unfortunate sufferers from an unjust law.

CHAPTER ELEVEN

Silent Stares, Smut, Censorship and Surgical Stores: the Makings of Popular Sexual Knowledges

It is only with the advent of the twentieth century that it has become at all possible to glean much evidence about what 'ordinary people' (as opposed to the occasional literate and articulate exception, usually of a social elite), thought about sex, and how their sexual knowledge might have been created. In the context of a mass reading public, Marie Stopes and agony aunts received pleas for help of an explicitness (edited, but at least expressed, in the published versions) seldom, if ever, encountered before on such a scale: the mass of correspondence upon which the probably spurious testimonials of quack advertising literature may (or may not) have been based does not survive. While potentially generating a sense that sex was an area fraught with problems, Stopes's correspondence and writings indicate a responsiveness to audience demands even while she imposed her own agendas. The response of her readers to her particular vision of marriage has already been discussed. A mass of confusion seems to have been desperately awaiting the enlightenment that *Married Love* shed on so many, even if what kind of individuals wrote to her and how representative they may have been are impossible to assess. It is, however, probable that those who wrote to Stopes were only the determined and literate tip of an iceberg of bewilderment about sexual phenomena.

Oral history can supply rich qualitative material, although questions about the reliability of memory, the construction of narrative, the relationship between interviewee and interviewer must influence how it is interpreted. Steve Humphries addressed some of these problems when describing the origins of *A Secret World of Sex*. He found almost total silence on sexual matters in existing British life-story collections (and sometimes deliberate censoring interviewer intervention). A pilot survey ran into problems as a result of prurient press reporting. He himself was aware of powerfully resonant taboos on talking about sex with those of his parents' or grandparents' generation. His final selection of subjects, based on the criteria of 'experience of sex before marriage, a vivid memory of the experience and a willingness to talk openly and honestly about it', raises considerable questions about typicality. The thorny ethical problem of seeking out 'the most private and intimate story of a person's life', with all the emotional freight this might have for that individual, remained a troubling thought.[1]

The question of self-selection does not apply to the Mass Observation (MO) surveys, at least as regards the street samples, though one may wonder what conscious or unconscious criteria influenced observers to approach specific individuals. The data were structured by the terms of reference of the questionnaire, and the tendency of those approached to give what were perceived as 'correct' answers was noted by MO, as already discussed. However, with the Mass Observation data, as indeed with the Stopes letters, the frequent recurrence of particular themes itself suggests the prevalence of certain attitudes or preoccupations.

These sources have to be treated with some caution, yet in spite of being generated by different approaches and needs they demonstrate some remarkable consistencies. The evidence they supply is impressionistic and suggestive, rather than 'hard' and quantitative. Nevertheless, they make it possible to essay a reconstruction of the 'ordinary person''s relationship to forms of sexual knowledge during a period of rapid social change and allegedly increasing sexual enlightenment.

Few people were engaged in overt self-conscious attempts to gain sexual knowledge, still fewer endeavoured to participate in the making of it, in the way groups such as the British Sexology Society did. For many, any sexual knowledge was the product of a combination of blind ignorance and sordid misinformation. How did ordinary individuals acquire such knowledge or misinformation as they had about sex, and how easy was it for them to gain the information?

In some cases the introduction to sex was coarse, brutal and direct: for example through 'a servant girl who used to play with my sexual organs' or the 20-year-old maidservant who induced a 12-year-old boy to have intercourse with her.[2] Other boys encountered sexual initiation at school involving force and reluctance rather than mutual adolescent exploration: 'degraded at the age of six at a high-class boarding-school', 'thrust on me in my sleep by a master!'[3] Humphries's oral material suggests similar loveless initiations for both sexes in more lower-class circles.[4] Besides such direct encounters, children and adolescents might be exposed to sexual behaviour between others (though actual prostitution was much less visible). The National Vigilance Association

recommended increasing the number of park-keepers to curb suggestive activities by courting couples in parks, though they seem also to
be alluding very inexplicitly to 'flashers'.[5] Humphries's respondents,
however, described deliberate group voyeurism, as well as 'I'll show you
mine if you show me yours' games.[6] Reminiscences of life in rural
Lincolnshire in the 1930s collected by Maureen Sutton record a mix-
ture of naive childhood curiosity, and furtive investigations of genitalia.[7]
Nevertheless, women in particular, and numbers of men as well,
managed to preserve high levels of innocence.

Entering the forces exposed many men to encounters with sexual
topics they would not necessarily have come across already, and might
even have avoided: as one man told Mass Observation, 'I never found
out anything till I went in the Army [in] 1914.'[8] It was impossible to
avoid coarse male talk once in the army, or to resist 'the infection of
impurity' whereby men came to 'do or think things which are obscene
and brutal'.[9] A 'constant flow of filthy language'[10] kept 'sexual suggestion before their minds' in all-male communities, far from their
homes.[11] War by its very nature bred 'vice and venereal',[12] while many
young men, tempted to 'keep pace with or copy coarse-minded men',
were ruined by the 'conversation, behaviour with women, and drinking
habits' of older men or superiors.[13] Military authorities persistently
assumed that men would indulge themselves, anxious only to preserve
them from disease.[14] The men themselves argued that 'sexual indulgence is natural and therefore legitimate',[15] while measures such as
provision of licensed brothels implied entitlement to sexual relief, even
its necessity. Though women in *maisons tolerées* were 'horribly brutalised
in manner and appearance', and the general atmosphere 'too sordid,
and the transaction too mechanical and degrading for men to tolerate
long', this institutionalized provision 'encouraged and incited' the
seeking out of women 'a grade higher'.[16] Thus, 'some of the finest
middle- and lower-middle-class stock in the Kingdom' who in peace
would 'have hesitated to line up outside a music hall' queued at
ablution clinics for venereal disease prevention as moral standards
were eroded.[17]

In spite (or because) of this exclusively, even perniciously, masculine
culture, it seems that Marie Stopes's *Married Love* (first published in
February 1918) was avidly read in army messes and barracks during the
final months of the war and in the peacetime army, with copies either
left lying about or exchanged among men. One private in the Army's
School of Instruction for clerks saw a colleague – 'ordinary . . . maybe a
City Council Education' – reading *Married Love*. An officer in the Middle East found a copy in North Persia left behind by another officer
going up the line. Another 'lent the book to several married brother

officers', who were 'one and all deeply impressed'. Reasons for the book's presence were not necessarily highminded: one army captain 'found your book in the mess . . . being read by boys with the idea of finding anything "Baudy" [*sic*]'. A captain in the Indian Army felt that comments on Stopes's works in the 'chiefly masculine gatherings' he frequented were 'not at all pleasant'.[18]

Stopes's male correspondents sometimes mentioned picking up such sexual information as they had had prior to reading her book in terms evoking the aura of the unpleasant and furtive or coarse associated with this male subculture: what one described as 'the usual talk one had to get accustomed to in the Army'. Such information was often perceived as of dubious value: one man mentioned his 'very limited knowledge of sexual matters – mostly gathered from smutty tales, or talks with men one meets on the daily path' and another the 'knowledge which is more or less common property' from sources 'such that I have grave doubts as to the advisability of making use of it'.[19]

Some men mentioned the contribution of prostitution to their amorous education. This was seldom such a deliberate act as accompanying a 'girl . . . of the professional class' to a hotel while in New York (well away from home) out of 'curiosity to know first hand something of sexual matters'; 'the only incident of the kind in my life,' the man claimed. Another, as a young man during the war, 'went four times to a prostitute'. 'During five years in India . . . few opportunities of promiscuous intercourse with white girls' (formerly a habit) presented themselves; although 'the idea of deliberately going with a prostitute' filled this man with disgust, he had 'on four occasions gone with prostitutes . . . when . . . somewhat under the influence of alcohol'.[20] Some men seem to have managed to come by quite a considerable amount of 'promiscuous intercourse': one man, following sexual initiation with a 'harlot', then a mistress of his own class, claimed to have lived with four women and slept with some thirty others, by the time he wrote to Stopes.[21] A man of 48 had had relationships with five or six women (none of them virgins), three of the relationships extending over periods of some years.[22] Others, however, did not enumerate with how many partners they had pursued a 'wild life'.[23]

Women, it would seem, were able to preserve their innocence uncontaminated for much longer. Some did pick up misinformation: 'the reason for my dislike to the thought of the physical side of love was that when I was at school I got such a hideous idea of things'. One woman heard 'such tales' about men, presumably from workmates and other companions, that she was quite nervous of going out with them, but did not say of what such tales had consisted. Another had only recently learnt (after two years' engagement) about the physical side of mar-

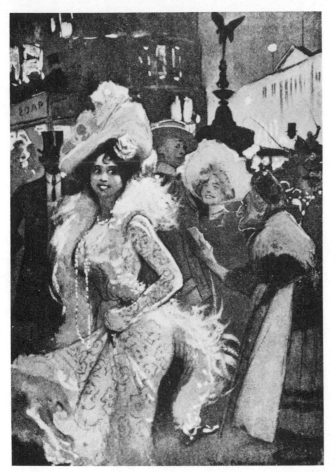

30 Piccadilly Circus at midnight in the early 1900s.

riage, 'in such a way that the idea was very repugnant to me'.[24] Many women were completely ignorant on their wedding night, a situation that, retrospectively at least, they found deplorable. Some engaged girls considered their 'ideas on marriage . . . of the haziest', having 'received no sex information from [their] parents'. Parents sometimes proceeded on the belief that 'a girl should learn all that is necessary when she is married', with the result that, as one woman said, 'until I recently read your books I had not any knowledge of what the words "marriage rite" meant'. 'Very much in the dark as to the physical side of marriage', women married with 'the vaguest idea as to what it was'.[25]

It was often assumed that mothers should enlighten their daughters, but many found their mothers 'very reserved on these matters': they were probably shy or ignorant rather than deliberately withholding information. Intelligent, articulate and informed women like those in

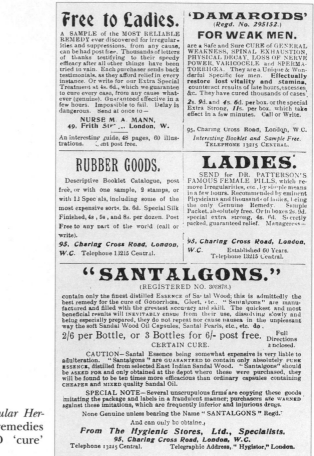

31 Advertisements from *The Popular Herbal*: rubber goods, abortifacients, remedies for male weakness and the VD 'cure' Santalgons.

the Women's Cooperative Guild found conveying sex information problematic; as one told Virginia Woolf,

> She had had to get a friend to explain the period to her own daughter, & she still feels shy if the daughter is in the room when sexual subjects are discussed. She's 23 years old.[26]

Occasionally mothers did make attempts to inform their daughters but too late, or later than the daughters would have liked: 'my mother told me that before I was married she would get me a doctor's book but I felt I wanted something now'.[27] The information provided by mothers may have been part of the problem rather than its solution: a Lincoln woman's mother told her of 'certain things your husband will require from you. It's not nice and you'll just have to put up with it.'[28] Even 'advanced' mothers did not necessarily get it right. Edith Lanchester, the centre of a *cause célèbre* of the 1890s, certified insane by her middle-class family when she left home to live with a young railway clerk of socialist views, endeavoured to enlighten her daughter by a 'prophylactic plumbing approach', but this was 'agony to her and left me with a disgust about how I must have been created'.[29]

Sometimes knowledge came to women abruptly as a nasty shock. Among Sutton's rural Lincolnshire informants, one reported a sister running back home on her wedding night because her husband 'tried to do something terrible to her', and a woman of Haxey, marrying at the late age of forty during the 1930s, went to the vicar to 'get unwed' the day after the wedding because her new husband had attempted ' "something very rude" '.[30] Educational level seems to have made no difference (as Stopes's own case confirmed): for a former teacher aged 30 'my first few days of married life were a nightmare'. 'The daughter of a scientist' was 'as ignorant . . . on matters of sex and birth as it is dangerous to be'.[31] Her experience echoes that of Naomi Mitchison, scion of a family of scientists and intellectuals and sister of J. B. S. Haldane – with whom she conducted breeding experiments on guinea pigs – whose own ignorance of human sexuality was dispelled by reading *Married Love* when already a mother.[32]

Sutton's informants additionally mentioned women conceiving out of sheer ignorance of the mechanism of the sex act, a vicar's wife whose notion of contraception was 'sticking plaster over her belly button', and women who went into labour with no idea, or the wrong idea, of where the baby was going to emerge from.[33] 'Not knowing where the baby was going to come out', 'suddenly knowing the child would have to come out of there' and being 'so shocked and frightened', and 'not even told it was painful' before going into childbirth were not uncommon experiences for women.[34]

The married seem to have been unwilling to enlighten unmarried friends, male or female, even when information was specifically sought. They tended to give 'rather evasive and not at all helpful replies', if not 'a blank stare or silence', and one man complained that 'they joke about things and give one no help at all'.[35] Possibly they were concealing their own relative ignorance. Fiancés seem to have played a major role in any enlightenment women received, sometimes with the aid of Stopes's works: 'My fiancé and I have read your book *Married Love* together . . . I had practically no knowledge of sex matters until I read your book'; 'I have gradually and carefully conveyed the invaluable information and advice they contain to my fiancée'; 'my fiancé heard of your two books and after reading them all my doubts and worries disappeared'; 'my boy has bought me two books'.[36]

There was a whole subculture of sexual misinformation and folklore. One woman asked Stopes: 'does every woman the first time she as conection [*sic*] bleed and faint are there cases when they don't', and the idea was still prevalent that children by a husband could resemble a former lover. One couple had been 'repeatedly told by different persons that a woman cannot conceive while she is breastfeeding an infant', but were now 'sadder and wiser persons'.[37] Sutton's Lincolnshire informants recounted confused ideas about sex and reproduction, negating notions that nature study and country life provided healthy sex education. Strange theories as to the cause of pregnancy (making bread, the phase of the tide in coastal areas, a Morris man putting his hat on the woman's head) blended into a web of superstition and folklore, such as the belief in the contraceptive properties of stealing a penny from a dead man.[38] Beliefs about maternal impressions were still prevalent in Lincolnshire up to the 1950s; similar anxieties about events and behaviour during pregnancy (drinking vinegar would cause the baby to be a boy, seeing a dead body meant the baby would be born dead) were expressed to 'The Family Doctor' in the magazine *Lucky Star* (and published) at least as late as 1941.[39] Other old wives' tales occasionally stimulated anxious queries to the problem pages of women's magazines, for example fears of the consequences of cousin marriage: 'my mother and father are first cousins, and I have heard several times that when cousins marry their children are imbeciles ... I was told that maybe this curse would pass over us and fall on our children.'[40]

It is possible that traditional networks for the communication of 'the facts of life' had irretrievably broken down in the face of social change. However, the above accounts suggest that the existence of a pre-lapsarian 'uncorrupted knowledge' is very questionable, as Leap and Hunter found when they investigated traditional midwifery practices: there was no 'treasure-chest of forgotten skills', but 'meddlesome, even dangerous practices', and handywomen were no more empathetically woman-centred than the professionalized midwives who superseded them.[41] Were people seeking new 'scientific' knowledge from manuals like Stopes's because of the new authority accorded it as 'modern' as opposed to traditional and old-fashioned, or were they desperate for any information at all that might shed light on the murky area of sexual functioning?

Fears and anxieties about the deleteriousness of masturbation (almost entirely among men) continued even as sex education rhetoric moved towards a position that viewed the fear as worse than the actual practice.[42] Men declared that 'I was a victim (through my own weakness of will and lack of knowledge of the consequences) of self-abuse'; 'I abused myself, not realising the damage I was doing'; 'I was a slave to the vile practice of masturbation'; 'too late, too late, it seems have I been pulled up in my abominable habit of "masturbation"'.[43] Such very negative attitudes persisted into the 1940s: 'From the age of 18 (I am

now 28) until 2 months ago I was foolish enough to masturbate';
'excessive masturbation, a habit which has continued from adolescence
in spite of many efforts to combat it'.[44] The idea of masturbation as
dangerous was also mentioned occasionally to the Mass Observation
survey,[45] although the report itself, written by those doubtless priding
themselves on being thoroughly up to date with the latest thinking,
pointed out that there was little rational basis for believing masturbation to be especially harmful.[46]

Mass Observation noted the 'haphazard, surreptitious passing on of
information': 'as many as one in twenty claimed marriage as their sex
instructor'. Most contemporary adults ' "picked up" their sex knowledge
– off the street-corner, from workmates, from other children, from
whatever literature, "respectable" or otherwise, they could lay their
hands on, or just by keeping their eyes and ears open'. Such information was often extremely bitty: 'knowledge of one aspect may or may not
be accompanied by ignorance of another', and some respondents had
not in fact realized until a relatively late age that there was anything to
learn (most startlingly, the midwife who had not realized the role of
fathers in procreation). A statistical breakdown of sources of information (some respondents gave more than one) reported that 25 per cent
had 'picked it up', 13 per cent had learnt from other children, 12 per
cent said that it 'came naturally' or by experience, 11 per cent (probably
mostly girls) had been instructed by their mothers, 8 per cent had
found out through reading, 6 per cent (probably more likely to have
been boys) had been told by their fathers, 6 per cent by a teacher, 6 per
cent learnt from workmates, 5 per cent by getting married, 4 per cent in
the armed forces, and 10 per cent from other sources. The older
respondents were more likely to claim knowledge of 'natural' origin.[47]

A selection of actual responses included: 'keeping eyes open and
experience'; 'natural I suppose'; 'haphazard fashion'; 'instinct'; 'picked
it up'; 'nature brought it on . . . and other chaps'; 'just came naturally';
'instinct and being nosy'; 'various sources often erroneous'; 'in a very
horrible and rotten manner'; 'by doing the wrong thing'; 'suppose it
just happens – in fact when I was having my first baby I didn't know what
was going to happen'; 'sort of second nature it came to you. I knew I was
a boy and my sister knew she was a girl'; 'read different books'; 'I don't
– I keep myself to myself'; 'self-taught'; 'found out for myself as best I
could'.[48] For many, especially men, their first knowledge was bound up
with negative associations: 'school lavatories and school desks. . . in
dark corners and lewd ways'; 'begins through filth – you hear a dirty
story and you begin then rightly or wrongly'; 'in the gutter more or
less'.[49] One man, describing the 'wrong way' he had learnt about
sex, detailed the usual tale of schoolboy smut and added, 'finally by

deliberately having sexual intercourse',[50] which would appear rather rare, although numbers seem to have learnt in marriage or engagement what they had not previously known. Deliberately requesting information was very uncommon, though one man did say he had found out 'by enquiry' and another at the public library.[51] Most however seem to have learnt from whatever sources they could lay hands on. One 'as a messenger boy at a chemist's shop . . . picked up knowledge from books on sex that were kept there'.[52] Some members of the older age groups believed that contemporary young people knew too much about the subject.[53]

Reading as the instructor of a mere 8 per cent of the respondents perhaps underestimates the extent to which it might have supplemented or corrected information derived from other sources. It may well have provided material, both practically and on an emotional level – a welcome contrast to the verbal (and indeed, non-verbal) sources of information or misinformation available. Slater and Woodside in *Patterns of Marriage* reported that 'books on sex have helped, and create a mental background which favours attempts at a planned adaptation',[54] citing instances of books being exchanged between the couple. Eustace Chesser, in his study of the English woman, similarly noted that 'the highest proportion of those who experience a lot of satisfaction (one-half) is among those who obtained their sex education mainly from books and pamphlets'. Such reading 'helped to allay fears and anxieties' and could indicate 'a desire to know more in order to find greater enjoyment in the sexual relationship', as well as suggesting 'more satisfactory sexual techniques'. In contrast, the women least satisfied with their sexual life within marriage were those who had obtained such sex education as they had had from other children, from which Chesser deduced the significant influence of 'the way in which sex education is gained in adolescent years'.[55] This may have borne some relation to social class.

The texts from which Mass Observation's respondents had gleaned sexual knowledge ranged from the Bible to daily papers, encyclopaedias, dictionaries, household medical books, Shakespeare, Bertrand Russell, Aldous Huxley, Freud, Havelock Ellis and Marie Stopes. L. N. Fowler, the nineteenth-century phrenological writer, was cited at least once. Among the works or authors cited more than an odd one or two times were the Bible, Havelock Ellis, Marie Stopes, Freud, Kenneth Walker, and books generally on natural history and biology.[56] The survey amassed a quantity of information and literature likely to fall into 'unspecialised hands', mostly on the ill-effects of masturbation. Advertisements in 'sex interest periodicals' preyed on anxieties about 'loss of

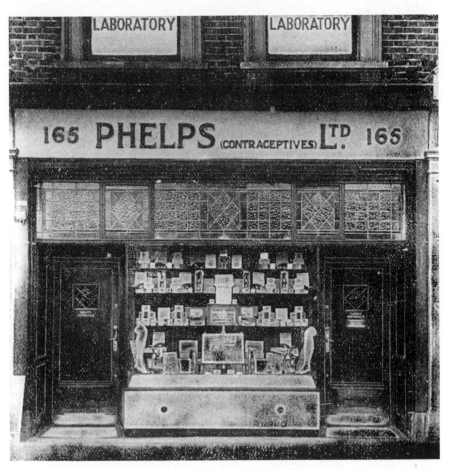

32   Phelps Contraceptives Ltd, 165 High Road, South Tottenham, London, N.15: a rare picture of a rubber goods shop, *c.* 1930s, with separate entrances for 'ladies' and 'gentlemen'.

"youthful vigour"', offered literature on birth control, and proffered cures for sexual difficulties and fears, in particular 'glandular' remedies,[57] though the old tradition of 'electrical belts' was continued in 'The Blakoe Energiser'.[58] Anxiety-making was still a prevalent register in many available materials about sex, at least at this commercial level.

Even for those who would naturally seek information from books, it required considerable determination to obtain reliable and helpful information about sex. Sex literature often had to be sought in sordid 'rubber-goods' shops, which no one would visit unless driven to: for example 'an "unsavoury" little establishment . . . with a window devoted to cheap rubber goods and pornographic fiction'.[59] One investigated by the National Vigilance Association was 'a singularly unattractive, dirty shop run by dirty people'. 'Suggestive literature' was 'partly an ordinary "sell"', which 'must be very disappointing to the purchaser'.[60] A rather different, positively idyllic, picture of surgical goods store as value-free provider of alternative sexual information is presented by one of Steve Humphries's interviewees, whose family ran one.[61]

The trade in contraception in the inter-war years was very largely run by rubber-goods shops, and mail-order companies who 'regularly circularised' respectable married couples 'after the arrival of their firstborn'. Even those distant from large towns with, allegedly, birth control devices 'exhibited freely in shop windows' were made aware that 'measures against conception can be taken';[62] these were also advertised in low-class papers 'practically unknown to ordinary people' (at least to those giving evidence to the Select Committee on Patent Medicines).[63] Sir William Arbuthnot Lane claimed that retail chemists were far more knowledgeable than doctors about contraception,[64] but reports of being regarded 'as if I were a libertine',[65] and feeling 'diffidence about ordering the appliances' in local chemists' shops,[66] suggest that many respectable chemists shared medical disdain for birth control. Not all rubber-goods businesses were exclusively aimed at making a sleazy fast buck; while 'malthusian devices' was a general code for birth control requisites, some operations were run by convinced Malthusians and social reformers.[67]

Social purity organizations perceived a menacing tide of filth about to swamp the nation: 'indiscriminate circulation of undesirable literature dealing in an unwholesome way with crimes, with birth control and with sexual matters', having 'a most undesirable effect on the minds of young people'.[68] American magazines full of 'vulgarity and indecent suggestiveness . . . entirely occupied with sex', were available in Woolworth's.[69] The London Public Morality Council in 1929 bewailed the 'tide of corruption pouring out of publishing houses lately' consisting of books 'dealing with birth-control, translations, such as the Decameron, and books of a pseudosociological or scientific character'. Frank Briant, MP had observed 'two capable, gentlemanly looking lads' browsing among such works in a bookshop, though if such material was so widely available one wonders why they needed to.[70]

Contrary views to this perception of pervasive obscenity were put forward by some members of the British Sexology Society. H. C. Booth was involved in the sunbathing movement (strongly associated with naturism), and thus had 'had some encounters with Scotland Yard and [knew] something of the workings of the official mind', which had 'heard nothing later than the fulminations of tabues [sic] of the Victorian epoch'. Even when they knew that they had no legal power to suppress, the police practised 'a sort of inverted blackmail' by threatening publicity, 'for most people something like social ruin'. 'The great majority of judges and magistrates are of the same type,' Booth added – devoid of understanding of people who did not conform to their ideas.[71] In obscenity cases offenders were usually persuaded to plead guilty at a summary trial without jury, with conviction almost certain (especially if the Director of Public Prosecutions was concerned), in return for a comparatively low penalty and little publicity. A case such as that of Eustace Chesser's *Love without Fear* in 1942 (discussed below) tested the limits of the law, but at the risk of adverse publicity and professional stigma.[72]

Even those seeking serious and reputable books about sex had to obtain them from insalubrious sources. Suggestions to local libraries to buy, for example, Stopes's works, tended to be 'instantly vetoed',[73] although in 1934 the chairman of the public library of the Bromley Borough Council produced a list of books available in that library on matters of sex education, alleging that nothing in Dr Norman Haire's *Encyclopaedia of Sexual Knowledge* was not available from that source.[74] But if libraries did purchase works on sex, they were likely to keep them under special conditions, such as in the librarian's office, as a deterrent to the reader (admittedly readers were always more likely to steal sex books because of shame over checking them out formally).[75]

The British Museum, of course, held 'all the standard works on the subject . . . in a receptacle called the Private Case', along with 'works subversive of loyalty to the throne, and others which may be described as filth'. The extent of these holdings, excluded from the catalogue, could only be discovered by 'personal application to the Reading Room Superintendent', a measure to prevent idle persons becoming a nuisance.[76] The British Society for the Study of Sex Psychology found when trying to compile a bibliography of works on sexology that material in the Private Case was practically inaccessible. Appreciating the wish of the librarians not to be 'plagued by enquirers after pornographic literature', they themselves, not involved in 'any such dubious enterprise', arranged a meeting with the trustees to discuss the matter. The satisfactory results of negotiations were subsequently reported.[77]

Even, or perhaps particularly, when stocked by reputable booksellers, works on sex were regarded as not for every eye. Many were published with a warning that they were issued for the medical and allied professions and serious students of the subject only,[78] though how sincerely booksellers adhered to these provisos seems to have varied widely. D. A. Thomas, wealthy colliery owner and Liberal MP, was unable to purchase Havelock Ellis's *Studies in the Psychology of Sex* (recommended by his daughter after reading them in the Cavendish Bentinck Library at the International Women's Suffrage Club) without a 'signed certificate from a doctor or lawyer'.[79] Walter Gallichan, a self-proclaimed 'life-long

student of sexual psychology . . . the writer of twelve books on the subject', claimed of an attempt to purchase Wilhelm Stekel's *Sexual Frigidity
in Women*, that he was 'not permitted to buy the work of another
psychologist'. He was in the 'ludicrous' situation of having to 'obtain a
letter from a medical man, professing that he desired to purchase the
volume'.[80] One of Stopes's readers, endeavouring to purchase her textbook *Contraception* (1923) at Denny's in the Strand, was told: 'the
assistant . . . had orders to sell the book only on production of a medical
or law degree certificate'. The work was subsequently obtained without
difficulty at Lewis's in Gower Street.[81] Medical students in the 1930s
gained popularity among their friends because of their ability to purchase works on sex from medical bookshops such as Lewis's.[82] The
reluctance of individuals to dare even to approach booksellers for works
on sex is testified to by Fifield the publisher's comments about the
immense and unusual proportion of direct mail inquiries for *Married
Love*.[83]

Writers themselves, and publishers, proceeded cautiously in the face
of the dangers of prosecution still threatening even serious and
highminded writers on sexual matters. When Isabel Hutton endeavoured to get *The Hygiene of Marriage* published, one colleague felt 'the
public should not know too much', another believed she would 'wear a
crown of thorns', and solicitors seemed to fear that her work was
unprintable. The Oxford University Press thought that the manuscript
'would be very difficult to place.' Even after the work had been accepted
by Heinemann's Medical Publications, Hutton 'had many a spasm of
apprehension in the watches of the night', envisaging 'street posters
announcing "Suppression of Woman Doctor's Marriage book"'. In
1923, the year of the Marie Stopes/Halliday Sutherland libel trial furore, ignominious suppression must have seemed a real risk. The book
received some favourable notices in the medical press, but 'was not
advertised in the Press nor did any of the lay papers or periodicals
acknowledge it' and an editor of a 'popular daily newspaper' wrote
'"you must know that we never touch sex stuff"'.[84]
    Many of the works available to the inquiring reader were of dubious
informative value. The numerous books and pamphlets distributed
widely through religious organizations and youth movements were seldom likely to have been of much practical assistance to anyone in search
of usable information about the sexual act. Suggestive material from
rubber-goods shops often proved 'a sell'. Alluringly titled works on
marriage and sex might be informative about the sex life of the amoeba
and/or bizarre marriage customs in exotic parts of the world, but

remarkably laconic about the average couple on the Clapham omnibus.[85] Stopes told a correspondent in 1919: 'if you can find another book on sex in which so little about savages and the lower animals appears, I will give you 6d!'; she herself wasted no space on 'primitive customs which have no bearing on our needs'.[86]

Though by 1930 increasing numbers of more explicit books were being published for the lay public by reputable publishers, for sale in respectable bookshops rather than backstreet rubber-goods shops, there was still some discontent about such books as were available, even for the medical profession. The continuing stigma on writing about sex meant that even those legitimately entitled to call themselves 'Doctor' adopted concealing pseudonyms. Maurice Newfield published as 'Michael Fielding', Norman Haire used the *nom de plume* 'Wyckham Terris' (mainly for journalism), and Joan Malleson employed the pseudonym 'Medica': this may have related to restrictions on advertising by doctors. According to the *Lancet*, works available for the enlightenment of the doctor were 'translated into English from foreign languages'. If English originals, they were timidly 'overladen with apologies for dealing with the topic' and exhortations to the reader 'to purge himself of prejudice', or conversely abounded in 'dubious anecdotes' and the advocacy of 'ultra-modern views on sexual reform'. Havelock Ellis's *Psychology of Sex*, if not necessarily suitable for public consumption, did fulfil the pressing need for a manual on the subject for medical students.[87] It seems probable that much of what the average person – or even doctors[88] – might learn, often with considerable difficulty, about sex was either mystifying, misleading or irrelevant.

As late as the 1940s Eustace Chesser's *Love without Fear* bore on the dustflap the statement that 'The author has written this book for those who are married or about to be married, and in this connection the bookseller's cooperation is requested.'[89] Whether such gestures of restriction were a mere matter of form, or whether they did operate as a barrier to the dissemination of these works is an open question. The large sales of many of the books, and their constant reprinting, suggests that people did manage to bring themselves to buy them by some means or other.

In spite of this precaution, *Love without Fear* was prosecuted in 1942 (after selling 5,000 copies) as 'an alleged obscene book', although it was a serious marriage manual by a practising doctor (specializing in gynaecology and psychology), largely composed of quotations from works already in circulation. 'Hortative and rather startling' in style, *Love without Fear* was aimed at 'ordinary men and women without any special knowledge of the subject or remarkable scholastic achievement'. It was sold by 'reputable booksellers' (such as 'Harrods and W. H. Smith's'), at a price of 12s. 6d. (£0.63), which was intended to 'keep it out of younger people's hands, such as typists and others'. Chesser pleaded the enormous amount of suffering caused by sexual difficulties he had seen in the industrial town of Salford as well as in his London practice. Three doctors testified to having recommended it to patients. The Common Serjeant summarized the defence position: 'in the year 1942, it is ridiculous and absurd to suggest that the discussion of sex and sex relationship in a book is obscene', and said that 'all this hush-hush and secrecy' had done a great deal of harm. The determination of guilt or innocence was entrusted to the 'common sense' of the jury, who returned the verdict of 'Not Guilty' after less than an hour's delibera-tion. Chesser did expurgate certain passages particularly objected to by the prosecution from subsequent editions.[90] Even so, the July 1942 edition (subsequent to the trial) still included the passage describing prostitutes in continental brothels parading in 'a silken sash which hides one breast but leaves the other exposed . . . long silk stockings and high-heeled shoes', and descriptions of homosexuality, lesbianism and sadomasochism.[91]

The foreman and another juror at the Chesser trial raised questions of distribution and the danger of such works finding their way into the wrong hands. This was a persistent issue in obscenity trials of the period. Books specified as being for the medical profession and students of physiology were being circulated with no restriction on the borrowers, or without ensuring that they were over 21. Precautions taken to pre-vent young people getting hold of the books, such as a declaration of majority, might be 'an additional inducement to adolescents'. Accused booksellers or library-owners might plead that customers included 'a number of doctors and clergymen', 'medical men and psychologists', or the mitigating circumstance of a shop's location 'in a quiet street well away from the front'.[92] Lending libraries circulating such literature made rather disingenuous claims for the serious and scientific rel-evance of their enterprise. The Direct Book Supply Co. of London NW9, a mail-order lending library operating around 1950, informed intending subscribers to their 'Exclusive Library' that it was intended solely for the 'PERSONAL use of members of the professions, psycholo-gists, social workers, students of psychology and responsible adults, for the purpose of serious study'. A declaration to this effect had to be signed.[93]

The library offered a bizarre but revealing selection (some 'VERY SCARCE'). Serious works of sexology by Havelock Ellis, Wilhelm Stekel and so on, sexual advice manuals by Marie Stopes, Eustace Chesser, Norman Haire, Van de Velde and other standard writers, anthropologi-cal classics such as Malinowski's *Sex and Repression in Savage Society* and

Margaret Mead's *Coming of Age in Samoa*, and banned novels such as D. H. Lawrence's *Lady Chatterley's Lover*, were listed in close proximity to works of a more specialized appeal, not merely the 'Leafless Eves' Library' but *Tortures and Torments of the Christian Martyrs, The History of Torture throughout the Ages, The Whip and the Rod, Slavery in the Roman Empire*, and other works 'of absorbing interest to students of torture and flagellation'. Other books were 'curious' or promised 'many strange illustrations'. Highminded works of seriously intended instruction and aid were juxtaposed not only with volumes verging upon the, if not wholly, pornographic, but also with works which were part of the problem they had been written to combat. Some of these had been circulating for many years: *The Superb Virility of Manhood* (originally entitled *The Virile Powers of Superb Manhood*) by Bernarr Macfadden, first issued during the 1890s and containing detailed accounts of the dangers of male debility, Huhner's *Disorders of the Sexual Function in the Male and Female*, first published before the First World War, Gardner's nineteenth-century treatise on *The Conjugal Relationship as regards Personal Health*, R. T. Trall's contemporaneous *Sexual Physiology and Hygiene*, and Walling's gruesome *Sexology*[94] were all listed in the catalogue without any comment on their age or reliability as guides. Readers did not necessarily realize that these were (or ought to be) what the sex educator Cyril Bibby described in 1946 as 'amusing museum relics'.[95] A continued association between the informative sex manual and pornography throughout this period can be deduced.

Large numbers of people learnt about sex from the general press. Thomas Boyle has explored sensationalism in the mid-Victorian press, and Richard Davenport-Hines has cited recurrent press panics around homosexuality and sexually transmitted diseases,[96] but the role of the press in both reflecting and creating popular sexual knowledge and attitudes needs a good deal of further study.[97] A contorted moral agenda underlay much popular-press writing about sexual matters: the 'story they said should not be told . . . full details on inner pages' syndrome, a combination of sensationalism and prurience.

One example of the ambiguous role of the press was the furore drummed up by James Douglas in the *Sunday Express* about Radclyffe Hall's novel on the plight of 'the female invert', *The Well of Loneliness*. The book had initially been published in a highly priced limited edition and sent for review only to 'the reputable and serious sections of the press', in which it had received 'amazing sympathy and understanding'. Nonetheless it was in a second printing (and displayed in W. H. Smith's window), when the 'hysterical commands of a rag . . . well known for

engineering stunts' for the Home Office to suppress it drew the attention of a wider public, and made it the book most in demand in
circulating libraries, until its condemnation for obscenity in a court
of law. The depositions of distinguished literary figures, doctors and
scientists as to the book's merits were not cited at the trial, and none of
the defenders was called to testify. Chief-Inspector John Prothero, who
had seized the book, declared under cross-examination that the 'whole
theme and treatment are objectionable. . . . The subject is physical relationship, a problem usually dealt with by scientists.' The counter-claims
that if Hall's book was indecent and obscene so were (among other
things) the *Sunday Express* itself and the Book of Leviticus did not get a
hearing.[98]

A recurrent source of, no doubt circulation-boosting, press panics was
'White Slavery'. Social purity organizations in the inter-war years took
the drily sober view that almost all reputed cases (girls shanghaied by
mysterious, often apparently helpful, strangers while shopping, at the
cinema, etc., in order to be sold into foreign brothels) were spurious:
what would now be described as urban folklore. The National Vigilance
Association (NVA) line on 'periodical scare stories (hypodermic
syringes, drugs, etc.)' was that 'such cases simply do not occur. They
generally turn out to be what somebody has told someone else or,
alternatively, a girl running away from her home for purely private
reasons', and the tales led 'nowhere, as . . . the police could confirm'.
Letitia Fairfield, senior medical officer of the London County Council,
pointed out in a letter to *The Times* in 1952 the practical difficulties of
injecting someone in the street and having a semi-conscious girl on
one's hands. A schoolteacher 'looking forward to the opportunity of
answering questions from some of the older girls who are leaving school
on the White Slave Traffic' was repressively told by the NVA to 'concentrate on the questions of modesty and decency rather than the
questions of brothels and white slave traffic'. White slave scaremonger-
ing met the 'Red Menace' in the imaginings of a 'Mr Henry Lawrence',
who contacted the NVA offering his services to investigate the recruit-
ment of 'Bolshevik sex slaves'.[99]

Marie Stopes found the popular press an ambivalent but nonetheless
useful ally in propagating her message, in particular her libel case
against Halliday Sutherland. One woman declared: 'I have treasured a
piece of paper because it is worth reading and that paper is the "Daily
Sketch" dealing with the action you has against Dr Halliday [*sic*].' Her
articles in *John Bull* also gained a mass audience: one woman who had
'longed to get into communication' with Stopes mentioned reading
there that she would enter into correspondence. Articles for and
against birth control in the *Penny Magazine* during 1922 had given one

Glasgow woman Stopes's name.[100] Clare Davey has demonstrated that working-class women were much more likely to have heard of Stopes through a mass circulation magazine than through her books.[101]

It is sometimes assumed that as they were instructing women in how to cope with the new technology of domesticity, women's magazines were also instructing them in the new techniques of love and marriage. It is impossible to generalize about a class of publications in which individual titles were targeted at particular audiences and pursued specific editorial policies. Nonetheless, they did come into the hands of many who had no other obvious sources of sexual information, though the information gleaned was not usually acquired directly. The relatively persistent woman might at least manage to gain a private recommendation to 'write to Dr. Stopes'; a number of her correspondents mentioned having been advised to do so by the 'Nurse' or 'Doctor' of some magazine. 'Nurse Crawford' of *Mother* advised one woman to consult Stopes 'to learn in some way more about the physical side of marriage'.[102] While the magazines might run articles about the new companionate marriage and modern 'frank and free' relationships between the sexes, this was not usually accompanied by explicit sexual information.[103]

The agony columns contained some, usually highly allusive and oblique, comments on sex and changing mores. The 'Heart-to-Heart Chat' column of *Woman's World* extended considerable practical sympathy to unmarried mothers, perhaps connected with the rising illegitimacy rates during the war; this was seen to a large extent as understandable and forgivable, if not exactly to be encouraged. The hope was expressed that these women would find some 'good and true man', and the women were encouraged to go to court for paternal contributions to the child's upkeep so that they could keep the child. A woman who had clearly led a dramatically rackety life, including marriage to a bigamist, a drink problem, war heroism, and promiscuity, was advised to put the past behind her, and to trust in the good man who loved her (and in God).[104] An increasing level of marital breakdown was also reflected, though policy seems to have been to encourage couples to remain together. A girl of $16\frac{1}{2}$ whose parents were divorcing was advised to try and reconcile them. Separation was a drastic step, but might bring an erring husband to his senses; if finally necessary, legal separation with maintenance should be sought.[105]

Sympathy might be extended to women who had lapsed from chastity, and those in marital difficulty, but the main tenor of advice was to fortify women in premarital restraint, and in endurance of adverse marital circumstances. A 'pure-hearted, self-respecting girl who has won through' against a 'young fellow who has insulted [her] terribly', was advised that her influence would surely help him to 'find that better self of his'. 'Courage and good sense to guard' oneself were praised, while girls who 'cheapened' themselves were rebuked: '[it] is the greatest mistake for any girl not to keep a boy in his proper place'. 'What a girl must expect nine times out of ten with a boy of this sort' was that after she had succumbed 'he would soon have wearied of you, and then gone off and left you'. 'Mrs Marryat' of *Woman's Weekly* advised that a girl was not wise even 'to get herself talked about as "unladylike"'.[106] Sex was something that men wanted and women might be inveigled into giving; something they allowed, or consented to, rather than something they might want themselves. Long engagements were 'much more of a trial to a man'.[107] (A widespread attitude, even in very different circles: heads of women's colleges and medical schools were horrified by McCance's inclusion of sexual feelings on his survey forms on female periodicity, considering that 'sexual feeling was abnormal in unmarried women students'.)[108] The expression for premarital sex employed in both answers and questions was 'do wrong';[109] this may be editorial rewriting, of course.

The journal *Modern Woman* aimed to be just that. Its problem page was 'From One Woman to Another: Leonora Eyles invites you to discuss your troubles with her'. Eyles was a writer and journalist associated with the Labour movement, and (after early qualms) a proponent of birth control; she also wrote works of sex education.[110] Her modest radicalism is suggested by her comment in this column that one of the commonest problems arose from 'woman's fatal capacity for sacrifice' and subsequent disillusionment. Even for her there were some problems she could help with, but not in print. Her modernity, or at least command of the latest catchphrases, was apparent: 'you just have to wait while a man gets rid of his various little complexes'. She conceded some independent sexual feeling to women: 'in the 'teens it is so easy to let one's emotions get on top, and even if social disaster is not the result, a girl is cheapened and spoilt by such an affair'. If girls remembered 'that their caresses and kisses are something beautiful, which some day they will want to give to a man they adore, they would find it easier to master these emotions'.[111]

Advertisements in these magazines might also supply information: those for 'Rendell's Pessaries' (a contraceptive), however, made no mention of what they were intended to do, while appearing in magazines which made no allusion to birth control and in which the kiss was the ultimate sexual act. Besides direct advertisements by publishers such as Health Promotions for books on sexually related matters (such as *What Every Woman Ought to Know, Advice to a Wife [Mother], Healthy Wedded Life*), firms promoting products such as nerve pills and abdominal belts might offer booklets containing information for women. The advertisements and titles such as 'Nature's Warning' constructed women as in danger of serious consequences at every stage of life ('weakness, and illnesses peculiar to women', 'a woman's health handicaps her always'), and in constant need of preserving their health. Menstruation was a boon to advertisers, who offered, besides the relatively new invention of sanitary towels, various remedies for pain and discomfort during periods (but at this period sanitary towel manufacturers do not seem to have been producing informative leaflets). Abortifacients were also promoted, in coded language.

Work is beginning to appear on the fiction in women's magazines and the sexual messages it conveyed. Billie Melman has investigated certain genres of the 1920s,[112] and Joseph McAleer has analysed the 'story' magazines as well as popular romance literature.[113] Little work has been done generally on changing messages about sexuality in fiction. The scientist Julian Huxley remarked in his unused deposition in defence of *The Well of Loneliness*: 'novels are the chief method for the average man and woman to get knowledge of life', and was 'strongly of the opinion that no subject should be taboo as a subject, if properly treated'.[114] The banning of several works now regarded as literary classics from British publication for many years – most notably James Joyce's *Ulysses* and D. H. Lawrence's *Lady Chatterley's Lover* – is well known; other works, not perhaps regarded as major literary achievements but of a certain sociological interest – for example *Her Privates We* by Frederic Manning, and *The Mint* by T. E. Lawrence writing as Aircraftman Shaw – were deemed too explicit for publication *in extenso* prior to the 1960s. Radclyffe Hall's *The Well of Loneliness* has already been mentioned: it was not, perhaps, the fact that it dealt with 'female inversion' as such that caused scandal but that it treated it neither as sick and evil (as did Clemence Dane's *Regiment of Women*) nor as comic (along the lines of Compton Mackenzie's *Extraordinary Women*).[115]

This double standard for the treatment of sexual themes in literature also characterized stage censorship. J. B. Fagan, who had tried to mount a British production of the reforming French play about venereal disease, *Damaged Goods*, complained to the Association of Moral and Social Hygiene Committee of Enquiry into Sexual Morality in 1919 that 'a subject of social or national importance . . . treated seriously and frankly spoken about' was denied licensing, while 'innuendo and any amount of improper suggestions' passed the censors. Censorship ignored the distinction between 'a work of art . . . which treats a subject which ought to be treated, in a decent manner' and 'a prurient exhibition' and licensed 'any amount of improper, or quasi-improper plays', such as *A Little Bit of Fluff,* described by Fagan as a 'dreadful play and full of improper suggestions from end to end'.[116] Marie Stopes raised similar points when her play *Vectia,* based on the débâcle of her marriage to Ruggles Gates, was banned 'at a time when plays and reviews of prodigious filthiness were being staged with the approval of the Lord Chamberlain's Department'. Current morality was a 'filthy and disgusting farce', a 'sanctimoniously indecent' man-made (and here 'man' bore gendered significance) code of pseudo-morality. 'Masculine over-sexuality and callous dominance and feminine frigidity, yet frailty' were 'approved, unthinkingly accepted, and consequently... not banned'. Comic portrayal of sexual themes was permissible, but the 'serious writer's portrayal of sound realism' was not, while intonation and stage 'business', not submitted to the Lord Chamberlain's office, often supplied obscenity to an innocuous text.[117]

As newspapers could deal titillatingly with 'vice' by being careful to deplore it, much popular fiction managed both to have its cake and eat it. Perhaps public morality paid less attention to popular fiction than it did to 'literature'. Rebecca West remarked that a sight to fill 'the heart of any serious English writer with wistfulness' was the 'old ladies reading their Ethel Dells' on 'the esplanade of any watering-place'. West recounted with sardonic glee the plot of one of Dell's novels, involving 'a middle-aged voluptuary', a girl disguised as a page-boy, 'the peculiar intercourse that takes place' (including an incident in which he 'beats her with a riding switch') when the voluptuary penetrates, though concealing his knowledge, the girl's disguise when she stows away on his yacht. After her sex is revealed there is extensive speculation as to 'whether the girl is or is not a virgin'. The voluptuary marries her but the marriage is unconsummated. . . .[118] The bestselling blend of the melodramatically preposterous with a strong vein of the sadomasochistic (seen also in the desert romance, typified by E. M. Hull's *The Sheikh*), is of considerable sociological interest.[119]

The crushing censorship of explicitly sexual texts has been recounted and the sexual subtexts of canonical literature have been explored in scholarly works too numerous to name. Even bestselling 'trash' has been the subject of either a retrospective gaze of amusement (as in Cockburn's *Bestseller*) or more nuanced analysis, such as that undertaken by Melman and McAleer.[120] But rather more overt depictions of sexuality, and reflections of current sexual mores, were now appearing in serious (and less serious) literature. Aldous Huxley's collusive knowingness about the sex-manners of Bohemia sometimes elides into prurience: good characters, like the Lawrentian Rampion in *Point Counter Point,* by implication having healthy life-affirming sex, contrast with baddies like Burlap, who have sleazy sordid exploitative perverse sex, in rather more detail.

A plethora of serious women writers (some of them now enjoying a Virago renaissance) employed fiction to speak about women's experiences. Eileen Arnot Robertson may have the distinction of being the first to mention menstruation in a fictional context, and even PMT. She also dealt with spontaneous female desire separate from love; shrinking from sex as the result of assault; the subversive possibility that a woman might find a second lover more satisfactory than the first since she would have no lingering associations of the pain of loss of virginity; and turned a cool eye on the rise of 'petting'.[121] A writer more often remembered for the gentle humour of her *Provincial Lady* books, E. M. Delafield in other works tackled stronger themes, including couples whose financial survival depended on the complaisance of the wife towards wealthy admirers, the unawakened wife (a recurrent theme), or the woman desperately grabbing lovers from fear of ageing.[122] There were limits, however. Naomi Mitchison found that the explicitness, which clad in wolfskins or togas in her historical novels had been quite acceptable to her publishers and her public, was frowned upon in dealing with modern themes and settings. *We Have Been Warned* (1935) dealt with female desire, contraception, abortion as at least able to be considered, adultery, and included a deeply unpleasant and unromantic rape, presented from the female point of view and the outcome at least in part of social misunderstandings rather than simple brute desire; homosexuality in artistic and bohemian circles was mentioned non-judgmentally. As a result she had difficulty in placing the book and even when she did found that extensive cuts were demanded.[123]

An intersection between the theatre of public sexual messages in the law courts and the novel was the Edith Thompson case of 1922. Thompson's lover murdered her husband during an encounter in the street; there is very little evidence of Thompson's implication. But she too was hanged, since letters read at the trial showed that she had, at least, fantasized about poisoning her husband. The most recent work on this subject points out that her self-administration of an abortifacient was considered too appalling even to cite in court.[124] At least two novels were closely based on this case: E. M. Delafield's *A Messalina of the Suburbs* (1924) and F. Tennyson Jesse's *A Pin to See the Peepshow* (1934). The idea that a woman who had transgressed societal norms of sexual behaviour was capable of any crime also underlies Harriet Vane's predicament at the beginning of Dorothy Sayers's *Strong Poison* (1930): her having lived with Philip Boyes outside of marriage is taken almost as a presumption of her guilt for his murder. Sexual innocence and virtue in women continued to be equated. Even Marie Stopes, although endowing her character Vectia with an urge for maternity and healthy natural desires for the normal sex life denied her by her impotent husband, could not depict her as coming to the recognition of her plight as she herself had done, through her own efforts. Instead, Vectia was enlightened by her neighbour, Heron (a good friend, not a lover, the text emphasized) as to the exact state of affairs, and where exactly her husband fell short.[125] Romance literature contrasted, and still does, the innocent 'good girl' heroine with the 'vampish sophisticated charm' of her rival; indeed the 'heroine must not even understand sexual desire, for knowledge entails guilt'.[126]

What of the cinema as agent for the transmission of sex information? Censorship codes in the movies have been mocked ('one foot on the floor at all times') though the very restriction of erotic interaction to kissing may have provided useful hints about this skill. It may have been less the content of films seen in cinemas which provided sex education than the provision of warm, dark privacy for sexual exploration (for which a Mickey Mouse cartoon would do quite as well).

The general public, in spite of the lacunae in their sexual knowledge, or perhaps because of it, seems to have been, as Mass Observation discovered, a good deal less prudish than legislators and opinion-makers supposed.[127] Homosexual cases were recurrently thrown out of court because the jury either didn't think it possible, or didn't think it mattered.[128] In obscenity prosecutions trial by jury, though risky, meant the possibility of the verdict being influenced by the defendant's sincerity or 'a healthy man-in-the-street knowledge of life': a risk vindicated, for example, in the notorious case of *Lady Chatterley's Lover*.[129] Reservations were still being registered, however, even in the context of the 'commonsense' attitudes of the Chesser jury and the Mass Observation Sex Survey respondents, about the dangers of material on sexual matters falling into the wrong hands and about the potential misuse of sex. The associations of danger and pathology lingered, while ignorance continued rife. Alex Comfort's 1950 claim that 'sex education of the public in England has almost certainly outstripped sex education of doctors' was an indictment of professional ignorance rather than an assertion about sexual enlightenment.[130]

Conclusion

Towards the present

By the 1950s most of the elements which continue to make sexual knowledge were already in place. There was vast social change to come, but the ways of making sexual knowledge were basically similar. Although they developed, and were perhaps more widely disseminated, with their content becoming more explicit, it can be argued that there has been no major conceptual change comparable to those that took place early in the nineteenth century or during the 1890s.

Yet again there was recourse to commissions and committees to deal with potentially explosive (at least in the government's eyes) subjects: the Wolfenden Committee on Homosexual Offences and Prostitution, the Lane Committee of Inquiry into the Working of the Abortion Act. Nonetheless, legislation spread out over a period of nearly twenty years from the mid-1950s to the mid-1970s achieved considerable reforms, all of which had been on the agenda of earlier British sex reformers. However, if one result of the Wolfenden Report was to create a climate of opinion leading to the final revocation of the notorious 'black-mailer's charter' of Labouchère's amendment to the 1885 Criminal Law Amendment Act, it removed once more from prostitutes the recognition of certain civil rights finally achieved a few years previously. Gays have protested against and historians have recorded the continuing heavy policing of male homosexual activity in any location which can be defined as 'public', while the advent of AIDS led to a resurgence (or a drumming up) of vicious homophobic motifs.[1] Continuing public anxieties concerning homosexuality were demonstrated by the furore caused by the attempt to lower the gay age of consent early in 1994; while the age limit was reduced from 21, the highest in Europe, it went down only to 18, the age of majority, not 16 to give equity with the heterosexual age of consent.

The passing of an Abortion Law Reform Act in 1967, twenty-one years after the foundation of the Abortion Law Reform Association, and still falling short of its full aim of abortion on the grounds of the woman's choice, led to the emergence of a self-conscious and vocal anti-abortion movement. So controversial was the Act that the Lane Committee was appointed after its first few years of operation to investigate its workings, and it has been subjected to recurrent, if largely ineffective, attempts to restrict, if not wholly repeal, the rights to abortion it established in 1967. So far the British opponents of abortion have not committed the excesses of the US 'pro-lifers', who have on occasions shot doctors known to perform abortions and who harass pregnant women who work in abortion clinics; but American anti-abortionists have already made attempts to bring their tactics to the UK.

In 1974 when contraception became free under the National Health Service, it seemed as if attempts of activists since the 1920s to make access to birth control a right for all women had achieved final success. However, the closure of specialist clinics was not necessarily a good thing. Not all women, particularly younger women, want to take such matters to their general practitioner, even if their GP is trained in contraceptive techniques.[2] Now, in the 1990s, health authority birth control clinics are being closed as 'soft targets' in a time of financial stringency, while some authorities no longer accept NHS abortions under the 'social clause' of the 1967 Act.[3] The Family Planning Association took new directions in the 1970s, in the belief that the work of providing contraception to the consumer was in safe hands, and no longer provides a safety network of clinics.

Heated arguments about the physical basis of sex, in particular over physical causes of sexual preference, still continue, as the media furore every time some scientist alleges 'proof' demonstrates. Recent examples include Simon LeVay's claim that there are discernible differences in the brains of gay men, and the suggestion by another scientist that there is a maternal genetic linkage to homosexuality in the male.[4] Surveys of sexual attitudes and behaviour are still conducted under similar constraints – 'too often political rather than scientific'.[5] The British survey of sexual behaviour that would have been so valuable in the era of AIDS, was refused government funding in 1989 after an initial pilot study – apparently on the personal say-so of Margaret Thatcher – and finally conducted with funding from the Wellcome Trust. In spite of Thatcher's alleged concern about the intrusion into areas of individual privacy, the researchers found, rather like the earlier Mass Observers working on 'Little Kinsey', 'beyond a peradventure . . . most members of the public will accept and cooperate' with a project of this kind.[6] This survey is noticeably in the already established mode of dry and unarousing presentation of statistical data and graphs, determinedly avoiding sensationalism, though it has not, even so, escaped criticism.[7]

If there are no longer active voluntary moral policing bodies like the National Vigilance Association, individuals and smaller groups can cause disruption and media agitation, however small their basis of support may be: the National Viewers' and Listeners' Association appears to have been almost a one-woman band run by Mrs Mary Whitehouse.[8] One mother, Victoria Gillick, conducted a high-profile media campaign in pursuit of assurances that her daughter would not be prescribed birth control while still under age, creating a dangerously persistent though misguided belief that doctors will and must inform the parents of an under-16-year-old if they are asked for contraception. Sex education continues to be a contested issue. Although a statutory element in education, how it is actually conducted relies very much on individual schools and their governing authorities, and is subject to constraint by the vocal protests of individuals drumming up moral panic.[9] Recurrent tension and anxiety were exemplified in March 1994 on both a local and a national level in the uproar over the sex educator who, in response to class questions, defined 'blow-job' for a class of 10 to 11-year-olds, and the withdrawal of a Health Education Authority guide to sex aimed at a teenage audience, described as 'smutty and not suitable' by the Health Minister. Initiatives to promote awareness of contraception and the prevention of sexually transmitted diseases among a vulnerable group clash with the commitment to 'moral values'.[10]

Sex is still considerably marginalized, with contraceptive and abortion services under the NHS regarded as prime targets for financial cutbacks. Marital counselling remains in the hands of the voluntary body Relate, despite lip-service paid by the authorities to the need for family values and the preservation of the family unit.[11] Debates continue over government intervention in areas such as AIDS prevention and sex education.[12]

While the rise of psychosexual medicine might be viewed as a new development, it can be argued that this directly influences relatively few individuals, though ideas generated in this field may have percolated into advice literature (or other media). It is still very much a marginal speciality within the National Health Service, and emerges from the existing attitude to marriage as subject to problems which need to be worked on, rather than simply endured.[13]

If the modern trend in marriage advice is through videos rather than the printed word, this is still offered as a support for legitimate monogamy, and to dispel ignorance. Monogamy, of course, is no longer linked indissolubly to the legal status of marriage, with increasing

numbers of couples choosing to live together unmarried, and with relationships dissolving and reforming in a serial fashion rather than
continuing 'till death us do part'. It may however be argued – and there
is strong evidence in the findings of the Wellcome Survey – that most
people do believe in the importance of some kind of central, monogamous relationship, and while premarital sex is far more acceptable
than it used to be, cheating on a partner is not.[14] This could account for
some of the animus expressed over sex scandals early in 1994 among
politicians involving extramarital entanglements. While there may be
an increased emphasis on the desirability of personal, individual, self-
fulfilment through good sex, even one's right to this, sex is still being
presented in terms suggesting that the best sort consists of mutual
pleasure and satisfaction in a meaningful relationship. The Wellcome
Survey found considerable agreement with the proposition that sex
improves with longer acquaintance.[15]

   There are questions as to how 'educational' some videos are: is this
really a cover for pornography – who uses them and how? – questions
which reflect back on to the texts discussed earlier. Did couples read
Stopes or Van de Velde not only for instruction but for arousal? The
persistent use of some version of the formula 'for the married only' for
explicit sexual material does suggest assumptions about the place of sex
within a monogamous unit, even if this may need spicing up – from Van
de Velde's carefully numbered and defined variant positions through
The Joy of Sex's (1972) advocacy of consensual bondage for fun. This
should perhaps be seen in the context of the claim by a majority of
respondents to the Wellcome Survey that sex was not necessarily the
most centrally important factor in a successful marriage.[16]

   Debates on pornography have burgeoned, and while pornographic
motifs have surfaced in material of much wider circulation, such as
Madonna's notorious *Sex* package, Paul Ferris for one suggests that
much material marketed as 'explicit' is as spurious as the 'sealed
packets' documented by Mayhew, encouraged by the continuing 'sly
and underhand' British approach to erotica.[17]

   Two factors which may have changed ways of making sexual knowledge since the 1950s are the so-called 'sexual liberation' of the 1960s
and, even more importantly, the resurgence of a 'second wave' of
feminism since that date.[18] While it can be argued that these were the
surfacing of ideas which had been around for a great deal longer (the
underlying thesis of such works as Paul Robinson's *The Modernization of
Sex*)[19] they had important consequences for the making of sexual knowledge. By the significance it gave to sex as a human activity, the 'sexual
revolution' made possible, even encouraged, the historical study of

sexual behaviour and attitudes as something other than a branch of pornography (though this had of course been prefigured by, for example, Havelock Ellis and Iwan Bloch). If the early works in this school now sometimes appear simplistic in their Whiggish enthusiasm for sexual liberation, and their uncomplicated model of Victorian repression, they laid the necessary foundations for investigation and debate.

Feminism since the 1960s and the ideas it has generated and debated are such an enormous subject that it is scarcely possible to summarize them in a few lines. This 'second wave' has paid enormous attention to excavating the work of feminist forebears, and has resurrected old arguments which are seen to pertain to still unresolved (and probably never to be resolved!) questions about female sexuality, indeed human sexuality as a whole.[20] It has emphasized the need to bring a gender-sensitive awareness to any analysis of sexual discourses. How it has contributed to a remaking of sexual knowledges is a subject for books: an early venture in this direction, in the US context, was Barbara Ehrenreich, Elizabeth Hess and Gloria Jacobs's *Re-Making Love: The Feminization of Sex* (1986).[21]

A Specifically British Sexual Knowledge?

Looking backwards, we can perceive various persisting motifs in the specifically British making of sexual knowledge. A consistent perception of sex as beautiful and sacred has been continually intertwined with its representation as dirty, disgusting and dangerous, so much so that it is tempting to be universalist and essentializing and conclude that the nature of sex is such that it is capable of generating these very different emotions.

In the depiction of sex and sexuality, the two themes of moral earnestness and prurient titillation sometimes seem particularly 'British'. This is especially noticeable when the tone shifts from defenders of one position to the other. No one could surpass Havelock Ellis in the moral earnestness stakes, and the tone of 'high seriousness' resonates throughout *Studies in the Psychology of Sex*, yet, after the *Sexual Inversion* débâcle, its volumes were published abroad and have never, in their entirety, been published in the United Kingdom. However, his antagonist (as far as we may judge from 'LORD DAWSON MUST GO' (for his advocacy of birth control, see p. 237) and his furious attack on *The Well of Loneliness*), James Douglas, self-acclaimed defender of moral and family values, employed the devices of prurient sensationalist journalism to defend these values (or possibly just towards boosting sales?) in a mass-circulation newspaper for 'family' reading.

Implicated in the salacious journalistic discourse was a deep class bias, the assumption of a respectable middle-class tut-tutting over aristocratic (initially *Roman*) debauchery and the feckless, immoral poor. Josephine Butler assigned an aristocratic status to doctors that is hard to substantiate objectively, associating their involvement in applying the Contagious Diseases Acts with a tradition of upper-class vicious perversity. W. T. Stead, in 'The Maiden Tribute of Modern Babylon' plaited together these two motifs, depicting the collusion of aristocratic vice with the unnatural avarice of the lowest classes in the trade in young virgins, to the (profitable) horror of the respectable. In March 1994 'vice in high places', in particular among Tory politicians, has provided the press with a field-day, with cases of the old staples of adultery and bizarre sexual practices (autoerotic strangulation and cross-dressing).

Perhaps connected with this class bias is the persistent assignment of titillating overtones to the concept of the 'French': the upper classes, after all, were the ones most likely to seek an erotic education in Paris, and the ones for whose delectation, it was alleged, foreign prostitutes skilled in techniques literally foreign to good English girls were being imported. This is an area in which further study of different nationalities might be helpful: is it always the nearest foreign nation (and traditional enemy) to which is attributed what the British used to call the 'French pox' ('Italian disease' to the French), and the use of 'French letters' (the 'capote anglais') and other vices, or is there some other factor? (For example, the Renaissance designation of sodomy as the 'Italian vice' – a country at an even greater distance than France?)[22] Foreigners were blamed for unnatural vices in the eighteenth century; respondents to the Mass Observation venereal disease survey of 1942–3 attributed the spread of these diseases to an undifferentiated class of 'all these foreigners', while in the post-war period 'Yanks' took the rap for general moral decline. To what extent are other nations imagined to be liberal/immoral merely because their strictures are different (and not necessarily experienced and perceived as either liberal or immoral by their natives)? Moreover, the moral strictures of a culture are unlikely to afflict the transient or even resident foreigner. Conversely, other nations may be judged by the behaviour of footloose travellers, soldiers passing through and so on.

Is there anything specifically British about the recurrent urge (ever since the Reformation of Manners societies of the 1690s) for private individuals to associate for the moral policing of society? There has also been persistent resistance to such 'smut-hunting' and interference, summed up in the famous phrase 'I don't care what people do so long as they don't do it in the street and frighten the horses.' This creed of tolerance, however, coexists with the recurrent phenomenon of 'the British public in one of its periodical fits of morality' – 'no spectacle so ridiculous' – and suggests a haphazard and unpredictable oscillation between the two. The actual operation of social purity organizations requires closer attention than they have yet received: perusal of the files of the National Vigilance Association indicates that as well as imposing their own standards of purity on literature and advertising, the Association was appealed to by the general public not merely when its sensibilities were offended by obscene graffiti and nude sunbathing but in cases relating to the protection of women and children in which the law could not or would not intervene.

From the seventeenth century, marriage recurs as a central element in discussions of sexuality. Emphasis on marriage may represent a concession to moral norms: 'for the married only' can cover a multitude of explicit sexual detail, as in Chesser's *Love without Fear*, and as in recent sex education videos; presented as being for the benefit of the married, in fact a sound support for monogamy in a dangerous age. But this appeal to the centrality of marriage may have been as much market driven as imposed, if we can trust McAleer's account of the materials found most acceptable in romance literature of the inter-war period. Mills and Boon authors were able to present 'fantastic, even shocking' situations, providing that 'lovemaking was "honourable" and ended in marriage', and 'in all circumstances the primacy of marriage and marital vows was asserted'. The attitude of these books to erotic love within marriage was 'encourag[ing] . . . often described in vaguely mystical terms . . . a kind of wonderful prize obtainable only through marriage', which sounds very similar to Marie Stopes's *Married Love*.[23] The D. C. Thomson Group story papers appealed to a readership which liked 'the spicy thing', which meant not sex, but murder – far more acceptable than adultery.[24]

This attitude towards marriage is perhaps associated with perceptions of the normal: as mentioned in an earlier chapter, there is a ready elision from nature as instinct to nature as normative concept. Replies of respondents to the Mass Observation 'Little Kinsey' were largely in tune with the attitudes depicted in romance literature of the period: sex was 'natural, but only insofar as it is also reasonably orthodox', and reservations were largely registered in terms of 'infringement of conventional ethics'.[25] There was also anxiety about 'sex "getting a hold on you" ' and about the danger of overindulgence: men both thought that 'over-frequent sex relations' could be dangerous, and that prostitutes fulfilled an important role in meeting men's sexual needs.[26] While sex was insistently defined as 'natural' there were also fears of 'uncontrolled' sex.[27]

It is tempting to assume that the 'British school' of sexology had the particularly 'English' characteristic of an amateur quality. Certainly, far from being a pathway to professional success, too obvious an interest in sex was likely to prove a barrier to advancement. This is perhaps the more noticeable for occurring at a time when science as a whole was becoming more professionalized. The marginalization of sexual questions within medicine was apparent, with venereology continuing to be stigmatized even as it became more scientific and efficacious and gained a defined foothold in the medical system.[28]

While the British occasionally looked longingly to other countries in order to criticize local arrangements, since some kind of 'Victorian' era was found in nearly all Western, industrialized, capitalist societies it is by no means certain that interest in sex was something that brought professional kudos in any country, though it might prove profitable. The Dutch sexologist, Van de Velde, took up the speciality after his elopement, when he was a married man, with a married patient from his gynaecological practice. The scandal had forced him to leave the Netherlands altogether and live abroad, even after the union had been sanctified by marriage, while the Belgian researcher Lanval worked in fear of police raids.[29] Early resistance to Freud among his countrymen has been well documented. Kinsey's work was greeted with establishment outrage (although it also became a popular bestseller), and political pressure led to the termination of funding by the Rockefeller Foundation.[30] Even in the AIDS era efforts to organize surveys comparable to that undertaken by the Wellcome Trust in Britain have been thwarted in the USA, Sweden and Switzerland, and the French survey 'encountered some testing hurdles'.[31]

While the study of sex in England is certainly redolent of the fine old English tradition of the eccentric amateur, it was perhaps not quite so unique in its peripherality as it seems at first. This is an area in which differing national and cultural norms could usefully be compared and contrasted. While generalization may be misleading, a nuanced study of the different emphases of 'repression' and 'liberation' in different cultures would be valuable.[32]

Texts and the Making of Sexual Knowledge(s)

How did individuals read the texts discussed in the previous chapters, and how, ultimately, did they make their own sexual knowledge? We can gain some sense of how they read Marie Stopes from the copious correspondence she received, but how far can this be generalized? While *Married Love* seems to have supplied a language for what previously could not be articulated, it could be argued that the use of Stopes's own terminology was a strategy employed by her correspondents in seeking her assistance, and that they might not have used it in other circumstances. It would be helpful, though probably records no longer survive, to find out whether correspondents to women's magazine agony aunts employed their standard rhetoric (did anyone really write 'my boy wants me to do wrong'?), or whether letters had to be heavily rewritten in 'house style'. It is unfortunately not entirely clear from Barret-Ducrocq's *Love in the Time of Victoria* whether the women applying to place their babies in the Foundling Hospital actually used the term 'crim. con.' for sexual intercourse (as in 'crim. con. took place'), or whether this was editorial intervention by the committee members. Or was 'crim. con.' perceived by the women in question as appropriate terminology for this particular context?[33]

Apart from the question of language, how were these books used? (Quite distinct from any pornographic function they may have served!) Did people swallow works of sexual advice whole, or did they pick about in them for what seemed relevant to their own predicament? How did they read them, given the other sexual messages that were around – whispers of smutty folklore, media scandals, romances?

It is possible to hypothesize that the books may have been used differently, and had different meanings, according to context – *Married Love* was surely being read differently when it was being passed round the barrack room than when it was given as a loving present to enlighten a fiancée's ignorance. It may also have served differing purposes for the individual: the one who demonstrated his sexual knowingness by sniggering in a public context might furtively return to it in private for sorely needed assistance. Do those who giggle over agony columns never write, or feel at least the temptation to write, to them themselves? Reviewers of Rusbridger's in itself mocking *History of the Sex Manual* were perhaps over-concerned to make it clear that they were not among those sad, sick failures who – perish the thought – *needed* to consult a sex manual.[34]

Sex advice is only one, rather extreme case of a type of literature the use of which has been very little studied: the self-help or advisory manual (itself shelved alongside that first of all advice manuals, the Bible). Does the mere acquisition of such a book represent an aspiration to some particular state (sexual bliss, gourmet cooking, social know-how, psychological well-being) or even a magical identification with such a state? Are such works occasionally consulted to help with some specific need: a sudden marital difficulty, the need to give a dinner party, an invitation to a function perceived as socially threatening, or an emotional crisis? Or are they read and their instructions carried out in detail, in order to *become* a happy married lover, gourmet cook, socially confident or psychologically well-integrated person? We do not know, although it may be guessed that different individuals fall into different groups, and that of all copies acquired, some will sit on a shelf (or in a corset-drawer), some will be infrequently referred to, some will be read through thoroughly once, and some will be repeatedly referred to, or at least specific passages, like a favourite recipe, may be returned to again and again.

Another model which may be pertinent is that of the medical dictionary or home health manual, which fulfils some of the same functions as any work of popular advice. There is also, however, a potential morbid attraction to reading medical dictionaries, and indeed the associated tendency to believe that one has every ailment detailed, like the narrator of Jerome K. Jerome's *Three Men in a Boat* (1889), who discovered, upon reading a medical dictionary, that he had everything but housemaid's knee. This taste for the morbid was surely a motive for visiting 'anatomical museums', and there even might be a certain doom-laden enjoyment to be obtained from perusing the awful warnings of doctors, quacks and sex educators about the dangers of spermatorrhoea and self-abuse. Did people read such works with the same sort of scary *frisson* that they obtained from reading, for example, *Dracula*? Or, again, did they giggle over them in some contexts and return to them with furtive anxiety in others?

Forms of sexual knowledge around in any given historical context should perhaps be regarded not as discrete packages or competing systems, but as a buffet from which individuals make their own selections of the items which seem to fit their own circumstances (which, perhaps, seem to them 'natural'?). Particular social contexts will favour the selection of particular choices from those available: sex as dangerous and threatening for many Victorians, married eroticism as mystic union for the 1920s readers of Marie Stopes.

Angus McLaren in *A History of Contraception* (1991) has shown how individuals and couples throughout history have endeavoured to gain at least the sense of control over reproduction, but how greatly this has varied in specific historical contexts, from the promotion of a fertility perceived as endangered to the restraint of fertility perceived as superabundant.[35] While technological changes had a part to play, they were not the sole determinants for behaviour and attitudes, as early historians of the development of contraception have suggested.[36] Economic and social changes also had a key part to play, as Wally

Seccombe demonstrates in his powerful study of changing family structures since the Industrial Revolution, *Weathering the Storm* (1993).[37] Debates about female sexuality, and the possibility of separating the sexual act from motherhood, needed not only the availability of effective contraception, but also major changes in the social and economic opportunities open to women.

A question which has to be asked in the era of AIDS is how far the awareness of sexually transmitted diseases has influenced sexual knowledge in general. It is noticeable that Victorian sex advice was directed far less against avoiding catching venereal disease than against the solitary vice, and there is just enough evidence for one to be unable to quite dismiss as apocryphal the tales of copulation being recommended as the 'cure' for masturbation. The perception of sex as potentially dangerous and causative of disease may be present alongside complete myths about the causation of the supposed disease. This perhaps needs to be considered alongside other popular concepts of disease aetiology, with the proviso that the very lack of, or furtiveness of, information about venereal disease might lead to the lengthy persistence of such folk beliefs as the curative power of intercourse with a virgin.

Even those who seem to have the most up-to-date information on the subject may have ideas and theories wildly at variance with it. The respondents to Mass Observation's VD survey, so recently exposed to a massive, if, in its final form, expurgated government-sponsored press campaign of enlightenment (see pp. 241–2), very largely saw sexually transmitted disease either as something pervasive and impersonally transmitted, avoided by eschewing contact with lavatory seats and keeping oneself 'clean' (a deeply loaded term), or as inhabiting particular stigmatized bodies – of foreigners (especially Americans)[38] or of those perennial scapegoats, 'little cheap loose-living girls'[39] – which, presumably, could be identified and avoided. It was a rare respondent who remarked that the venereally diseased looked like anyone else: 'you'd be surprised seeing the nice looking fellows going there' (the Covent Garden VD clinic).[40] A more typical response may have been that of a self-admitted prostitute that if, despite her care, she contracted a venereal disease 'I should put my head in the gas oven',[41] or the reply of the woman who was so anxious that (without any given reason for imagining she might have it) 'I keep thinking I've got it every pain I have'.[42]

Even before the government press campaign and the MO survey, the National Society for the Prevention of Venereal Disease received numbers of letters from the general public (in response to their small ads) requesting information as to how they might prevent VD. The very words 'venereal disease' were regarded as dangerous and contaminating; Mr Lewis, secretary to the NSPVD, told the British Sexology Society in 1940 that 'the bank manager had expressly desired that the VD should not be mentioned on the cheques, for the sake of the "purity" of the clerks at his bank'.[43] However, those soliciting its advice presumably had ideas about the transmission of VD attuned to 'modern' theories of the disease as opposed to vague fears of lavatory seats, though their letters do not reveal what their ideas were.[44] Whether they acted on the information supplied is of course unknowable; the relationship between 'knowing' and any kind of action is extremely hard to assess. The Wellcome Survey investigated whether individuals were making behavioural changes in their sex lives as a result of AIDS, but evidence appears somewhat ambiguous, with a relatively low proportion claiming this – under 20 per cent of men and less than 15 per cent of women – and contradictions between such statements and reports of actual sexual practices.[45]

It may be doubted how coherent and self-consistent have ever been and are the ideas about sex held by any one person at a given time. The capacity of individuals to hold competing and contradictory ideas should not be underestimated. Since, unperceived by the writers at the time of writing, contradictions can be traced even in thought-out and self-conscious texts, how much more must this be the case in the unarticulated ideas about sex that most of us carry around.

A further question is why particular individuals do write about/ investigate sex. Certainly those who have dared to venture upon the subject in Britain, at least from the time of such Enlightenment individuals as James Graham, appear to have some pre-existing eccentricity, or some grounds of exclusion from 'normal' life, before they embarked on the subject. Edward Carpenter, as well as Laurence Housman and many of the other founders of the British Society for the Study of Sex Psychology, was homosexual at a time of legal penalization and social stigma. Havelock Ellis's peculiarities have been documented.[46] As mentioned in Chapter 7, Geddes felt himself excluded by wider theoretical differences from the biologists who would normally have constituted his professional peer group. Norman Haire, though he had a successful Harley Street practice in gynaecology and sexual medicine, was Australian, homosexual and Jewish, which must have militated against him in medical circles.[47]

Even those who wrote for 'the normal' were not themselves entirely 'normal'. Marie Stopes came to write *Married Love* after a failed love affair with a Japanese colleague and a disastrous first marriage to a Canadian botanist.[48] Isabel Hutton had undergone the shock of the decision to marry at a point in her life at which she may have considered herself wedded to her medical career, followed by (apart from any problems of adjustment, which may be reflected in *The Hygiene of Marriage*; see pp. 213–14) the very real trauma of finding her career stalemated at every turn by formal or informal marriage bars.[49] The autobiography of E. F. Griffith indicates a troubled questing spirit, whose recourse to Jungian analysis in the 1940s represented the culmination of pre-existing dissatisfactions with his life.[50]

Marie Stopes, the British Society for the Study of Sex Psychology, and other individuals and organizations received unsolicited letters expressing thoughts and theories about sex which individuals had worked out or puzzled about for themselves. These letters are sometimes rather (even extremely) strange: the papers of reproductive biologist Sir Alan Parkes include one file entitled by him 'Screwball Letters', several of which deal with sexual matters,[51] and it is tempting to place the writers of these letters in the same class as those who write to the well-known to communicate their theories about the cause or cure of cancer and messages dictated by the devil.

But the writers of these letters were trying to express ideas perhaps not so much weirder than those held by many who did not even attempt to make an effort to work them out into any kind of system. Unlike Geddes, Ellis, Carpenter or Stopes, they were not writers and communicators of ideas with some access to the means of disseminating them; all of these authors additionally wrote on subjects other than sex, and were used to organizing and presenting ideas for a specified audience. Given that some unknown, 'ordinary' person was capable of cogently arguing his or her sexual system, would they have had the kind of outlet for their writing that was available either to outright hacks like 'Courtney Beale', or to a genuine Harley Street practitioner like Eustace Chesser? Would they even have dared to think of publication?

This book has drawn a rather coarse diagram to indicate some of the kinds of ideas floating around at particular historical moments in a particular national context upon which individuals have drawn to make up their own 'sexual knowledge', their sense of the 'facts of life'. But posterity condescends if it imagines that the ideas of Acton, of Ellis, of Stopes, were the sole shaping force of the sexual knowledge even of the individuals who read their texts, as opposed to those who gleaned some vague apprehension of their existence through rumour or press reports. Mechling has suggested that mothering is learnt not from advice books but from the experience of being mothered, at a pre-verbal stage of existence. While his account, suggesting that patterns are passed on without change for generations, fails to consider modifications in child-rearing practices over time, it reminds us that we learn from other sources than texts, that there are bodily responses and social practices which are by no means so accessible to the historian.[52] If it is hard enough to read texts as they might have been read by their contemporaries, how much harder it is to reconstruct their extra-textual context.

Notes

Introduction: Histories of Sex

1. D'Arcy Power, *The Foundations of Medical History* (Baltimore, Md.: Johns Hopkins University Press, 1931), Lecture vi, '*Aristotle's Master-Piece*', 147.
2. 'Victorian' is highly problematic: see Michael Mason, *The Making of Victorian Sexuality* (Oxford: Oxford University Press, 1994). For 'Victorian' fear of sex, see N. Perrin, *Dr Bowdler's Legacy – A History of Expurgated Books in England and America* (London: Macmillan, 1970).
3. There is a rapidly growing literature on topics such as these, barely mentioned in this book, and it would be pointless to attempt a bibliography here. See listings of new works in the *Journal of the History of Sexuality*.
4. For a recent attempt see Richard Davenport-Hines, *Sex, Death and Punishment: Attitudes to Sex and Sexuality in Britain since the Renaissance* (London: Collins, 1990); older surveys include Nina C. Epton, *Love and the English* (Cleveland, NY: World Publishing; London: Cassell, 1960) and Gordon Rattray Taylor, *Sex in History* (New York: Vanguard, 1954; Harper and Row, 1973).
5. See Irving Singer, *The Nature of Love*, 3 vols (Chicago: University of Chicago Press, 1984–7).
6. See for instance Rita Goldberg, *Sex and Enlightenment. Women in Richardson and Diderot* (Cambridge: Cambridge University Press, 1984); Alan Bold (ed.), *The Sexual Dimension in Literature* (London: Vision Press, 1982; Totowa, NJ: Barnes and Noble, 1983) P. Webb, *The Erotic Arts* (London: Secker and Warburg, 1975); Susan Rubin Suleiman (ed.), *The Female Body in Western Culture: Contemporary Perspectives* (Cambridge, Mass.: Harvard University Press, 1986); L. Nead, *Myths of Sexuality: Representations of Women in Victorian Britain* (Oxford: Basil Blackwell, 1988).
7. See Lawrence Stone, *The Family, Sex and Marriage in England, 1500–1800* (London: Weidenfeld and Nicolson, 1977); R. Trumbach, *The Rise of the Egalitarian Family: Aristocratic Kinship and Domestic Relations in Eighteenth Century England* (New York: Academic Press, 1978); Alan Macfarlane, *Marriage and Love in England: Modes of Reproduction, 1300–1840* (Oxford: Basil Blackwell, 1986); Frank Mort, *Dangerous Sexualities: Medico-Moral Politics in England since 1830* (London and New York: Routledge and Kegan Paul, 1987); John C. Fout (ed.), *Forbidden History: The State, Society, and the Regulation of Sexuality in Modern Europe* (Chicago: University of Chicago Press, 1992).
8. Thomas W. Laqueur, *Making Sex. Gender and the Body from Aristotle to Freud* (Cambridge, Mass.: Harvard University Press, 1990); Sander Gilman, *Sexuality: An Illustrated History* (New York: Wiley, 1989); Ornella Moscucci, *The Science of Woman: Gynaecology and Gender in England,*

1800–1929 (Cambridge: Cambridge University Press, 1990); Cynthia Eagle Russett, *Sexual Science: The Victorian Construction of Womanhood* (London and Cambridge, Mass.: Harvard University Press, 1989).

9. As will become obvious, 'Britain' will largely be England, with a little on Scotland.

10. Kaye Wellings, Julia Field, Anne Johnson and Jane Wadsworth, with Sally Bradshaw, *Sexual Behaviour in Britain. The National Survey of Sexual Attitudes and Lifestyles* (Harmondsworth: Penguin, 1994).

11. For popular culture, see Peter Burke, *Popular Culture in Early Modern Europe* (London: Temple Smith, 1978); John M. Golby and A. W. Purdue, *The Civilization of the Crowd: Popular Culture in England, 1750–1900* (London: Batsford Academic and Educational, 1984).

12. For these themes see J. Donnison, *Midwives and Medical Men: A History of Interprofessional Rivalries and Women's Rights* (London: Heinemann Educational, 1977); A. Eccles, *Obstetrics and Gynaecology in Tudor and Stuart England* (London: Croom Helm, 1982); Adrian Wilson, *A Safe Deliverance* (London: University College Press, forthcoming 1995).

13. W. F. Bynum, 'Treating the Wages of Sin: Venereal Disease and Specialism in Eighteenth-Century Britain', in W. F. Bynum and R. Porter (eds), *Medical Fringe and Medical Orthodoxy, 1750–1850* (London: Croom Helm, 1987), 5–28; A. Fessler and R. S. France, 'Syphilis in Seventeenth-Century Lancashire', *British Journal of Venereal Disease*, ii (1945), 177–8. A key contemporary work was Jean Astruc, *A Treatise of the Venereal Disease*, trans. W. Barrowby (London: W. Innys and R. Manby, 1737).

14. Jay Mechling, 'Advice to Historians on Advice To Mothers', *Journal of Social History*, ix (1975–6), 46–63; Roger Chartier, *Cultural History. Between Practices and Representations* (Ithaca: Cornell University Press; Cambridge: Polity Press, 1988).

15. John Money, 'Teaching in the Market-Place, or "Caesar adsum jam forte aderat": The Retailing of Knowledge on Provincial England during the Eighteenth Century', in John Brewer and Roy Porter (eds), *Consumption and the World of Goods* (London and New York: Routledge, 1993), 335–79; Patricia Cline Cohen, *A Calculating People: The Spread of Numeracy in Early America* (Chicago: University of Chicago Press, 1982); idem, 'Reckoning with Commerce: Numeracy in Eighteenth-Century America', in John Brewer and Roy Porter (eds), *Consumption and the World of Goods* (London and New York: Routledge, 1993), 320–34.

16. Some evidence is adduced *passim* in Lawrence Stone, *The Road to Divorce, England 1530–1987* (Oxford: Oxford University Press, 1990); idem, *Uncertain Unions: Marriage in England 1660–1753* (Oxford: Oxford University Press, 1992); idem, *Broken Lives: Separation and Divorce in England 1660–1857* (Oxford: Oxford University Press, 1993). Stone draws upon testimony presented before various ecclesiastical and common law courts.

17. Peter Gay, *The Bourgeois Experience: Victoria to Freud*, Vol. II: *The Tender Passion* (Oxford and New York: Oxford University Press, 1986) has discussion, for example, of the intimate sexual secrets of Charles Kingsley and his wife.

18. Edward Le Comte, *Milton and Sex* (London: Macmillan, 1978), for instance, has nothing on Milton's intimate sex life.

19. Lesley A. Hall, *Hidden Anxieties. Male Sexuality, 1900–1950* (Cambridge: Polity Press, 1991); Steve Humphries, *A Secret World of Sex: Forbidden Fruit, the British Experience 1900–1950* (London: Sidgwick and Jackson, 1988); Maureen Sutton, *We Didn't Know Aught* (Stamford: Paul Watkins, 1992). It hardly needs emphasizing that no claim is here being made that sex advice books *per se* were uniquely important within the print culture of sex. Pulp novels may have had a greater impact. In any case, as 'little histories' and oral histories like Maureen Sutton's suggest, sexual attitudes and practices were probably regulated far more through oral transmission than through print.

20. Iwan Bloch, *Sex Life in England Illus-*

trated: As Revealed in its Obscene Litera-ture and Art, trans. Richard Deniston (New York: Falstaff, 1934); *idem, A History of English Sexual Morals*, trans. William H. Forstern (London: Francis Aldor, 1936); *idem, Sexual Life in England Past and Present*, trans. William H. Forstern (London: Arco, 1958).

21. Alan Rusbridger, *A Concise History of the Sex Manual, 1886–1986* (London and Boston: Faber and Faber, 1986).

22. See, for instance, issues of the *Journal of the History of Sexuality*.

23. Michel Foucault, *Histoire de la sexualité*, Vol. I, *La Volonté de savoir* (Paris: Gallimard, 1976), trans. Robert Hurley, *The History of Sexuality: Introduction* (London: Allen Lane, 1978; New York: Vintage Books, 1985); for discussion see Jonathan Dollimore, *Sexual Dissidence: Augustine to Wilde, Freud to Foucault* (Oxford: Clarendon Press, 1991); I. Diamond and L. Quinby (eds), *Feminism and Foucault: Reflections on Resistance* (Boston, Mass.: Northeastern University Press, 1988); Lois McNay, *Foucault and Feminism: Power, Gender and the Self* (Cambridge: Polity Press, 1992); Roy Porter, 'Is Foucault Useful for Understanding Eighteenth and Nineteenth Century Sexuality?', *Contention*, i (1991), 61–82; and the fine chapter, 'Foucault on Sexuality', by Anthony Giddens in his *The Transformation of Intimacy. Sexuality, Love and Eroticism in Modern Societies* (Cambridge: Polity Press, 1992). For the related issue of the understanding of the body, see Dorinda Outram, *The Body and the French Revolution: Sex, Class and Political Culture* (New Haven, Conn.: Yale University Press, 1989); Bryan S. Turner, *The Body and Society: Explorations in Social Theory* (Oxford: Basil Blackwell, 1984); *idem*, 'The Practices of Rationality: Michel Foucault, Medical History and Sociological Theory', in R. Fardon (ed.), *Power and Knowledge: Anthropological and Sociological Approaches* (Edinburgh: Scottish Academic Press, 1985), 193–213; and *idem, Medical Power and Social Knowledge* (Beverly Hills, Calif.: Sage Publications, 1987).

24. Hence the very constitution of the sexual is itself hotly debated: is it pos-sible to draw clear lines between the erotic and, more broadly, gender identity or the sensual? See Stephen Heath, *The Sexual Fix* (New York: Schocken; London: Macmillan, 1982); Lynda Birke, *Women, Feminism and Biology: The Feminist Challenge* (Brighton: Wheatsheaf Books, 1986); Ludmilla Jordanova, *Sexual Visions* (Hemel Hempstead: Harvester, 1989). On the recent collapse of sexual boundaries see Giddens, *Transformation of Intimacy*; Judith Butler, *Bodies that Matter: On the Discursive Limits of 'Sex'* (London: Routledge, 1993).

25. Roland Barthes, *Mythologies*, trans. Annette Lavers (London: Cape, 1972); *idem, The Fashion System*, trans. Matthew Ward and Richard Howard (New York: Hill and Wang, 1983).

26. For discussion see 'Introduction' to Roy Porter and Mikuláš Teich (eds), *Sexual Knowledge, Sexual Science: The History of Attitudes to Sexuality* (Cambridge: Cambridge University Press, 1994), 1–28. For the denial of the traditional notion of science as 'dis-covery', see Barry Barnes and Steven Shapin (eds), *Natural Order: Historical Studies of Scientific Culture* (Beverly Hills, Calif. and London: Sage Publica-tions, 1979); Barry Barnes, *Interests and the Growth of Knowledge* (London: Routledge and Kegan Paul, 1977); D. Bloor, *Knowledge and Social Imagery* (London: Routledge and Kegan Paul, 1976); Harry Collins, *Changing Order: Replication and Induction in Scientific Practice* (Beverly Hills and London: Sage Publications, 1985); H. M. Collins and T. J. Pinch, *Frames of Meaning: The Social Construction of Extra-ordinary Science* (London: Routledge and Kegan Paul, 1982); R. M. Young, 'Science *is* Social Relations', *Radical Science Journal*, v (1977), 65–129. A good survey is provided by Barry Barnes, 'Sociological Theories of Sci-entific Knowledge', in R. C. Olby, G. N. Cantor, J. R. R. Christie and M. J. S. Hodge (eds), *Companion to the History of Modern Science* (London: Routledge, 1990), 60–76.

27. For such histories, see Wayland Young, *Eros Denied: Studies in Exclusion* (London: Weidenfeld and Nicolson, 1965); for this climate of opinion, see Paul A. Robinson, *The Modernization of*

Sex: Havelock Ellis, Alfred Kinsey, William Masters and Virginia Johnson (London: Elek, 1976; New York: Harper and Row, 1976); and for debates within the development of American sexology, revealing its complex politics, see Janice M. Irvine, *Disorders of Desire: Sex and Gender in Modern American Sexology* (Philadelphia: Temple University Press, 1990).

28. Russett, *Sexual Science*.

29. For valuable basic feminist studies see Mary Jacobus, Evelyn Fox Keller and Sally Shuttleworth (eds), *Body/Politics: Women and the Discourses of Science* (New York: Routledge, 1990); Nead, *Myths of Sexuality*; Martha Vicinus (ed.), *Suffer and Be Still: Women in the Victorian Age* (Bloomington: Indiana University Press, 1972), and her 'Sexuality and Power: A Review of Current Work in the History of Sexuality', *Feminist Studies*, viii (1982), 133–56; D. Gorham, *The Victorian Girl and the Feminine Ideal* (London: Croom Helm, 1982); Carroll Smith-Rosenberg, 'The Hysterical Woman: Sex Roles and Conflict in Nineteenth-Century America', *Social Research*, xxxix (1972), 652–78; and her 'Puberty to Menopause: The Cycle of Femininity in Nineteenth-Century America', in M. Hartman and L. Banner (eds), *Clio's Consciousness Raised* (New York: Harper and Row, 1974), 23–37; see also her *Disorderly Conduct: Visions of Gender in Victorian America* (New York: Knopf, 1985), and Carroll Smith-Rosenberg and Charles Rosenberg, 'The Female Animal: Medical and Biological Views of Woman and Her Role in Nineteenth-Century America', *Journal of American History*, lx (1973), 332–56; Mary Poovey, ' "Scenes of an Indelicate Character": The Medical "Treatment" of Victorian Women', *Representations*, xiv (1986), 152; and her 'Speaking of the Body: Mid-Victorian Constructions of Female Desire', in Mary Jacobus, Evelyn Fox Keller and Sally Shuttleworth (eds), *Body/Politics: Women and the Discourses of Science* (New York and London: Routledge, 1990), 29–46; John S. Haller Sr., 'From Maidenhead to Menopause: Sex Education for Women in Victorian America', *Journal of Popular Culture*, vi

(1972), 49–69; John Christie, 'Feminism in the History of Science', in R. Olby, G. Cantor, J. R. R. Christie and M. J. Hodge (eds), *Companion to the History of Modern Science* (London: Routledge, 1990), 100–9.

30. B. Dijkstra, *Idols of Perversity: Fantasies of Feminine Evil in Fin-de-Siècle Culture* (Oxford and New York: Oxford University Press, 1986).

31. For the gendering of authorial personae, see S. Gilbert and S. Gubar, *The Madwoman in the Attic: The Woman Writer and the Nineteenth-Century Imagination* (New Haven and London: Yale University Press, 1979).

32. These matters are further discussed in the 'Introduction' to Porter and Teich (eds), *Sexual Knowledge, Sexual Science*, 1–28.

33. Barbara Ehrenreich, Elizabeth Hess and Gloria Jacobs, *Remaking Love: The Feminization of Sex* (Garden City, NY: Anchor Press/Doubleday, 1986).

34. Sheila Jeffreys, *The Spinster and Her Enemies: Feminism and Sexuality, 1880–1930* (London: Pandora Press, 1985); *idem, Anti-climax: A Feminist Perspective on the Sexual Revolution* (London: Women's Press, 1990); Andrea Dworkin, *Intercourse* (London: Secker and Warburg, 1987). See the critique in Camille Paglia, *Sexual Personae* (New Haven: Yale University Press, 1990).

35. It may be argued, for instance, that Germaine Greer's *The Female Eunuch* (London: MacGibbon and Kee, 1970) played into male hands with its rather straightforward advocacy of sexual permissiveness; and that her later writings – for instance *The Change* (London: Hamish Hamilton, 1991) – have backtracked from that position, aware of how sexual permissiveness may tend towards the exploitation of women.

36. Eva Cantarella, *Bisexuality in the Ancient World*, trans. Cormac Ó'Cuilleánain (New Haven and London: Yale University Press, 1992); John Boswell, *Christianity, Social Tolerance, and Homosexuality: Gay People in Western Europe from the Beginning of the Christian Era to the Fourteenth Century* (Chicago: University of Chicago Press, 1980); Aline Rousselle, *Porneia: On Desire and the Body in Antiquity*, trans. Felicia Pheas-

ant (New York: Basil Blackwell, 1988); John J. Winkler, *Constraints of Desire: The Anthropology of Sex and Gender in Ancient Greece* (New York: Routledge, Chapman and Hall, 1990); John Boardman, *Eros in Greece* (London: John Murray, 1978); Kenneth J. Dover, *Greek Homosexuality* (Cambridge, Mass.: Harvard University Press, 1978; updated with a new postcript 1989); Eva Keuls, *The Reign of the Phallus: Sexual Politics in Ancient Athens* (New York: Harper and Row, 1985). For more modern times, see David F. Greenberg, *The Construction of Homosexuality* (Chicago: University of Chicago Press, 1988); Mandy Merck, *Perversions: Deviant Readings* (London: Virago, 1993).

37. Michel Foucault, *Histoire de la sexualité*, Vol. II: *L'Usage des plaisirs* (Paris: Gallimard, 1984), trans. Robert Hurley, *The Use of Pleasure* (New York: Random House, 1985; London: Viking, 1986; Harmondsworth: Penguin, 1987); *idem, Histoire de la sexualité*, Vol. III: *Le Souci de soi* (Paris: Gallimard, 1984), trans. Robert Hurley, *The Care of the Self* (New York: Pantheon Books, 1986; Random House, 1987).

38. J. Culler, *On Deconstruction* (London: Routledge and Kegan Paul, 1983); *idem, Framing the Sign: Criticism and Its Institutions* (Norman: University of Oklahoma Press, 1988); Dollimore, *Sexual Dissidence*; Michael Worton and Judith Still (eds), *Textuality and Sexuality: Reading Theories and Practices* (Manchester: Manchester University Press, 1993). Illuminating on language are Dale Spender, *Man Made Language* (London: Routledge and Kegan Paul, 1980), and Mary Daly, *Gyn/ecology* (Boston, Mass.: Beacon Press, 1978; London: Women's Press, 1984).

39. W. E. Houghton, *The Victorian Frame of Mind 1830–1870* (New Haven: Yale University Press, 1957); Fraser Harrison, *The Dark Angel: Aspects of Victorian Sexuality* (London: Sheldon Press, 1977).

40. Steven Marcus, *The Other Victorians: A Study of Sexuality and Pornography in Mid-Nineteenth Century England* (New York: Basic, 1964; London: Weidenfeld and Nicolson, 1966).

41. Peter Gay, 'Victorian Sexuality: Old Texts and New Insights', *American Scholar*, xlix (1980), 372–7; *idem, The Bourgeois Experience – Victoria to Freud*, Vol. I: *Education of the Senses* (London and New York: Oxford University Press, 1983); *idem, The Bourgeois Experience – Victoria to Freud*, Vol. II: *The Tender Passion* (London and New York: Oxford University Press, 1986).

42. K. V. Thomas, 'The Double Standard', *Journal of the History of Ideas*, xx (1959), 195–216.

43. Françoise Barret-Ducrocq, *L'amour sous Victoria: sexualité et classes populaires à Londres au XIX siècle* (Paris: Plon, 1989); trans. John Howe, *Love in the Time of Victoria: Sexuality, Class, and Gender in Nineteenth-Century London* (London and New York: Verso, 1991); Mason, *Making of Victorian Sexuality*.

44. The seamy side of Restoration sex has been illuminated by Stone's *Broken Lives*.

45. David Foxon, *Libertine Literature in England 1660–1745: with an Appendix on the Publication of John Cleland's 'Memoirs of a Woman of Pleasure', Commonly Known as 'Fanny Hill'* (New York: University Books, 1965); Peter Wagner, *Eros Revived: Erotica of the Enlightenment in England and America* (London: Secker and Warburg, 1988).

1   Contexts: from the Restoration to the Accession of Queen Victoria

1. For examples see A. Lloyd, *The Wickedest Age* (Newton Abbot: David and Charles, 1971); Morton M. Hunt, *The Natural History of Love* (New York: Knopf, 1959; London: Hutchinson, 1960); Reay Tannahill, *Sex in History* (New York: Stein and Day, 1980). The puritan reaction is documented in Edward J. Bristow, *Vice and Vigilance: Purity Movements in Britain since 1700* (Dublin: Gill and Macmillan, 1977).

2. Maurice J. Quinlan, *Victorian Prelude: A History of English Manners, 1700–1830* (London: Cass; New York: Columbia University Press, 1941); Muriel Jaeger, *Before Victoria: Changing Standards*

and Behaviour, 1787–1837 (London: Chatto and Windus, 1956): F. K. Brown, *Fathers of the Victorians: The Age of Wilberforce* (Cambridge: Cambridge University Press, 1961).

3. Alan Macfarlane, *Marriage and Love in England: Modes of Reproduction, 1300–1840* (Oxford: Basil Blackwell, 1986); Mary Abbott, *Family Ties: English Families 1540–1920* (London and New York; Routledge, 1993); Lawrence Stone, *The Family, Sex and Marriage in England, 1500–1800* (London: Weidenfeld and Nicolson, 1977); David Levine, *Family Formation in an Age of Nascent Capitalism* (New York: Academic Press, 1977); Michael Anderson, *Approaches to the History of the Western Family, 1500–1914* (London: Macmillan, 1980); John R. Gillis, *For Better, For Worse: British Marriages, 1600 to the Present* (New York and Oxford: Oxford University Press, 1985); Randolph Trumbach, *The Rise of the Egalitarian Family: Aristocratic Kinship and Domestic Relations in Eighteenth Century England* (New York: Academic Press, 1978).

4. Keith Wrightson and David Levine, *Poverty and Piety in an English Village: Terling 1525–1700* (New York and London: Academic Press, 1979); Rosalind Mitchison and Leah Leneman, *Sexuality and Social Control: Scotland 1660–1780* (Oxford: Basil Blackwell, 1989); Martin Ingram, *Church Courts, Sex and Marriage in England, 1570–1640* (Cambridge: Cambridge University Press, 1987); G. R. Quaife, *Wanton Wenches and Wayward Wives: Peasants and Illicit Sex in Early Seventeenth Century England* (London: Croom Helm, 1979); John Addy, *Sin and Society in the Seventeenth Century* (London and New York: Routledge, Chapman and Hall, 1989); John R. Gillis, 'Married but Not Churched: Plebeian Sexual Relations and Marital Nonconformity in Eighteenth-Century Britain', in R. P. Maccubbin (ed.), *Unauthorized Sexual Behaviour during the Enlightenment* (Williamsburg, Va.: College of William and Mary, 1985), 31–42; Paul Hair (ed.), *Before the Bawdy Court: Selections from the Church Court and Other Records Relating to the Correction of Moral Offences in England, Scotland and New England, 1300–1800* (London: Paul Elek, 1972); *idem*, 'Bridal Pregnancy in Britain: The Limits of "Establishment" Social Control?', in Ad van der Woude (ed.), *The Role of the State and Public Opinion in Sexual Attitudes and Demographic Behaviour* (Paris: International Commission of Historical Demography, 1990), 35–48.

5. This was for idealistic reasons – that is, moral improvement, but also, as the cynical Mandeville noted, for the mercenary reason of keeping the price up. For the moral ambiguities of the era see Lee Davison, Tim Hitchcock, Tim Keirn and Robert B. Shoemaker (eds), *Stilling the Grumbling Hive: The Response to Social and Economic Problems in England, 1689–1750* (Stroud: Alan Sutton; New York: St Martin's Press, 1992).

6. Admirably brought out in Angus McLaren, *Reproductive Rituals: The Perception of Fertility in England from the Sixteenth to the Nineteenth Century* (London and New York: Methuen, 1984); *idem*, 'Clever Practices: Fertility Control Methods from the 18th to 20th Centuries', in Ad van der Woude (ed.), *The Role of the State and Public Opinion in Sexual Attitudes and Demographic Behaviour* (Paris: International Commission of Historical Demography, 1990), 425–40.

7. Peter Earle, *The Making of the English Middle Class: Business, Society and Family Life in London, 1660–1730* (London: Methuen, 1989).

8. Stone, *Family, Sex and Marriage*; *idem*, *The Road to Divorce, England 1530–1987* (Oxford: Oxford University Press, 1990); *idem*, *Uncertain Unions: Marriage in England 1660–1753* (Oxford: Oxford University Press, 1992); *idem*, *Broken Lives: Separation and Divorce in England 1660–1857* (Oxford: Oxford University Press, 1993).

9. All these ideas are contentious but considerable evidence is adduced for them in Janet Todd, *Sensibility: An Introduction* (London: Methuen, 1986); Patricia Meyer Spacks, *The Female Imagination: A Literary and Psychological Investigation of Women's Writing* (New York: Knopf, 1975; London: Allen and Unwin, 1976); G. J. Barker-Benfield,

The Culture of Sensibility: Sex and Society in Eighteenth-Century Britain (Chicago: University of Chicago Press, 1992); Jean H. Hagstrum, *Sex and Sensibility. Ideal and Erotic Love from Milton to Mozart* (Chicago and London: University of Chicago Press, 1980); Gordon Rattray Taylor, *The Angel-Makers: A Study in the Psychological Origins of Historical Change* (London: Heinemann, 1958; New York: E. P. Dutton, 1974). For a contemporary view, see W. Alexander, *The History of Women from the Earliest Antiquity to the Present Times*, 2 vols in 1 (London: W. Strahan and T. Cadell, 1779).

10. Stella Tillyard, *Aristocrats* (London: Chatto and Windus, 1994) – a superb study of the emotional, personal, sexual and marital lives of the four Lennox sisters, their husbands and children.

11. For separate spheres see Leonore Davidoff and Catherine Hall, *Family Fortunes: Men and Women of the English Middle Class, 1780–1850* (London: Hutchinson, 1987; London: Routledge, 1987); L. Davidoff, 'The Family in Britain', in F. M. L. Thompson (ed.), *The Cambridge Social History of England 1750–1950*, Vol. II (Cambridge: Cambridge University Press, 1990).

12. See Stone, *Broken Lives*. For sexual shenanigans in the American colonies, see also Thomas H. Johnson, 'Jonathan Edwards and the "Young Folks' Bible"', *The New England Quarterly*, v (1932), 37–54.

13. For the Enlightenment in England and in Scotland, see Roy Porter and Mikuláš Teich (eds), *The Enlightenment in National Context* (Cambridge: Cambridge University Press, 1981).

14. J. H. Plumb, *The Commercialization of Leisure in Eighteenth Century England* (Reading: University of Reading Press, 1973); *idem, Georgian Delights* (London: Weidenfeld and Nicolson, 1980).

15. Edward Shorter, *The Making of the Modern Family* (New York: Basic Books, 1975); P. Branca, *Women in Europe since 1750* (London: Croom Helm, 1978). For critique, see C. Fairchilds, 'Female Sexual Attitudes and the Rise of Illegitimacy: a Case Study', *Journal of Interdisciplinary History*, viii (1978), 627–67.

16. For discussions, see Stone, *Family, Sex and Marriage*, ch. 12, and Roger Thompson, *Unfit for Modest Ears: A Study of Pornographic, Obscene and Bawdy Works Written or Published in England in the Second Half of the Seventeenth Century* (London: Macmillan, 1979), 214. See also F. Bottomley, *Attitudes to the Body in Western Christendom* (London: Lepus Books, 1979).

17. Community control of individual sexual behaviour had been stressed by Peter Laslett, most notably in *The World We have Lost* (London: Methuen, 1965), and by Laslett, Karla Oosterveen and Richard M. Smith (eds) in *Bastardy and its Comparative History* (London: Edward Arnold, 1980). See also Wrightson and Levine, *Poverty and Piety*. Of course, controls were much laxer in big towns such as London. There Francis Place thought that in the late eighteenth century 'want of chastity in girls was common'; M. Thale (ed.), *The Autobiography of Francis Place* (Cambridge: Cambridge University Press, 1972), 57. Villages always had sexually easygoing women: Quaife, *Wanton Wenches and Wayward Wives*. Mobile men like soldiers notoriously sowed wild oats.

18. I. Bloch, *A History of English Sexual Morals*, trans. William H. Forstern (London, Francis Aldor, 1936), ch. 8; Stone, *Family, Sex and Marriage*, 530ff.

19. Thompson, *Unfit for Modest Ears*, 210.

20. C. Strachey (ed.), *The Letters of the Earl of Chesterfield to his Son*, 2 vols, 3rd edn (London: Methuen, 1932), Vol. II, 133. For introductions to this slant of moral thought, see L. A. Selby-Bigge, *British Moralists*, 2 vols (Oxford: Oxford University Press, 1897); D. D. Raphael, *British Moralists 1650–1800*, 2 vols (Oxford: Oxford University Press, 1969); J. Passmore, *The Perfectibility of Man* (London: Duckworth, 1970), esp. chs 7–10; and E. Halévy, *The Growth of Philosophic Radicalism*, trans. M. Morris (London: Faber and Faber, 1928). In *Memoirs of a Woman of Pleasure* (London, 1749; edn quoted, Mayflower Books, London, 1977) John Cleland has the prostitute heroine Fanny Hill say that though she knew that as a whore she was engaging in vice, yet 'to say the plain truth, the

dissipation and diversion I began to find in this new acquaintance' cured her of anxieties (p. 83).

21. Quoted in N. Smith, 'Sexual Mores in the Eighteenth century: Robert Wallace's "Of Venery"', *Journal of the History of Ideas*, xxxix (1978), 419–33, p. 426.

22. F. Pottle (ed.), *Boswell's London Journal 1762–1763* (London: Heinemann, 1950; New York: McGraw-Hill, 1950), 84.

23. Erasmus Darwin, *Zoonomia*, 2 vols (London: J. Johnson, 1794–6), Vol. I, 147.

24. David Hume: *A Treatise of Human Nature*, ed. L. A. Selby-Bigge (Oxford: Clarendon Press, 1978), 486.

25. For the rise of individualist hedonism in the context of the wider European Enlightenment see L. Crocker, *An Age of Crisis: Man and World in Eighteenth Century French Thought* (Baltimore, Md: Johns Hopkins University Press, 1959); R. Mauzi, *L'idée du bonheur dans la littérature et la pensée françaises au XVIIIᵉ siècle* (Paris: Colin, 1960); F. E. and F. P. Manuel, *Utopian Thought in the Western World* (Cambridge, Mass.: Belknap Press of Harvard University Press, 1979), ch. 22: 'New Faces of Love'. Crocker controversially sees the movement culminating in De Sade.

26. Quoted in M. Williford, 'Bentham on the Rights of Women', *Journal of the History of Ideas*, xxxvi (1975), 167–76, p. 172. Bentham claimed that sex was a legitimate pleasure in its own right and denounced moralists who argued that 'a man is to convert the highest enjoyment that kind nature has bestow'd upon him into a mechanical operation to make children': Bentham papers, University College, Box 74, fol. 8.

27. Cleland, *Memoirs*, 10. For Cleland's debts to the *philosophes*, sec Leo Braudy, '*Fanny Hill* and Materialism', *Eighteenth Century Studies*, iv (1970–1), 21–40, and also W. H. Epstein, *John Cleland, Images of a Life* (New York: Columbia University Press, 1974), ch. 6. What actual, as distinct from fictional, women of pleasure thought is a totally separate issue: see Randolph Trumbach, 'Modern Prostitution and Gender in *Fanny Hill*: Libertine and Domesticated Fantasy', in G. S.

Rousseau and Roy Porter (eds), *Sexual Underworlds of the Enlightenment* (Manchester: Manchester University Press, 1987), 69–85.

28. Cleland, *Memoirs*, 33.

29. *Ibid.*, 36. Cf. 51: 'I did what I did because I could not help it'.

30. *Ibid.*, 57.

31. *Ibid.*, 68.

32. *Ibid.*, 81. Cf. 122: 'O how powerful are the instincts of nature! How little is there wanting to set them in motion!'

33. *Ibid.*, 114.

34. Pottle (ed.), *Boswell's London Journal*, 116.

35. S. Moravia, 'The Enlightenment and the Sciences of Man', *History of Science*, xviii (1980), 247–68; A. Vartanian, *La Mettrie's L'Homme Machine* (Princeton, NJ: Princeton University Press, 1960).

36. Darwin, *Zoonomia*, Vol. I, 146. Fanny Hill by contrast refers to the male genitals as the 'originals of beauty', objects 'above all the imitation of art': Cleland, *Memoirs*, 59.

37. Cleland, *Memoirs*, 36. See also Braudy, '*Fanny Hill* and Materialism'.

38. See D. King-Hele, *Doctor of Revolution* (London: Faber and Faber, 1977), 255; *idem, The Essential Writings of Erasmus Darwin* (London: MacGibbon and Kee, 1968), 81.

39. Cleland, *Memoirs*, 33.

40. Erasmus Darwin, *Phytologia* (London: J. Johnson, 1800), 103.

41. Erasmus Darwin, *The Temple of Nature* (London: J. Johnson, 1803), canto ii, lines 245–6. See Londa Schiebinger, *Nature's Body: Gender in the Making of Modern Science* (Boston, Mass.: Beacon Press, 1993).

42. Erasmus Darwin, *The Botanic Garden* (London: J. Johnson, 1791), canto i, lines 61–2. Janet Browne, 'Botany for Gentlemen: Erasmus Darwin and *The Loves of the Plants*', *Isis*, lxxx (1989), 593–612. In his *Essay on Woman* (London: privately printed, 1763), John Wilkes expressed this cosmic philosophy of sex in summary form: 'Life can little else supply/But a few good fucks and then we die.'

43. King-Hele, *Doctor of Revolution*, 242ff.

44. Boswell expounded to Belle de Zuylen, how, within marriage, he would expect to be free to pursue his sexual appetites where they took him.

When she replied she would expect the same freedom, he termed her a 'frantic libertine'. F. Pottle (ed.), *Boswell in Holland 1763–1764* (London: Heinemann, 1952), 279. Boswell remained deeply troubled as to how to square his desire for sexual freedom with his Christianity: see C. Ryskamp and F. A. Pottle (eds), *Boswell: the Ominous Years 1774–1776* (London: Heinemann, 1963; New York: McGraw-Hill, 1963), 74.

45. Williford, 'Bentham on the Rights of Women', 167–76, p. 171.
46. Quoted in Taylor, *The Angel Makers*, 7.
47. A. McLaren, *Birth Control in Nineteenth Century England* (London: Croom Helm, 1978), ch. 1; J. Blackman, 'Popular Theories of Generation: the Evolution of *Aristotle's Works*. The Study of an Anachronism', in J. Woodward and D. Richards (eds), *Health Care and Popular Medicine in Nineteenth Century England. Essays in the Social History of Medicine* (London: Croom Helm, 1977), 56–88. Francis Place reported reading *Aristotle's Master-piece* while at school: Thale (ed.), *Autobiography of Francis Place*, 45:

> I had read a book at that time openly sold, on every stall, called Aristotles Master Piece, it was a thick 18 mo, with a number of badly drawn cuts in it explanatory of the mystery of generation. This I contrived to borrow and compared parts of it with the accounts of the Miraculous Conception in Matthew and Luke.

48. Plentiful evidence can be found in books such as Bloch, *History of English Sexual Morals*; Hunt, *Natural History of Love*; N. C. Epton, *Love and the English* (Cleveland, NY: World Publishing; London: Cassell, 1960); G. Rattray Taylor, *Sex in History*, new edn (London: Thames and Hudson, 1959).
49. D. Foxon, *Libertine Literature in England 1660–1745* (New York: University Books, 1965); Peter Wagner, *Eros Revived: Erotica of the Enlightenment in England and America* (London: Secker and Warburg, 1988).
50. R. Alter, '*Tristram Shandy* and the Game of Love', *American Scholar*, xxxvii

(1968), 316–23. F. Brady, '*Tristram Shandy*, Sexuality, Morality, and Sensibility', *Eighteenth Century Studies*, iv (1970–1), 41–56, where on p. 49 Brady writes of Sterne's 'hedonistic delight in the joys of the senses'.
51. D. A. Coward, 'Eighteenth-Century Attitudes to Prostitution', *Studies on Voltaire and the Eighteenth Century*, clxxxix (1980), 363–99; A. R. Henderson, 'Female Prostitution in London, 1730–1830' (PhD dissertation, University of London, 1992).
52. Pottle, *Boswell's London Journal*, 255. 'Armour' is a condom.
53. A. Spencer (ed.), *Memoirs of William Hickey*, 6th edn, 4 vols (London: Hurst and Blackett, 1923–5), Vol. I, 12.
54. Quoted in A. Parreaux, *Daily Life in England in the Reign of George III*, trans. C. Congreve (London: Allen and Unwin, 1969), 127.
55. Stone, *Broken Lives*, 39.
56. Thale (ed.), *Autobiography of Francis Place*, 71.
57. W. K. Wimsatt and F. A. Pottle (eds), *Boswell for the Defence, 1769–1774* (New York: McGraw Hill, 1959), 76. Of course, there were limits to tolerance: in 1792 Mrs Siddons took it very badly when her husband gave her the pox.
58. Quoted in Stone, *Family, Sex and Marriage*, 621.
59. J. Greig (ed.), *The Letters of David Hume*, 2 vols (Oxford: Clarendon Press, 1932), Vol. II, 319.
60. Quoted in Taylor, *The Angel Makers*, 191.
61. Thale (ed.), *Autobiography of Francis Place*, 81.
62. This point is well made by T. Gibson, *The English Vice: Beating, Sex and Shame in Victorian England and After* (London: Duckworth, 1978), 12. See for example this verse on a child's sampler of 1842, from the Doll's Museum, Warwick:

> How gracious and how wise
> Is our chastising God
> And Oh how much the blessings are
> Which blossom from his rod.
>
> He lifts it up on high
> With pity in His heart
> And every stroke his children feel
> May grace and peace impart.

63. Cleland, *Memoirs*, 138.
64. *Ibid.*, 141.
65. *Ibid.*, 115.
66. Quaife, *Wanton Wenches and Wayward Wives*; Addy, *Sin and Society*; Ingram, *Church Courts, Sex and Marriage*.
67. Groups such as the Evangelicals seeking to clean up public life did not particularly look to parliamentary legislation to serve their purposes. Public opinion remained hostile to bowdlerization. See N. Perrin, *Dr Bowdler's Legacy: a History of Expurgated Books in England and America* (New York: Atheneum, 1969; London: Macmillan, 1970). Chaucer was first expurgated in 1795 (US edn, p. 53).
68. Henry Fielding, *An Enquiry into the Causes of the Late Increase in Robberies* (London: A. Miller, 1751), 47.
69. H. F. B. Compston, *The Magdalen Hospital* (London: SPCK, 1917), 42–3. Of course, humanitarianism had its limits: in 1783 the hospital declined to admit a black woman (p. 200). See also J. Bettley, '*Post Voluptatem Misericordia*: The Rise and Fall of the London Lock Hospitals', *The London Journal*, x (ii) (1984), 167–75.
70. Bristow, *Vice and Vigilance*; see also J. Redwood, *Reason, Ridicule and Religion* (London: Thames and Hudson, 1976), 182 ff.
71. *Arminian Magazine*, xii (1789), 496.
72. For inequalities see K. Thomas, 'The Double Standard', *Journal of the History of Ideas*, xx (1959), 195–216; Patricia Meyer Spacks, ' "Ev'ry Woman is at Heart a Rake" ', *Eighteenth Century Studies*, viii (1974–5), 27–46. For Enlightenment upgrading of women, see E. Jacobs, W. H. Barber, J. H. Bloch, F. W. Leakey and E. Le Breton (eds), *Woman and Society in Eighteenth Century France* (London: Athlone Press, 1980); M. LeGates, 'The Cult of Womanhood in Eighteenth Century Thought', *Eighteenth Century Studies*, x (1976), 21–40; K. B. Clinton, 'Femme et Philosophe: Enlightenment Origins of Feminism', *Eighteenth Century Studies*, viii (1975), 283–300. For Mary Wollstonecraft, see C. Tomalin, *The Life and Death of Mary Wollstonecraft* (London: Weidenfeld and Nicolson, 1974).
73. C. McC. Weis and F. A. Pottle (eds), *Boswell in Extremes* (New York: McGraw-Hill, 1970), 180.
74. Taylor, *The Angel Makers*, 4.
75. For this retreat into primness see A. Wallas, *Before the Bluestockings* (London: Allen and Unwin, 1929); M. A. Hopkins, *Hannah More and her Circle* (New York: Longmans, Green, 1947); Elizabeth Kowaleski-Wallace, *Their Fathers' Daughters: Hannah More, Maria Edgeworth, and Patriarchal Complicity* (Oxford and New York: Oxford University Press, 1991).
76. A. Comfort, *The Anxiety Makers: Some Curious Preoccupations of the Medical Profession* (New York: Nelson, 1967); E. H. Hare, 'Masturbatory Insanity: the History of an Idea', *Journal of Mental Science*, cviii (1962), 1–25; R. H. MacDonald, 'The Frightful Consequences of Onanism: Notes on the History of a Delusion', *Journal of the History of Ideas*, xxviii (1967), 423–31.
77. L. DeMause, 'The Evolution of Childhood', in L. DeMause (ed.), *The History of Childhood* (New York: Psychohistory Press, 1974), 1–73; P. Coveney, *Poor Monkey: The Child in Literature* (London: Rockliff, 1957).
78. Kent Gerard and Gert Hekma (eds), *The Pursuit of Sodomy: Male Homosexuality in Renaissance and Enlightenment Europe* (New York: Harrington Park, 1989); H. Montgomery Hyde, *The Other Love* (London: Heinemann, 1970); A. L. Rowse, *Homosexuals in History* (London: Weidenfeld and Nicolson, 1977), where (p. 111) Rowse writes, 'Regency society was flagrantly shameless in its sex life, provided it was heterosexual'. A. D. Harvey, 'Prosecution for Sodomy in England at the Beginning of the Nineteenth Century', *Historical Journal*, xxi (1978), 939–48; A. N. Gilbert, 'Sexual Deviance and Disaster during the Napoleonic Wars', *Albion*, ix (1977), 98–113; Lesbianism seems to have been regarded by men with tolerant condescension. Emma Donoghue, *Passions between Women: British Lesbian Culture 1668–1801* (London: Scarlet Press, 1993).
79. Quoted in Taylor, *The Angel Makers*, 274.
80. Romantic friendships form an in-between case. See Lillian Faderman,

Surpassing the Love of Men: Romantic Friendship and Love between Women from the Renaissance to the Present (New York: Morrow, 1981); *idem, Scotch Verdict: Dame Gordon vs. Pirie and Woods* (New York: Morrow, 1983); Louis Crompton, *Byron and Greek Love: Homophobia in Nineteenth Century England* (Berkeley: University of California Press, 1985); G. S. Rousseau, 'The Pursuit of Homosexuality in the Eighteenth Century: "Utterly Confused Category" and/or Rich Repository?', *Eighteenth-Century Life,* ix (1985), 132–68.

81. W. Godwin, *Enquiry concerning Political Justice,* ed. I. Kramnick (Harmondsworth: Penguin, 1978), 756. On the basis of Enlightenment individualistic and libertarian principles Godwin pronounced marriage the 'worst of monopolies' (p. 762), and demanded emotional and sexual freedom.

82. Cleland, *Memoirs,* 207.

83. *Ibid.,* 135.

84. *Ibid.,* 117.

85. *Ibid.*

86. Advertisement taken from *A Collection of Cuttings . . . Referring to James Graham,* in the Library of the Wellcome Institute for the History of Medicine, London, Acc. No. 73143.

87. For the medico-physiological background see G. S. Rousseau, 'Nerves, Spirits and Fibres: Towards Defining the Origins of Sensibility; with a postscript, 1976', *The Blue Guitar,* ii (Rome, 1976), 125–53; *idem,* 'Science and the Discovery of the Imagination in Enlightened England', *Eighteenth Century Studies,* iii (1969), 109–35; *idem,* 'Psychology' in G. S. Rousseau and Roy Porter (eds), *The Ferment of Knowledge* (Cambridge: Cambridge University Press, 1980), 143–210; *idem,* 'Towards a Semiotics of the Nerve: The Social History of Language in a New Key', in Peter Burke and Roy Porter (eds), *Language, Self and Society: The Social History of Language* (Cambridge: Polity Press, 1991), 213–75.

88. Francis Hutcheson, *A System of Moral Philosophy,* 2 vols (Glasgow: published by his son F. Hutcheson, 1755), Vol. II, 151–2.

89. Cleland, *Memoirs,* 150.

90. *Ibid.,* 48.

91. *Ibid.,* 192.

92. *Ibid.,* 146.

93. Strachey (ed.), *Letters of Chesterfield,* Vol. II, 59.

94. M. Price, *To the Palace of Wisdom* (New York: Doubleday, 1964), 444; for the complexities of Blake's attitudes to the body see T. R. Frosch, *The Awakening of Albion: the Renovation of the Body in the Poetry of William Blake* (Ithaca, NY: Cornell University Press, 1974), and more broadly, J. Benthall, *The Body Electric* (London: Thames and Hudson, 1976).

95. See Taylor, *The Angel Makers,* Brown, *Father of the Victorians;* Quinlan, *Victorian Prelude;* Jaeger, *Before Victoria;* P. Fryer, *Mrs Grundy: Studies in English Prudery* (London: Dennis Dobson, 1963); E. Trudgill, *Madonnas and Magdalens: The Origins and Development of Victorian Sexual Attitudes* (New York: Holmes and Meier, 1976). Nineteenth-century sexual repression of course took the form of physical mutilation of manuscripts in order to expunge sexual passages, as happened to Francis Place's collections. David Vincent has pointed out how working-class autobiographers in the nineteenth century found it impossible to discuss their sex lives: 'Love and Death and the Nineteenth Century Working Class', *Social History,* v (1980), 223–48.

96. *The Works of Beilby Porteus, Late Bishop of London: With His Life by Robert Hodgson,* new edn, 6 vols (London: T. Cadell and W. Davies, 1811), Vol. II, 217.

97. *Evangelical Magazine,* i (1793), 79.

98. John Styles, *An Essay on the Character, Immoral and Antichristian Tendency of the Stage* (London: printed for the author, 1806), 37.

2   *Medical Folklore in High and Low Culture:* Aristotle's Master-Piece

1. The best modern survey of the range of erotica is Peter Wagner, *Eros Revived: Erotica of the Enlightenment in England and America* (London: Secker and Warburg, 1988). It should be emphasized here that, while we draw upon

developments beyond Britain, we are principally investigating British authors and works published in Britain.

2. Gilbert D. McEwen, *The Oracle of the Coffee-House: John Dunton's 'Athenian Mercury'* (The Huntington Library, San Marino, Ca.: 1972).

3. Roger Thompson, *Unfit for Modest Ears: A Study of Pornographic, Obscene and Bawdy Works Written or Published in England in the Second Half of the Seventeenth Century* (London: Macmillan, 1979). Apart from Culpeper, other roughly contemporary works containing miscellaneous sexual advice include [Anon.], *Marriage Promoted. In a Discourse of its Ancient and Modern Practice, Both under Heathen and Christian Common-Wealths* (London: printed for R. Baldwin, 1690); John Maubray, *The Female Physician* (London: J. Holland, 1724); Jane Sharp, *The Complete Midwife's Companion: or, the Art of Midwifery Improv'd* (London: J. Marshall, 1724). Immensely valuable on all the contextual issues covered in this chapter is Patricia Crawford, 'Sexual Knowledge in England, 1500–1750', in Roy Porter and Mikuláš Teich (eds), *Sexual Knowledge, Sexual Science: The History of Attitudes to Sexuality* (Cambridge: Cambridge University Press, 1994), 82–106.

4. C. J. S. Thompson, *The Mystery and Lore of Monsters* (London: Williams and Norgate, 1930); Dudley Watson, *Signs and Portents: Monstrous Births from the Middle Ages* (London and New York: Routledge, 1993); K. Park and L. J. Daston, 'Unnatural Conceptions: The Study of Monsters in Sixteenth Century France and England', *Past and Present*, xcii (1981), 20–54.

5. Helkiah Crooke, *Microcosmographia* (London: W. Jaggard, 1615). For the genre of popular anatomies and books of health, see Andrew Wear, 'The Popularization of Medicine in Early Modern England', in Roy Porter (ed.), *The Popularization of Medicine, 1650–1850* (London: Routledge, 1992), 17–41. For disputes about the interpretation of the body at this time, see Emma U. H. Seymour, 'Bodying Forth the Mind: Mind, Body and Metaphor, 1590–1640' (PhD thesis, University of Cambridge, 1993) and Gail Kern

Paster, *The Body Embarrassed: Drama and the Disciplines of Shame in Early Modern England* (Ithaca, NY: Cornell University Press, 1993); Jonathan Sawday, *The Mirror and the Knife: The Renaissance Culture of Dissection* (London: Routledge, forthcoming).

6. H. J. Norman, 'John Bulwer and his *Anthropometamorphosis*', in E. Ashworth Underwood (ed.), *Science, Medicine and History. Essays on the Evolution of Scientific Thought and Medical Practice*, Vol. II (Oxford: Oxford University Press, 1953), 80–99.

7. Jacques Ferrand, *A Treatise on Lovesickness*, trans. and ed. Donald A. Beecher and Massimo Ciavolella (Syracuse, New York: Syracuse University Press, 1990).

8. For an introduction to Burton see L. Babb, *Sanity in Bedlam: A Study of Robert Burton's 'Anatomy of Melancholy'* (East Lansing: Michigan State University Press, 1959). The modern scholarly edition contains a first-rate discussion of the sources of Burton's learning: see Robert Burton, *The Anatomy of Melancholy*, Vol. I: *Text – 'Democritus Junior to the Reader' and 'The First Partition'*, ed. Thomas C. Faulkner, Nicolas K. Kiessling and Rhonda L. Blair (Oxford: Oxford University Press, 1989).

9. Three excellent works now survey medieval philosophical and medico-academic works on this area: Joan Cadden, *Meanings of Sex Difference in the Middle Ages: Medicine, Science and Culture* (Cambridge and New York: Cambridge University Press, 1993); Pierre J. Payer, *The Bridling of Desire: Views of Sex in the Later Middle Ages* (Toronto: Toronto University Press, 1993), and Danielle Jacquart and Claude Thomasset, *Sexualité et savoir médical au Moyen Age* (Paris: Presses Universitaires de France, 1985), trans. Matthew Adamson as *Sexuality and Medicine in the Middle Ages* (Cambridge: Polity Press, 1989). For discussion of texts, see Brian Lawn (ed.), *The Prose Salernitan Questions* (London: Oxford University Press, 1979). Also well worth consulting are Alexandre Leupin, *Barbarolexis: Medieval Writing and Sexuality*, trans. Kate Cooper (Cambridge, Mass.: Harvard Univer-

sity Press, 1989); Helen Rodnite Lemay, 'Human Sexuality in Twelfth through Fifteenth Century Scientific Writings', in Vern L. Bullough (ed.), *Sexual Practices and the Medieval Church* (Buffalo, NY: Prometheus, 1982), 187–205; Renate Blumenfeld-Kosinski, *Not of a Woman Born: Representations of Caesarean Birth in Medieval and Renaissance Culture* (Ithaca, NY: Cornell University Press, 1990); Caroline Walker Bynum, *Fragmentation and Redemption: Essays on Gender and the Human Body in Medieval Religion* (New York: Zone Books, 1991), which warns against anachronistic readings of what 'sex' was. See also James A. Brundage, *Law, Sex and Christian Society in Medieval Europe* (Chicago: University of Chicago Press, 1988); Vern L. Bullough and James Brundage, *Sexual Practices and the Medieval Church* (Buffalo, NY: Prometheus, 1982); Beryl Rowlands, *Medieval Woman's Guide to Health: The First English Gynecological Handbook* (Kent, Ohio: Kent State University Press, 1981); Jan Ziolkowski, *Alan of Lille's Grammar of Sex: The Meaning of Grammar to a Twelfth-Century Intellectual* (Cambridge, Mass.: Medieval Academy of America, 1985); Marie-Christine Pouchelle, *The Body and Surgery in the Middle Ages* (Cambridge: Polity Press, 1989). Recent scholarship conclusively destroys the canard that medieval learning or the medieval mind was somehow un-interested in matters sexual. For this, see William Eamon, *Science and the Secrets of Nature. Books of Secrets in Medieval and Early Modern Culture* (Princeton: Princeton University Press, 1994), 73ff.

10. R. Howard Bloch, *Medieval Misogyny and the Invention of Western Romantic Love* (Chicago: University of Chicago Press, 1991); Mary F. Wack, *Lovesickness in the Middle Ages: The 'Viaticum' and Its Commentaries* (Philadelphia: University of Pennsylvania Press, 1990); C. S. Lewis, *The Allegory of Love: A Study in Medieval Tradition* (London: Oxford University Press, 1959).

11. The most challenging study of this literature is Thomas W. Laqueur, *Making Sex. Gender and the Body from Aristotle to Freud* (Cambridge, Mass.: Harvard University Press, 1990). Laqueur is particularly concerned to recover the interpretative paradigm within which anatomical features and differences were understood. Many critics believe he presents too monolithic a reading of a situation typified by diversity of views. See also Johann L. Choulant, *History and Bibliography of Anatomic Illustration in its Relation to Anatomic Science and the Graphic Arts*, trans. Mortimer Frank (Chicago: University of Chicago Press, 1920; revised edn New York: Schuman's, 1945); K. B. Roberts, *The Fabric of the Body: European Traditions of Anatomical Illustration* (Oxford and New York: Clarendon Press, 1992); Londa Schiebinger, 'Skeletons in the Closet: The First Illustrations of the Female Skeleton in Eighteenth-Century Anatomy', in Catherine Gallagher and Thomas Laqueur (eds), *The Making of the Modern Body: Sexuality and Society in the Nineteenth Century* (Berkeley: University of California Press, 1987), 42–82; Sander Gilman, *Sexuality: An Illustrated History* (New York: Wiley, 1989).

12. See David Cressy, *Literacy and the Social Order: Reading and Writing in Tudor and Stuart England* (Cambridge: Cambridge University Press, 1980); idem, 'Literacy in Context: Meaning and Measurement in Early Modern England', in John Brewer and Roy Porter (eds), *Consumption and the World of Goods* (London and New York: Routledge, 1993), 305–19; R. A. Houston, *Literacy in Early Modern Europe: Culture and Education, 1500–1800* (London: Longman, 1988); Mary E. Fissell, 'Readers, Texts and Contexts: Vernacular Medical Works in Early Modern England', in Roy Porter (ed.), *The Popularization of Medicine 1650–1850* (London and New York: Routledge, 1992), 72–91; Margaret Spufford, *Small Books and Pleasant Histories: Popular Fiction and its Readership in Seventeenth-Century England* (London: Methuen; Athens: University of Georgia Press, 1981); Alain Boureau and Roger Chartier (eds), *The Culture of Print: Power and the Uses of Print in Early Modern Europe*, ed. Roger Chartier (Cambridge: Polity Press, 1989); idem, *The Order of*

Books, trans. Ludia M. Cochrane (Cambridge: Polity Press, 1993); Peter Burke, 'Popular Culture in Seventeenth Century London', *London Journal*, iii (1977), 143–62; *idem*, *Popular Culture in Early Modern Europe* (London: Temple Smith, 1978).

13. Neil McKendrick, John Brewer and J. H. Plumb, *The Birth of a Consumer Society: The Commercialization of Eighteenth-Century England* (London: Europa, 1982); Carole Shammas, *The Pre-Industrial Consumer in England and America* (Oxford: Clarendon Press, 1990); Lorna Weatherill, *Consumer Behaviour and Material Culture, 1660–1760* (London: Routledge, 1988); John Brewer and Roy Porter (eds), *Consumption and the World of Goods* (London: Routledge, 1993).

14. Fenella Childs, 'Prescriptions for Manners in Eighteenth Century Courtesy Literature' (DPhil dissertation, Oxford University, 1984); L. A. Curtis, 'A Case Study of Defoe's Domestic Conduct Manuals Suggested by *The Family, Sex and Marriage in England 1500–1800*', *Studies in Eighteenth Century Culture*, x (1981), 409–28.

15. Jeremy Black, *The English Press in the Eighteenth Century* (London: Croom Helm, 1986); I. Rivers (ed.), *Books and their Readers in Eighteenth Century England* (Leicester: Leicester University Press, 1982); D. Foxon, *Libertine Literature in England 1660–1745* (New York: University Books, 1965); J. Feather, 'The Commerce of Letters: The Study of the Eighteenth Century Book Trade', *Eighteenth Century Studies*, xvii (1984), 405–24.

16. J. H. Plumb, *The Commercialization of Leisure in Eighteenth Century England* (Reading: University of Reading Press, 1973). For popular medical advice, see Roy Porter (ed.), *The Popularization of Medicine, 1650–1850* (London: Routledge, 1992); *idem*, 'Lay Medical Knowledge in the Eighteenth Century: the Case of the *Gentleman's Magazine*', *Medical History*, xxix (1985), 138–68; *idem*, 'Laymen, Doctors and Medical Knowledge in the Eighteenth Century: The Evidence of the *Gentleman's Magazine*', in Roy Porter (ed.), *Patients and Practitioners: Lay Perceptions of Medicine in Pre-Industrial Society* (Cambridge:

Cambridge University Press, 1985), 283–314.

17. See S. Parks, *John Dunton and the English Book Trade: a Study of his Career with a Checklist of his Publications* (New York: Garland, 1976).

18. *Rare Verities: The Cabinet of Venus Unlocked, and Her Secrets Laid Open* (London: P. Briggs, 1657) was a partial translation of Sinibaldus's *Geneanthropeiae, sivi de Hominis Generatione Decateuchon* (Rome, 1642).

19. It is interesting that at a time when Aristotle's reputation in elite culture was waning, thanks to the 'ancients *v.* moderns' debate, his name evidently retained its talismanic quality within popular culture. For Aristotle's sexual views see J. Morsink, *Aristotle on the Generation of Animals: A Philosophical Study* (Washington, DC: University Press of America, 1982). For *Aristotle's Master-Piece*, see J. Blackman, 'Popular Theories of Generation: The Evolution of *Aristotle's Works*. The Study of an Anachronism', in J. Woodward and D. Richards (eds), *Health Care and Popular Medicine in Nineteenth Century England: Essays in the Social History of Medicine* (London: Croom Helm, 1977), 56–88; V. Bullough, 'An Early American Sex Manual; or Aristotle Who?', *Early American Literature*, vii (1973), 236–46; Angus McLaren, 'The Pleasures of Procreation', in W. F. Bynum and Roy Porter (eds), *William Hunter and the Eighteenth Century Medical World* (Cambridge: Cambridge University Press, 1985), 323–420.

20. A prolific medical writer, and perhaps without any formal medical education, William Salmon (1644–1713) was author, amongst other works, of *Synopsis Medicinae* (London: C. Jones, 1671); *Seplasium. The Compleat English Physician* (London: Gilliflower and Sawbridge, 1693); *The Country Physician, or A Choice Collection of Physick Fitted for Vulgar Use* (London: John Taylor, 1703); *Collectanea Medica, the Country Physician* (London: J. Taylor, 1703); *The Family-Dictionary* (London: H. Rhodes, 1696); and *Botanologia. The English Herbal* (London: N. Rhodes and J. Taylor, 1710). See R. L. Meade-King, 'Notes from a Seventeenth Century Textbook of Medicine', *British*

Medical Journal, ii (1906), 433–5. On the growth and style of popular medical writers after 1660, see Harold J. Cook, 'Sir John Colbatch and Augustan Medicine: Experimentalism, Character and Entrepreneurialism', *Annals of Science,* xlvii (1991), 495–6; *idem,* 'Good Advice and Little Medicine: The Professional Authority of Early Modern English Physicians', *Journal of British Studies,* xxxiii (1994), 1–31.

21. G. L. Simons, *Sex and Superstition* (London: Abelard-Schuman, 1973).

22. D'Arcy Power, *The Foundations of Medical History* (Baltimore, Md.: Johns Hopkins University Press, 1931), Lecture vi, *'Aristotle's Master-Piece'*, 147.

23. *Ibid.,* 168.

24. Otho T. Beall, Jr., *'Aristotle's Master-Piece* in America; a Landmark in the Folklore of Medicine', *William and Mary Quarterly,* 3rd series, xx (1963), 207–22, p. 220; P. -G. Boucé, 'Some Sexual Beliefs and Myths in Eighteenth Century Britain', in Boucé (ed.), *Sexuality in Eighteenth Century Britain* (Manchester: Manchester University Press, 1982), 28–46, p. 36. Boucé suggests the 'myths' contained in *Aristotle's Master-Piece* are redolent of 'pre-logical *mentalité'*, p. 30.

25. Blackman, 'Popular Theories of Generation', 56–88, p. 83. It is, she suggests, a 'substitute for thought' (p. 84).

26. For Enlightenment ideas on sexuality see the preceding chapter and J. Hagstrum, *Sex and Sensibility: Ideal and Erotic Love from Milton to Mozart* (Chicago and London: University of Chicago Press, 1980).

27. Compare Margaret Spufford's comment on sex in contemporary chapbooks: 'the whole tenor of the merry books conveys that seventeenth-century women enjoyed their own sexuality and were expected to enjoy it': *Small Books and Pleasant Histories,* 63; V. E. Neuburg, *Popular Literature; A History and Guide* (Harmondsworth: Penguin, 1977).

28. Version 3 will be quoted throughout from *Aristotle's Master-Piece* (London: 12th edn, early eighteenth century). This reference will be followed in brackets by a page number reference

to *The Works of Aristotle in Four Parts* (London: All the Booksellers, 1796). Thus: p. 32 (25).

29. *Ibid.,* 47 (40).

30. *Ibid.,* 40–41 (31–2).

31. *Ibid.,* 11 (7).

32. Version 2 will be quoted throughout from *Aristotle's Master-Piece* (London: printed for D. P., 1710). Figures in brackets give the page numbers of *The Works of Aristotle, the Famous Philosopher* (London, printed for Archibald Whisleton, Chiswell Street, n. d. but *c.* 1810). Thus: 9 (8).

33. Michel Foucault, *Histoire de la sexualité,* Vol. I: *La volonté de savoir* (Paris: Gallimard, 1976), trans. Robert Hurley, *The History of Sexuality: Introduction* (London: Allen Lane, 1978; New York: Vintage Books, 1985). For helpful warnings about the pitfalls of back-projecting modern sexology, see Jeffrey Weeks, *Sex, Politics and Society: The Regulation of Sexuality since 1800* (London: Longman, 1981); M. Ignatieff, 'Homo Sexualis', *London Review of Books,* 4–17 March, 1982, 8–9; S. Heath, *The Sexual Fix* (New York: Schocken; London: Macmillan, 1982); Paul Robinson, *The Modernization of Sex: Havelock Ellis, Alfred Kinsey, William Masters and Virginia Johnsom* (New York: Harper and Row, 1976).

34. Before there can be a modern sexual self, there must first be a modern self: see C. Taylor, *Sources of the Self. The Making of Modern Identity* (Cambridge: Cambridge University Press, 1989).

35. See Contents Lists reproduced in the Appendix, pp. 54–63.

36. James Graham, *Lecture on the Generation of the Human Species* (London: printed for the author, 1780).

37. *Aristotle's Master-Piece* (12th edn), 39 (31).

38. Venette and Graham would have agreed. See Roy Porter, 'The Sexual Politics of James Graham', *British Journal for Eighteenth Century Studies,* v (1982), 201–6.

39. *Aristotle's Master-Piece* (12th edn), 39 (30).

40. *Ibid.,* 45 (35).

41. Version 1 will be quoted throughout from *Aristotle's Master-Piece or the Secrets*

of Generation Display'd in all the Parts Thereof (London: J. How, 1690). See the Introduction: 'God, having created man added Allurements, and desire of mutual Embracing, so that they might in Procreation be sweetly affected and delighted by wonderous ways: For unless this was natural to all kinds of Creatures, they would be regardless of Posterity, and Procreation would cease; whereby Mankind would quickly be lost, and the Affairs of Mortals of no Continuance'. See also Aristotle's Master-Piece (1710), 9 (5).

42. Aristotle's Master-Piece: or The Secrets of Generation Displayed in All the Parts Thereof (London: F. L. for J. How, 1690).

43. Aristotle's Master-Piece (12th edn), 9 (5).

44. Ibid., Introduction, 9 (5). For the natural philosophy of organic growth – surviving, despite the mechanical philosophy of the Scientific Revolution – see Carolyn Merchant, The Death of Nature: Women, Ecology and the Scientific Revolution (New York: Harper and Row, 1980; London: Wildwood House, 1982); D. Hirst, Hidden Riches (London: Eyre and Spottiswoode, 1964).

45. Aristotle's Master-Piece (1690), Introduction.

46. Aristotle's Master-Piece (12th edn), 9 (5).

47. For discussions of homosexuality see P.-G. Boucé, 'Aspects of Sexual Tolerance and Intolerance in Eighteenth Century England', British Journal for Eighteenth Century Studies, iii (1980), 173–89; and idem, 'Some Sexual Beliefs and Myths', 36; and A. Bray, Homosexuality in Renaissance England (London: Gay Men's Press, 1982); Kent Gerard and Gert Hekma (eds), The Pursuit of Sodomy: Male Homosexuality in Renaissance and Enlightenment Europe (New York: Harrington Park, 1989); Jonathan Goldberg, Sodometries: Renaissance Texts, Modern Sexualities (Stanford, Calif.: Stanford University Press, 1992); Alan Graham Stewart, 'The Bounds of Sodomy: Textual Relations in Early Modern England' (PhD thesis, University of London, 1993).

48. For nymphomania or the furor uterinus, see G. S. Rousseau, 'Nymphomania, Bienville and the Rise of Erotic Sensibility', in P.-G. Boucé (ed.), Sexuality in Eighteenth Century

Britain (Manchester: Manchester University Press, 1982), 95–119, and M. D. T. de Bienville, Nymphomania, or, A Dissertation Concerning the Furor Uterinus (London: J. Bew, 1775).

49. No edition of Aristotle's Master-Piece jumped on to the bandwagon fear of masturbation, for which see Robert H. MacDonald, 'The Frightful Consequences of Onanism: Notes on the History of a Delusion', Journal of the History of Ideas, xxviii (1967), 423–31.

50. Aristotle's Master-Piece (1710), 76–7 (43). The counter-belief, that Venus and Bacchus didn't mix, became common amongst Enlightenment figures such as James Graham and Erasmus Darwin.

51. For relations between sex and the family see Jean-Louis Flandrin, Le Sexe et l'Occident (Paris: Seuil, 1981).

52. On Aristotle's Master-Piece and nineteenth-century Malthusianism, see Angus McLaren, Birth Control in Nineteenth Century England (London: Croom Helm, 1978), 28–9, 78–9, 84–5, 222–3, 238–9.

53. Aristotle's Master-Piece (1690), 1.

54. See E. A. Wrigley and R. S. Schofield, The Population History of England 1541–1871 (London: Edward Arnold, 1981).

55. Aristotle's Master-Piece (1690), ch. 7.

56. Ibid., 3. Medical measures such as purges were also suggested: p. 71ff. See also Aristotle's Master-Piece (12th edn), 30 (22); (1796), 22; and I. Loudon, 'Chlorosis, Anaemia and Anorexia Nervosa', British Medical Journal, cclxxxi (1980), 1–19; idem, 'The Diseases called Chlorosis', Psychological Medicine, xiv (1984), 27–36; Jean Astruc, A Treatise on all the Diseases Incident to Women (London: Cooper, 1743). 'Green sickness' was supposedly a wasting disorder of teenage girls. It might be seen as connected with what we would call anorexia nervosa.

57. Aristotle's Master-Piece (1690), 58. Barrenness is endlessly represented in the literature of the time as the punishment for sexual lewdness.

58. Aristotle's Master-Piece (12th edn), 27 (20).

59. Aristotle's Master-Piece (1690), 55.

60. Ibid., 10.

61. Ibid.; see also P. Crawford, 'Attitudes to Menstruation in Seventeenth Century

England', *Past and Present*, xci (1981), 47–73.

62. For menstruation as polluting, see E. Shorter, *A History of Women's Bodies* (London: Allen Lane, 1982; Harmondsworth: Penguin, 1983); Penelope Shuttle and Peter Redgrove, *The Wise Wound: Menstruation and Everywoman* (London: Gollancz, 1978); for monsters, see Marie-Hélène Huet, *Monstrous Imagination* (Cambridge, Mass.: Harvard University Press, 1993); Dudley Wilson, *Signs and Portents: Monstrous Births from the Middle Ages to the Enlightenment* (London: Routledge, 1993).

63. *The Works of Aristotle* (London: printed for Archibald Whistleton, Chiswell Street, n. d. but *c.* 1810), 43.

64. *Aristotle's Master-Piece* (1690), ch. 2; see Angus McLaren, *Reproductive Rituals: The Perception of Fertility in England from the Sixteenth to the Nineteenth Century* (London and New York: Methuen, 1984).

65. *Ibid.*, 8; cf. *Aristotle's Master-Piece* (12th edn), 41 (32); *The Works of Aristotle* (*c.* 1810), 8.

66. *Aristotle's Master-Piece* (12th edn), 37–43 (29–33).

67. *Aristotle's Master-Piece* (1690), 114; *Aristotle's Master-Piece* (12th edn), 55 (44).

68. *Aristotle's Master-Piece* (12th edn), 44 (34). For the body symbols of left and right see B. Turner, *The Body and Society: Explorations in Social Theory* (Oxford: Basil Blackwell, 1984).

69. Turner, *The Body and Society*, 37–50; *Aristotle's Master-Piece* (1690), 50.

70. *The Works of Aristotle* (1796), 50.

71. *Aristotle's Master-Piece* (12th edn), 48 (38); *Aristotle's Master-Piece* (1690), 16, 34. For backgrounds to contemporary embryology see F. J. Cole, *Early Theories of Sexual Generation* (Oxford: Clarendon Press, 1930); S. Roe, *Matter, Life and Generation* (Cambridge: Cambridge University Press, 1981).

72. *Aristotle's Master-Piece* (1690), ch. 2.

73. *Ibid.*, 94ff.; and see P. Darmon, *Le Mythe de la procréation à l'âge baroque* (Paris: J. J. Pauvert, 1977).

74. A brief discussion can be found in Adrian Wilson, *The Making of Man-Midwifery: Women and Men in English Childbirth, 1700–1770* (London: University College Press, forthcoming 1995).

75. See Audrey Eccles, *Obstetrics and Gynaecology in Tudor and Stuart England* (London: Croom Helm, 1982); J. Donnison, *Midwives and Medical Men: A History of Inter-Professional Rivalries and Women's Rights* (London: Heinemann Educational, 1977); A. Wilson, 'William Hunter and the Varieties of Man-Midwifery', in W. F. Bynum and Roy Porter (eds), *William Hunter and the Eighteenth Century Medical World* (Cambridge: Cambridge University Press, 1985), 343–69; Wilson, *The Making of Man-Midwifery*.

76. *The Works of Aristotle* (*c.* 1810), 12.

77. Shorter, *History of Women's Bodies*, and Barbara Ehrenreich and Deirdre English, *Complaints and Disorders* (Old Westbury, NY: Feminist Press, 1973; London: Compendium, 1974).

78. Another text that treats of barrenness at great length is Guillaume de la Motte, *A General Treatise of Midwifery* (London: J. Waugh, 1746); see especially ch. 4. See also Germaine Greer, *Sex and Destiny* (London: Secker and Warburg, 1984), ch. 3: 'The Curse of Sterility'; McLaren, *Reproductive Rituals*, 38.

79. Though brief advice is given for restoring 'flaggy yards': *Aristotle's Master-Piece* (1690), 7.

80. *Ibid.*

81. *Aristotle's Master-Piece* (12th edn), 45 (36).

82. *Ibid.*

83. *Aristotle's Master-Piece* (1690), 53, 118ff.

84. *Ibid.*, 44–5.

85. *Ibid.*, 30; *Aristotle's Master-Piece* (1710), 26 (15).

86. Park and Daston, 'Unnatural Conceptions'; Thompson, *Mystery and Lore of Monsters*; L. Fiedler, *Freaks* (New York: Simon and Schuster, 1978). See also the discussion in J. Sergeant, *Solid Philosophy* (London: R. Clavil, 1697), 352ff.

87. *Aristotle's Master-Piece* (1690), 52; for men-beasts see Keith Thomas, *Man and the Natural World* (London: Allen Lane, 1983).

88. *Aristotle's Master-Piece* (1690), 52. For the wider perspective on witchcraft see Keith Thomas, *Religion and the Decline of Magic* (London: Weidenfeld and Nicolson, 1971).

89. *Aristotle's Master-Piece* (1710), ch. 5;

Aristotle's Master-Piece (1690), 46.

90. *Aristotle's Master-Piece* (1690), 43. Compare this report in the *Gentleman's Magazine*, xvi (1746), 270:

> *Monday April 28*
>
> The wife of one Rich. Haynes of Chelsea, aged 35 and mother of 16 fine children, was deliver'd of a monster, with nose and eyes like a lyon no palate to the mouth, hair on the shoulders, claws like a lion, instead of fingers, no breastbone, something surprising out of the navel as big as an egg, and one foot longer than the other. – She had been to see the lions in the Tower, where she was much terrify'd with the old lion's noise.

91. See for instance J. Blondel, *The Strength of Imagination in Pregnant Women Examin'd* (London: J. Peele, 1727), who denied the teaching; and the excellent discussion by Philip Wilson: '"Out of Sight, out of Mind?": The Daniel Turner–James Blondel Dispute over the Power of the Maternal Imagination', *Annals of Science*, xlix (1992), 63–85; McLaren, *Reproductive Rituals*, 38.

92. *Aristotle's Master-Piece* (1710), ch. 3.

93. *Aristotle's Master-Piece* (1690), 20.

94. See Laurence Sterne, *The Life and Opinions of Tristram Shandy*, ed. C. Ricks (Harmondsworth: Penguin, 1967); for debates on female rationality, see Sylvana Tomaselli, 'The Enlightenment Debate on Women', *History Workshop Journal*, xx (1985), 101–24; Paul Hoffman, *La Femme dans la pensée des lumières* (Paris: Ophrys, 1977); Vivien Jones (ed.), *Women in the Eighteenth Century: Constructions of Femininity* (London: Routledge, 1990).

95. *Aristotle's Master-Piece* (London: F. L. for J. How, 1690), 19.

96. *Ibid.*, 87; *Aristotle's Master-Piece* (1710), ch. 3.

97. *Aristotle's Master-Piece* (12th edn), 34–5 (26).

98. *Ibid.*, 36 (28).

99. *Aristotle's Master-Piece* (1690), 65.

100. For different approaches to the flesh and the body see F. Bottomley, *Attitudes to the Body in Western Christendom* (London: Lepus Books, 1979); T. R. Frosch, *The Awakening of Albion: The Renovation of the Body in the Poetry of William Blake* (Ithaca, NY: Cornell University Press, 1974).

101. Ebenezer Sibly, *The Medical Mirror; or, Treatise on the Impregnation of the Human Female. Shewing the Origin of Diseases, and the Principles of Life and Death* (London, 1794).

102. Wrigley and Schofield, *Population History of England.*

103. Contrast the flowery language of John Armstrong's *The Oeconomy of Love* (London: T. Cooper, 1736; 3rd edn 1739), lines 181–91:

> Recline your Cheek, with eager Kisses press
> Her balmy Lips, and drinking from her Eyes
> Resistless Love, the tender Flame confess,
> Ineffable but by the murmuring Voice
> Of genuine Joy; then hug and kiss again
> Stretch'd on the flow'ry turf, while joyful glows
> Thy manly pride, and throbbing with Desire
> Pants earnest, felt thro' all the obstacles
> That intervene: but Love, whose fervid Course
> Mountains nor Seas oppose, can soon remove
> Barriers so Slight. . . .

104. For the literary stratagems perhaps in operation here, see Fissell, 'Readers, Texts and Contexts'.

105. *The Works of Aristotle* (1796), 123.

106. *Aristotle's Master-Piece* (1710), 44 (24).

107. *Ibid.*

108. *Ibid.*, 26. Compare James A. Secord, 'Newton in the Nursery: Tom Telescope and the Philosophy of Tops and Balls, 1761–1838', *History of Science*, xxiii (1985), 127–51, which shows, by way of parallel, that children's books, for their part, were routinely ostensibly aimed at higher social groups than their actual readership; such is the flattery of hegemony.

109. *Aristotle's Master-Piece* (1710), 44 (26).

110. *Aristotle's Master-Piece* (1690), title-page. For the dynamic interaction of popular and polite culture, the 'great' and 'little' traditions, see Burke, *Popular Culture.*

111. *The Works of Aristotle* (*c.* 1810), Introduction.

112. The versions of *Aristotle's Master-Piece* play elaborate games with 'Aristotle' as the author of the work. *Cf. Aristotle's Master-Piece* (1710), 'To The Reader'.

113. For mixed feelings about the Ancients see R. F. Jones, *Ancients and Moderns* (St Louis: Washington University Press, 1961); B. J. Shapiro, *Probability and*

Certainty in Seventeenth Century England (Princeton, NJ: Princeton University Press, 1983). See also *Aristotle's Master-Piece* (1710), 25–6 (14).

114. *Aristotle's Master-Piece* (1710), 89 (50).
115. See Peter Burke, 'Popular Culture between History and Ethnology', *Ethnologi Europaea*, xiv (1984), 5–13.
116. See L. J. Jordanova, 'Natural Facts: A Historical Perspective on Science and Sexuality', in C. MacCormack and M. Strathern (eds), *Nature, Culture and Gender* (Cambridge: Cambridge University Press, 1980), 42–69.
117. For 'viriculture' see B. Easlea, *Science and Sexual Oppression: Patriarchy's Confrontation with Women and Nature* (London: Weidenfeld and Nicolson, 1981).
118. Though there is mention of Lamia in *Aristotle's Master-Piece* (1690), 59–60; for misogyny see K. M. Rogers, *The Troublesome Helpmate* (Seattle: University of Washington Press, 1966).
119. Nancy F. Cott, 'Passionlessness: An Interpretation of Victorian Sexual Ideology, 1790–1850', *Signs: Journal of Women in Culture and Society*, iv (1978), 219–36; S. Delamont and L. Duffin (eds), *The Nineteenth Century Woman. Her Cultural and Physical World* (London: Croom Helm, 1978); G. J. Barker-Benfield, *The Horrors of the Half-Known Life: Male Attitudes toward Women and Sexuality in Nineteenth-Century America* (New York: Harper and Row, 1976).
120. *Aristotle's Master-Piece* (1690), 13.
121. *Ibid.*, 15.
122. For the sexual construal of women in the eighteenth century see P. M. Spacks, 'Ev'ry Woman is at Heart a Rake', *Eighteenth Century Studies*, viii (1974–5), 27–46; Tomaselli, 'Enlightenment Debate on Women'.
123. *Aristotle's Master-Piece* (1690), 22, notes that deformed children are the products of feeble desire. *Aristotle's Master-Piece* (12th edn), 47 (37), argues that 'the greater the woman's desire of copulation is, the more likely she is to conceive'. The text adds that women approach the marriage bed with 'equal vigour' to the man: 30.
124. *Aristotle's Master-Piece* (1690), 93. There is a rather similar discussion in Sharp, *Complete Midwife's Companion*, ch. 12.
125. *Aristotle's Master-Piece* (12th edn), 23

(18). For the doctrines underpinning such views, see Laqueur, *Making Sex.*
126. *Aristotle's Master-Piece* (12th edn); *ibid.*, 22 (17–18).
127. See Hagstrum, *Sex and Sensibility.*
128. But for the complexities of the ideological uses of the concept of Nature see also S. Shapin, 'The Social Uses of Science', in G. S. Rousseau and Roy Porter (eds), *The Ferment of Knowledge* (Cambridge: Cambridge University Press, 1980), 93–142; Ludmilla Jordanova (ed.), *Languages of Nature: Critical Essays on Science and Literature* (London: Free Association Books, 1986); *idem, Sexual Visions* (Hemel Hempstead: Harvester, 1989).
129. For growing confidence in 'Nature' see B. Willey, *The Seventeenth Century Background* (London: Chatto and Windus, 1934); *idem, The Eighteenth Century Background* (London: Chatto and Windus, 1940); A. O. Lovejoy, *The Great Chain of Being* (Cambridge, Mass.: Harvard University Press, 1936), chs 7–8.

3   Doctors and the Medicalization of Sex in the Enlightenment

1. This is to oversimplify, for it is widely supposed that *Aristotle's Master-Piece* was written by the physician William Salmon. But Salmon's authorship is a matter for conjecture; and he was, in any case, primarily a hack writer. Venette, by contrast, was a rather prominent physician, who wrote in the persona of a medical man. Although he hid the authorship of the first edition of his work under a pseudonym, his authorship quickly became well known.

This chapter draws on material earlier published in Roy Porter, 'Spreading Carnal Knowledge or Selling Dirt Cheap? Nicolas Venette's *Tableau de l'amour conjugal* in Eighteenth Century England', *Journal of European Studies*, xiv (1984), 233–55; and *idem*, 'Love, Sex and Medicine: Nicolas Venette and his *Tableau de l'amour conjugal*', in Peter Wagner (ed.), *Erotica and the Enlightenment* (Frankfurt: Lang, 1990), 90–122.

2. N. Venette, *La Génération de l'homme,*

new edn, 2 vols (Paris: no publisher, 1764), Vol. I, p. iv, 'Avis de l'Editeur'.

3. See Jean Flouret, *Nicolas Venette: Médecin Rochelais 1633–1698* (La Rochelle: Editions Rupella, 1992).

4. Guy Patin upheld Hippocratic theories against Harvey's double circulation theory. Because of the similarity between Venette's ideas of the *Tableau* and those of his teacher, the *Tableau* has sometimes been wrongly attributed to Guy Patin's son, Charles.

5. T. Zeldin, *France, 1848–1945. Ambition, Love, Politics* (Oxford: Clarendon Press, 1973), Vol. I, 296. Zeldin suggests that Venette's text may have been salutary, in reminding men 'that women had sexual demands that needed to be met'. Flouret, *Nicolas Venette*, is particularly strong on later editions.

6. P. Darmon, *Le Mythe de la procréation à l'âge baroque* (Paris: J. J. Pauvert, 1977).

7. See Roger Thompson, *Unfit for Modest Ears: A Study of Pornographic, Obscene and Bawdy Works Written or Published in England in the Second Half of the Seventeenth Century* (London: Macmillan, 1979); Peter Wagner, *Eros Revived: Erotica of the Enlightenment in England and America* (London: Secker and Warburg, 1988); Lynn Hunt (ed.), *The Invention of Pornography, 1500–1800* (New York: Zone Books, 1993); Jean-Marie Goulemot, *Reading the Erotic: The Uses of Pornographic Literature in Eighteenth-Century France* (Cambridge: Polity Press, 1994).

8. Angus McLaren, *Reproductive Rituals: The Perception of Fertility in England from the Sixteenth to the Nineteenth Century* (London and New York: Methuen, 1984), 36.

9. Audrey Eccles, *Obstetrics and Gynaecology in Tudor and Stuart England* (London: Croom Helm, 1982); Jean Donnison, *Midwives and Medical Men. A History of Inter-Professional Rivalries and Women's Rights* (London: Heinemann Educational, 1977); E. Shorter, *A History of Women's Bodies* (New York: Basic Books; London: Allen Lane, 1982; Harmondsworth: Penguin, 1983); B. This, *La Requête des enfants à naître* (Paris: Editions du Seuil, 1982); Adrian Wilson, *The Making of Man-Midwifery: Women and Men in English Childbirth, 1700–1770* (London: University College Press, forthcoming 1995).

10. J. Needham, *A History of Embryology* (Cambridge: Cambridge University Press, 1934); F. J. Cole, *Early Theories of Sexual Generation* (Oxford: Clarendon Press, 1930).

11. H. B. Adelmann, *Marcello Malpighi and the Evolution of Embryology*, 5 vols (Ithaca, NY: Cornell University Press, 1966). For venereal disease, see Jean Astruc, *A Treatise of the Venereal Disease*, trans. W. Barrowby (London: W. Innys and R. Manby, 1737).

12. Elizabeth Gasking, *Investigations into Generation, 1651–1828* (London: Hutchinson, 1967).

13. For example he speaks about men 'well hung' with large penises and 'swinging Parts' – they are nevertheless blockheads.

14. An English parallel is Robert Burton's *Anatomy of Melancholy*, ed. Thomas C. Faulkner *et al* (Oxford: Oxford University Press, 1989).

15. See M. C. Jacob, *The Radical Enlightenment* (London: Allen and Unwin, 1981); R. Darnton, *The Literary Underground of the Old Regime* (Cambridge, Mass.: Harvard University Press, 1982); Peter Burke, *Popular Culture in Early Modern Europe* (London: Temple Smith, 1978).

16. See A. Portal, *Histoire de l'anatomie et de la chirurgie* (Paris: Didot le Jeuen, 1770–3), Vol. IV, 202; 'l'anatomie est le dernier objet que cet Auteur se soit proposé. Il a rempli cet ouvrage d'histoires lascives et indécentes plus propres à corrompre la jeunesse qu'à l'instruire.' Venette's work received only one reference in *L'Encyclopédie* (SEMENCE, Vol. XIV, 940a, line 19). For these reasons, modern scholarship on Enlightenment medicine hardly mentions Venette. F. Duchesneau's *La Physiologie des lumières* (The Hague: M. M. Nijhoff, 1982) has no reference to him.

17. This fact is noted in Paul Hoffman, *La Femme dans la pensée des lumières* (Paris: Ophrys, 1977).

18. *Ibid.*

19. J. Hagstrum, *Sex and Sensibility: Ideal and Erotic Love from Milton to Mozart* (Chicago and London: University of Chicago Press, 1980).

20. F. Steegmuller (ed.), *The Letters of Gustave Flaubert*, Vol. I (Cambridge, Mass.: Belknap Press of Harvard University Press, 1980; London: Faber and Faber, 1981), 172 (Letter to Louise Colet, 22 Nov. 1852).

21. For the Dutch publishing history see H. F. Wijnman, '*Venus Minsieke Gasthuis*', in Herbert Lewandowski and P. J. van Dronen, *Beschavingson zedergeschiedenis van Nederland* (Amsterdam: N. V. Uitagevers-Maatschappy, 1983), 280–4. This valuable article must be used with some caution, however, as it too readily subscribes to a 'popularization spells corruption' reading. For example 'after which an enterprising publisher bought the remaining copies and replaced the old title page with a new ... : *The Minsieke Hospital of the Goddess of Love, or the Practices and Natural Properties of the Man and the Woman in the State of Marriage and the Gentle Sensation of the Embrace* (Alkmaar, 1797) 8°. So the completely out-dated book met an infamous end in this country; printed on low quality paper and fallen into the hands of a dubious publisher, nothing but unsavoury pornography remained' (p. 282). Dr A. Huussen of the Department of History at the State University of Groningen has been very helpful with this information.

22. In this respect it is characteristic of the age. See Darmon, *Le Mythe de la procréation à l'âge baroque*; Patricia Crawford, 'Sexual Knowledge in England, 1500–1750', in Roy Porter and Mikuláš Teich (eds), *Sexual Knowledge, Sexual Science: The History of Attitudes to Sexuality* (Cambridge: Cambridge University Press, 1994), 82–106.

23. Wagner, *Eros Revived*, 265–7.

24. See Roy Porter, 'The Sexual Politics of James Graham', *British Journal for Eighteenth Century Studies*, v (1982), 199–206; G. S. Rousseau, 'Nymphomania, Bienville and the Rise of Erotic Sensibility', in P.-G. Boucé (ed.), *Sexuality in Eighteenth Century Britain* (Manchester: Manchester University Press, 1982), 95–119; Peter Wagner, 'The Pornographer in the Courtroom; Trial Reports about Cases of Sexual Crimes and Delinquencies as a Genre of Eighteenth Century Erotica', *ibid.*, 120–40.

25. For such Renaissance paradoxes see R. Colie, *Paradoxia Epidemica* (Princeton, NJ: Princeton University Press, 1966).

26. *Ibid.*, 2.

27. For wider views see Iwan Bloch, *Sexual Life in England Past and Present*, trans. William H. Forstern (London: Arco, 1958); Morton M. Hunt, *The Natural History of Love* (New York: Knopf, 1959; London: Hutchinson, 1960); Nina C. Epton, *Love and the English* (Cleveland, NY: World Publishing; London: Cassell, 1960).

28. Lawrence Osborne, *The Poisoned Embrace: A Brief History of Sexual Pessimism* (London: Bloomsbury, 1993); Crawford, 'Sexual Knowledge in England'.

29. Vern L. Bullough and James Brundage, *Sexual Practices and the Medieval Church* (Buffalo, NY: Prometheus, 1982), 8:

> Saint Gregory of Nyssa in the fourth century AD dismissed marriage as a sad tragedy, while Saint Jerome (d. 420 AD) emphasized its inconveniences and tribulations. His views can perhaps be summarized in an oft-quoted passage: 'I praise marriage and wedlock, but I do so because they produce virgins for me. I gather roses from thorns, gold from the earth, and pearl from the shell.' Saint Ambrose (d. 397 AD) called marriage a 'galling burden', and urged all those contemplating matrimony to think about the bondage and servitude into which wedded love degenerated. With almost monotonous regularity, the Church Fathers argued that the wedded state was not as good as the single, celibate state. Though marriage was not quite evil, it could only count as thirty-fold, compared to the sixty-fold of widowhood and the hundred-fold of virginity.

30. Thompson, *Unfit for Modest Ears*; N. Davis, *Society and Culture in Early Modern France* (London: Duckworth,

1975); K. M. Rogers, *The Troublesome Helpmate. A History of Misogyny in Literature* (Seattle: University of Washington Press, 1966).

31. Lawrence Stone, *The Family, Sex and Marriage in England 1500–1800* (London: Weidenfeld and Nicolson, 1977); Edward Shorter, *The Making of the Modern Family* (New York: Basic Books, 1975; London: Collins, 1976); R. Trumbach, *The Rise of the Egalitarian Family: Aristocratic Kinship and Domestic Relations in Eighteenth Century England* (New York: Academic Press, 1978).

32. Hagstrum, *Sex and Sensibility.*

33. T. Tanner, *Adultery in the Novel* (Baltimore, Md.: Johns Hopkins University Press, 1979); Janet Todd, *Sensibility: An Introduction* (London: Methuen, 1986).

34. N. Venette, *The Mysteries of Conjugal Love Reveal'd* (London: S.N., 1712), Preface, 185. All subsequent quotations are from this edition unless otherwise indicated.

35. *Ibid.*, 136.

36. *Ibid.*, 91.

37. I. Maclean, *Woman Triumphant* (Oxford: Clarendon Press, 1977); Jean-Louis Flandrin, *Le Sexe et l'Occident* (Paris: Seuil, 1981); Edward le Comte, *Milton and Sex* (London: Macmillan, 1978).

38. Venette, *Mysteries of Conjugal Love Reveal'd*, 80.

39. For confidence in Nature see B. Willey, *The Seventeenth Century Background* (London: Chatto and Windus, 1934); idem, *The Eighteenth Century Background* (London: Chatto and Windus, 1940); A. O. Lovejoy, *The Great Chain of Being* (Cambridge, Mass.: Harvard University Press, 1936), chs 7–8.

40. Peter Brown, *The Body and Society: Men, Women and Sexual Renunciation in Early Christianity* (New York: Columbia University Press, 1988).

41. Marie Boas Hall, *Nature and Nature's Laws* (New York: Harper and Row, 1970).

42. Hagstrum, *Sex and Sensibility*; Hoffmann, *La Femme dans la pensée*; M. Delon, 'Le Prétexte anatomique', *Dix-Huitième Siècle*, xii (1980), 35–48.

43. For a specific example see W. Alexander, *The History of Women from the Earliest Antiquity to the Present Times*, 2 vols in 1 (London: W. Strahan and T. Cadell, 1779).

44. N. Bryson, *Word and Image* (Cambridge: Cambridge University Press, 1981); Lynda Nead, *The Female Nude: Art, Obscenity, and Sexuality* (New York: Routledge, 1992); P. Webb, *The Erotic Arts* (London: Secker and Warburg, 1975); J. B. Hess and L. Nochlin, *Women as Sex Objects* (London: Allen Lane, 1973); Roy Porter, 'The Exotic as Erotic: Captain Cook at Tahiti', in G. S. Rousseau and Roy Porter (eds), *Exoticism in the Enlightenment* (Manchester: Manchester University Press, 1989), 117–44.

45. Cf. E. Wind, *Pagan Mysteries in the Renaissance* (Harmondsworth: Penguin, 1967); F. Yates, *The Art of Memory* (London: Routledge and Kegan Paul, 1966); D. O'Keefe, *Stolen Lightning* (Oxford: Martin Robertson, 1982).

46. See R. F. Jones, *Ancients and Moderns* (St Louis: Washington University Press, 1961): Barbara J. Shapiro, *Probability and Certainty in Seventeenth Century England* (Princeton, NJ: Princeton University Press, 1983).

47. L. S. King, *The Road to Medical Enlightenment 1650–1695* (London: Macdonald, 1970); O. Temkin, *Galenism* (Ithaca, NY: Cornell University Press, 1973); I. Bernard Cohen, *Revolution in Science* (Cambridge, Mass.: Belknap Press of Harvard University Press, 1985); Roy Porter, 'The Scientific Revolution: a Spoke in the Wheel?', in R. Porter and Mikuláš Teich (eds), *Revolution in History* (Cambridge: Cambridge University Press, 1986), 290–316.

48. For French medical conservatism see T. Gelfand, *Professionalizing Modern Medicine* (Westport, Conn.: Greenwood Press, 1980).

49. For the 'modern mind' confronting superstition see Shorter, *History of Women's Bodies*; Burke, *Popular Culture*; Eccles, *Obstetrics and Gynaecology.*

50. K. Hutchinson, 'What Happened to Occult Qualities in the Scientific Revolution?', *Isis*, lxxiii (1982), 233–53; I. Couliano, *Eros and Magic in the Renaissance*, trans. Margaret Cook (Chicago and London: University of Chicago Press, 1987).

51. Darmon, *Le Mythe de la procréation*; I.

MacLean, *The Renaissance Notion of Woman: A Study in the Fortunes of Scholasticism and Medical Science in European Intellectual Life* (Cambridge and New York: Cambridge University Press, 1980).

52. Sander Gilman, *Sexuality: An Illustrated History* (New York: Wiley, 1989); Thomas W. Laqueur, *Making Sex. Gender and the Body from Aristotle to Freud* (Cambridge, Mass.: Harvard University Press, 1990).

53. Thomas Power Lowry (ed.), *The Classic Clitoris: Historic Contributions to Scientific Sexuality* (Chicago: Nelson-Hall, 1978).

54. Johannes Morsink, *Aristotle on the Generation of Animals: A Philosophical Study* (Washington, DC: University Press of America, 1982); Thomas W. Laqueur, 'Orgasm, Generation, and the Politics of Reproductive Biology', in C. Gallagher and T. Laqueur (eds), *The Making of the Modern Body* (Berkeley: California University Press, 1987), 1–41.

55. Gasking, *Investigations into Generation*; S. Roe, *Matter, Life and Generation* (Cambridge: Cambridge University Press, 1981); J. Roger, *Les Sciences de la vie dans la pensée Française du XVIIIe siècle* (Paris: Colin, 1963); P. J. Bowler, 'Preformation and Pre-existence in the Seventeenth Century: A Brief Analysis', *Journal of the History of Biology*, iv (1971), 221–44.

56. For the construction of gender stereotypes, see Ludmilla Jordanova, 'Natural Facts: A Historical Perspective on Science and Sexuality', in C. MacCormack and M. Strathern (eds), *Nature, Culture and Gender* (Cambridge: Cambridge University Press, 1980), 42–69; Londa Schiebinger, 'Mammals, Primatology and Sexology', in Roy Porter and Mikuláš Teich (eds), *Sexual Knowledge, Sexual Science: The History of Attitudes to Sexuality* (Cambridge: Cambridge University Press, 1994) 184–209.

57. G. J. Barker-Benfield, *The Horrors of the Half Known Life: Attitudes Toward Women and Sexuality in Nineteenth-Century America* (New York: Harper and Row, 1976).

58. Venette, *Mysteries of Conjugal Love Reveal'd*, 88.

59. *Ibid.*, 80.

60. *Ibid.* See Rousseau, 'Nymphomania, Bienville and the Rise of Erotic Sensibility'.

61. Venette, *Mysteries of Conjugal Love Reveal'd*, 98. *Cf.* C. Lougée, *Le Paradis des Femmes: Women, Salons and Social Stratification in Seventeenth Century France* (Princeton, NJ: Princeton University Press, 1976).

62. For the sexual construal of women see Vivien Jones (ed.), *Women in the Eighteenth Century: Constructions of Femininity* (London: Routledge, 1990); Patricia Meyer Spacks, ' "Ev'ry Woman is at Heart a Rake' ", *Eighteenth Century Studies*, viii (1974–5), 27–46; M. LeGates, 'The Cult of Womanhood in Eighteenth Century Thought', *Eighteenth Century Studies*, x (1976), 21–40; K. B. Clinton, 'Femme et Philosophe: Enlightenment origins of Feminism', *Eighteenth Century Studies*, viii (1975), 283–300; Sylvana Tomaselli, 'The Enlightenment Debate on Women', *History Workshop Journal*, xx (1985), 101–24.

63. Venette, *Mysteries of Conjugal Love Reveal'd*, 107.

64. For similar doctrines amongst other eighteenth-century writers see Roy Porter, 'Mixed Feelings: the Enlightenment and Sexuality in Eighteenth Century Britain', in P.-G. Boucé (ed.), *Sexuality in Eighteenth Century Britain* (Manchester: Manchester University Press, 1982), 1–27.

65. Venette, *Mysteries of Conjugal Love Reveal'd*, 203.

66. *Ibid.*, 204.

67. *Ibid.*, 196.

68. The influential American health reformer, William Alcott, recommended once-a-month sex. See J. Whorton, *Crusaders for Fitness* (Princeton, NJ: Princeton University Press, 1982).

69. For the heightened attention to venereal disease at that time, see Claude Quétel, *The History of Syphilis*, trans. Judith Braddock and Brian Pike (Oxford: Basil Blackwell, 1990).

70. Venette, *Mysteries of Conjugal Love Reveal'd*, 155. Belief that Venus and Bacchus did not mix became common in such Enlightenment writers as James Graham and Erasmus Darwin. See Porter, 'Sexual Politics of James Graham'.

71. Venette, *Mysteries of Conjugal Love Reveal'd*, 366.

72. Darmon, *Le Mythe de la procréation*; Shorter, *History of Women's Bodies*.

73. P. Darmon, *Le Tribunal de l'impuissance: virilité et defaillances conjugales dans l'Ancienne France* (Paris: Editions du Seuil, 1979).

74. Shorter, *History of Women's Bodies*.

75. [Anon.], 'Piss Pot Science', *Journal of the History of Medicine*, x (1955), 121–3.

76. Horace, *Odes*, 2.

77. Venette, *Mysteries of Conjugal Love Reveal'd*, 11, 76.

78. *Ibid.*, 84.

79. See Katherine Park and Lorraine J. Daston, 'Unnatural Conceptions: The Study of Monsters in Sixteenth Century France and England', *Past and Present*, xcii (1981), 20–54; C. J. S. Thompson, *The Mystery and Lore of Monsters* (London: Williams and Norgate, 1930).

80. Cf. Keith Thomas, *Religion and the Decline of Magic* (London: Weidenfeld and Nicolson, 1971).

81. Venette, *Mysteries of Conjugal Love Reveal'd*, 380.

82. *Ibid.*, 383.

83. *Ibid.*, Preface.

84. See Mary Douglas, *Purity and Danger* (London: Routledge and Kegan Paul, 1966); idem, *Implicit Meanings* (London: Routledge and Kegan Paul, 1975), 236; S. Shapin, 'History of Science and its Sociological Reconstructions', *History of Science*, xx (1982), 157–211.

85. Alex Comfort, *The Anxiety Makers: Some Curious Preoccupations of the Medical Profession* (London: Nelson, 1967).

86. G. L. Simons, *Sex and Superstition* (London: Abelard-Schuman, 1973).

87. Penelope Shuttle and Peter Redgrove, *The Wise Wound: Menstruation and Everywoman* (London: Gollancz, 1978); Patricia Crawford, 'Attitudes to Menstruation in Seventeenth-Century England', *Past and Present*, xci (1981), 47–73.

88. Venette, *Mysteries of Conjugal Love Reveal'd*, 25.

89. *Ibid.*, 27.

90. Comfort, *The Anxiety Makers*; Barbara Ehrenreich and Deirdre English, *Witches, Midwives and Nurses: A History of Women Healers*, 2nd edn (Old Westbury, NY: Feminist Press, 1973).

91. See Leo Braudy, 'Fanny Hill and Materialism', *Eighteenth Century Studies*, iv (1970–1), 21–40; W. H. Epstein, *John Cleland, Images of Life* (New York: Columbia University Press, 1974); G. Rudé, *Wilkes and Liberty* (Oxford: Clarendon Press, 1962), 31–5; Peter Wagner, 'The Discourse on Sex – or Sex as Discourse: Eighteenth Century Medical and Paramedical Erotica', in G. S. Rousseau and Roy Porter (eds), *Sexual Underworlds of the Enlightenment* (Manchester: Manchester University Press, 1987), 46–68.

92. David Foxon, *Libertine Literature in England 1660–1745: With an Appendix on the Publication of John Cleland's 'Memoirs of a Woman of Pleasure', Commonly Known as 'Fanny Hill'* (New York: University Books, 1965). John Marten, *Gonosologium Novum: Or, A New System of all the Secret Infirmities and Diseases, Natural, Accidental, and Venereal in Men and Women* (London: Crouch, 1709).

93. Marten, *Gonosologium Novum*, 1–2.

94. Sir Thomas Browne, *Religio Medici*, in C. Sayle (ed.), *The Works of Sir Thomas Browne*, 3 vols (Edinburgh, 1912), Vol. I, 100.

95. John Armstrong, *The Oeconomy of Love* (London, 1736; 3rd edn 1739). Cf. lines 181–91, quoted in note 103 to Chapter 2.

96. N. Venette, *Conjugal Love Reveal'd, In the Nightly Pleasure of the Marriage Bed and the Advantages of that Happy State, in an Essay Concerning Humane Generation, done from the French of Monsieur Venette, by a Physician*. Seventh Edition, Amor Omnibus Idem. London. Printed for the Author, and sold by Tho. Hinton, at the White Horse, in Water Lane, Blackfryars (tentatively dated *c.* 1720 by the British Library catalogue). This is approximately 4 inches × 3 inches in size, and runs to 202 pages. It contains an advertisement at the front: 'Just Published. The Adventures of the Priests and Nuns, containing many delightful Stories.'

97. N. Venette, *The Pleasures of Conjugal Love Explained in an Essay Concern-*

ing Human Generation, done from the French by a Physician. Amor Omnibus Idem. London. Printed for P. Meighan at Gray's Inn Gate, in Holborn, T. Griffiths at Charing Cross, T. Lapworth at the Anodyne Necklace without Temple Bar. Price One Shilling.

98. Darmon, *Le Tribunal de l'impuissance*.
99. See Park and Daston, 'Unnatural Conceptions'; Thompson, *Mystery and Lore of Monsters*; Thomas, *Religion and the Decline of Magic*.
100. N. Venette, *Conjugal Love; Or the Pleasures of the Marriage Bed Considered. In Several Lectures On Human Generation*. From the French of Venette, 20th edn (London: printed for the booksellers, 1750).
101. *Ibid.*, 38.
102. *Ibid.*, 141.
103. *Ibid.*, 38.
104. This shift chimes with wider developments in medicine. For the general reorientation from iatrophysics to a more biological or vitalistic medicine, see Lester King, *The Medical World of the Eighteenth Century* (New York: Kreiger, 1971); for the growing problematization of the operations of the psyche, see Roy Porter, 'Civilization and Disease: Medical Ideology in the Enlightenment', in J. Black and J. Gregory (eds), *Culture, Politics and Society in Britain 1660-1800* (Manchester: Manchester University Press, 1991), 154-83.
105. *Conjugal Love*, 20th edn, 49. The suggestion is that sex and marriage, far from being great sources of pleasure, or even Johnsonian triumphs of hope over experience, are indulged in only as part of the divine scheme of moral behaviour: p. 115, 'a little reflecting on the attractiveness of matrimony are [*sic*] only desirable . . . to keep us chaste and obedient unto God's commandments, who is desirous to fill heaven with blessed spirits' – a most un-Venettian sentiment!
106. *Ibid.*, 48.
107. *Ibid.*, 5.
108. *Ibid.*, 149.
109. *Ibid.*, 64-5.
110. *Ibid.*, 40.
111. *Ibid.*, 39-40.
112. *Ibid.*, 54.
113. *Ibid.*
114. A. F. M. Willich, *Lectures on Diet and Regimen* (London, 1799), 539.
115. *Conjugal Love*, 20th edn, 113. A parallel issue is the sexual nature of women. *Conjugal Love* still registers Venette's Hippocratic view that women are and should be sexually active. By contrast, authors such as Sibly and Graham view women as much more passive, since the new physiology had taught them that the active ingredient in procreation was the sperm. See Barker-Benfield, *Horrors of the Half-Known Life*.

4 Masturbation in the Enlightenment: Knowledge and Anxiety

1. Michel Foucault, *The History of Sexuality*, Vol. I, *Introduction* (London: Allen Lane, 1978; New York: Vintage Books, 1985), 23.
2. R. Latham and W. Matthews (eds), *The Diary of Samuel Pepys*, 11 vols (London: Bell and Hyman, 1970-83), Vol. IX, entry for 8 Feb. 1668.
3. For the roots of worries about authorship, see H. J. Chaytor, *From Script to Print* (Cambridge: Cambridge University Press, 1945).
4. For discussion of the history of the idea of forbidden knowledge, see Jean Delumeau, *Sin and Fear. The Emergence of a Western Guilt Culture, 13th-18th Centuries* (New York: St Martin's Press, 1990). For the lubricious see Roy Porter, 'A Touch of Danger: The Man-Midwife as Sexual Predator', in G. S. Rousseau and R. Porter (eds), *Sexual Underworlds of the Enlightenment* (Manchester: Manchester University Press, 1987), 206-32.
5. For Grub Street, see Pat Rogers, *Grub Street: Studies in a Subculture* (London: Methuen, 1972); Philip Pinkus, *Grub Street Stripped Bare* (London: Constable, 1980).
6. Lynn Hunt (ed.), *The Invention of Pornography, 1500-1800* (New York: Zone Books, 1993).
7. See G. S. Rousseau, 'The Sorrows of

Priapus: Anticlericalism, Homosocial Desire and Richard Payne Knight', in G. S. Rousseau and Roy Porter (eds), *Sexual Underworlds of the Enlightenment* (Manchester: Manchester University Press, 1987), 101–55; David Foxon, *Libertine Literature in England 1660–1745: with an Appendix on the Publication of John Cleland's 'Memoirs of a Woman of Pleasure', Commonly Known as 'Fanny Hill'* (New York: University Books, 1965).

8. On the relations between writing and authority, Brian A. Connery, 'Self-Representation, Authority, and the Fear of Madness in the Works of Swift', *Studies in Eighteenth-Century Culture*, xx (1990), 165–82 is stimulating.

9. John Marten, *Gonosologium Novum: Or, A New System of all the Secret Infirmities and Diseases, Natural, Accidental, and Venereal in Men and Women*, 6th edn (London: Crouch, 1709), A3.

10. John Marten, *A Treatise of all the Degrees and Symptoms of the Venereal Disease, in both Sexes*, 6th edn (London: S. Crouch, 1708), xxxiii. For the dialogues of quacks and regulars, see Roy Porter, *Health for Sale: Quackery in England 1650–1850* (Manchester: Manchester University Press, 1989).

11. W. Buchan, *Observations Concerning the Prevention and Cure of the Venereal Disease* (London: printed for T. Chapman, Fleet Street, and Mudie and Sons, Edinburgh, 1796), xvi–xvii. This piece of sexual folklore was still circulating in the late nineteenth century. Arthur P. Luff, *Textbook of Forensic Medicine and Toxicology* (London: Longmans, Green, 1895), 255:

> Rapes on young children are far more common than on adult women. There are many reasons to account for this, the most obvious being the comparative ease with which it may be attempted, owing to the ignorance and feeble powers of resistance of children. Another revolting reason for the commission of the crime is the erroneous superstition among some ignorant persons that an obstinate gonorrhoea or an attack of syphilis is cured by having sexual intercourse with a virgin.

Cf also George Vivian Poore, *A Treatise in Medical Jurisprudence* (London: John Murray, 1901), 322, re child rape:

> One reason is to be found in a very old tradition, mentioned in the mediaeval writings, that one way of curing obstinate venereal disease, notably gonorrhoea, was copulation with a virgin, there is no doubt that a great deal of rape has been perpetrated with that intent.

12. Buchan, *Observations Concerning the . . . Venereal Disease*, i–ii, xvi.

13. *Ibid.*, xxx. For the Enlightenment commitment to free knowledge see Peter Gay, *The Party of Humanity: Essays in the French Enlightenment* (New York: Norton, 1971); *idem, The Enlightenment: An Interpretation*, 2 vols (London: Weidenfeld and Nicolson, 1967 and 1969).

14. Nicholas Venette, *Conjugal Love; Or, The Pleasures of the Marriage Bed Considered. In Several Lectures On Human Generation*. From the French of Venette, 20th edn (London: printed for the booksellers, 1750), iii.

15. This was a line still convenient in Freud's day. Justifying his interrogation of 'Dora', Freud riposted,

> there is never any danger of corrupting an inexperienced girl. For where there is no knowledge of sexual processes even in the unconscious, no hysterical symptom will arise; and where hysteria is found, there can be no longer any question of 'innocence of mind' in the sense in which parents and educators use the phrase.

Sigmund Freud, 'Fragment of the Analysis of a Case of Hysteria', in *The Standard Edition of the Complete Psychological Works of Sigmund Freud*, trans. and ed. James Strachey *et al.* (London: Hogarth Press and the Institute of Psycho-Analysis, 1953–74), Vol. VII, 49.

16. *Onania, Or the Heinous Sin of Self-Pollution, And all its frightful Consequences, in both Sexes, Consider'd with Spiritual and Physical Advice to those, Who Have Already Injur'd Themselves by This Abominable Practice. And seasonable Admonition to the Youth of the Nation, (of both Sexes) and Those Whose Tuition They Are Under, Whether Parents, Guardians,*

Masters, or Mistresses. The Eighth Edition, Corrected, and Enlarg'd to almost as much again, as particulariz'd at the End of the Preface; and are all the Additions, that will be made to this Book, how often ever it may come to be Reprinted, pp. 130–2, 12. For earlier discussions about writing about the body as a source of embarrassment and corruption see Gail Kern Paster, *The Body Embarrassed: Drama and the Disciplines of Shame in Early Modern England* (Ithaca, NY: Cornell University Press, 1993).

17. Venette, *Conjugal Love*, 111.

18. For mealy-mouthedness after 1770, see Peter Fryer, *Mrs Grundy. Studies in English Prudery* (London: Dennis Dobson, 1963); Ronald Pearsall, *The Worm in the Bud: The World of Victorian Sexuality* (London: Weidenfeld and Nicolson, 1969; Harmondsworth: Penguin, 1971); N. Perrin, *Dr Bowdler's Legacy – A History of Expurgated Books in England and America* (New York: Atheneum, 1969; London: Macmillan, 1970).

19. S.-A.-A.-D. Tissot, *Onanism: or, a Treatise upon the Disorders Produced by Masturbation: or, the Dangerous Effects of Secret and Excessive Venery*. By M. Tissot, M.D. Fellow of the Royal Society of London. Member of the Medico-Physical Society of Basle, and of the Oeconomical Society of Berne. Translated from the last Paris Edition By A. Hume (London: printed for the Translator, sold by J. Pridden, 1761); See Ludmilla Jordanova, 'The Popularisation of Medicine: Tissot on Onanism', *Textual Practice*, i (1987), 68–80.

20. See Robert H. MacDonald, 'The Frightful Consequences of Onanism: Notes on the History of a Delusion', *Journal of the History of Ideas*, xxviii (1967), 423–31; J. Stengers and A. Van Neck, *Histoire d'une grande peur: la masturbation* (Brussels: University of Brussels Press, 1984); H. Tristram Engelhardt Jr, 'The Disease of Masturbation: Values and Concept of Disease', *Bulletin of the History of Medicine*, xlviii (1974), 234–48; E. H. Hare, 'Masturbatory Insanity: The History of an Idea', *Journal of Mental Science*, cviii (1962), 1–25; Thomas W. Laqueur,

'The Social Evil, the Solitary Vice and Pouring Tea', in Paula Bennett and Vernon A. Rosario II (eds), *Eros and Masturbation: The Historical, Theoretical and Literary Discourses of Autoeroticism* (London: Routledge, forthcoming).

21. *Onania, Or the Heinous Sin of Self-Pollution*, 8th edn, 3.

22. *Ibid.*, A/A.

23. *Ibid.*

24. *Ibid.*

25. *Ibid.*

26. *Ibid.*, 3.

27. *Ibid.*

28. *Ibid.*, 4.

29. *Ibid.*, A/A.

30. Alain Boureau and Roger Chartier (eds), *The Culture of Print: Power and the Uses of Print in Early Modern Europe* (Cambridge: Polity Press, 1989); Elizabeth Eisenstein, 'On Revolution and the Printed Word', in Roy Porter and Mikuláš Teich (eds), *Revolution in History* (Cambridge: Cambridge University Press, 1986), 186–205.

31. *Onania, Or the Heinous Sin of Self-Pollution*, 8th edn, A/A.

32. *Ibid.*

33. Marten, *Gonosologium Novum*, A4v.

34. *Onania, Or the Heinous Sin of Self-Pollution*, 8th edn, ch. 2, opening.

35. Venette, *Conjugal Love*, Preface.

36. *Onania, Or the Heinous Sin of Self-Pollution*, 8th edn, 3.

37. Jean Frédéric Osterwald, *Traité contre l'impureté* (Amsterdam: T. Lombrail, 1707; translated as *The Nature of Uncleanness Consider'd ... to which is added A Discourse Concerning the Nature of Chastity and the Means of Obtaining it* (London: R. Bonwicke, 1708).

38. *Onania, Or the Heinous Sin of Self-Pollution*, 8th edn, 4. Compare Josiah Woodward's *Rebuke of the Sin of Uncleanness* (London: printed and sold by Joseph Downing, 1704), and see Peter Wagner, 'The Veil of Science and Mortality: Some Pornographic Aspects of the ONANIA', *British Journal for Eighteenth Century Studies*, iv (1983), 181.

39. Quoted in *Onania, Or the Heinous Sin of Self-Pollution*, 8th edn, 5.

40. Venette, *Conjugal Love*, 114.

41. Not surprisingly, since the problems of sexual speech and sexual silence in many ways replicated traditional dilemmas regarding religious blaspheming,

profaning, cursing and swearing. See Geoffrey Hughes, *Swearing. A Social History of Foul Language, Oaths and Profanity in English* (Oxford: Basil Blackwell, 1991). Such issues were later at the core of Freud's notion of repression and the talking cure.

42. Jordanova, 'Popularisation of Medicine'; Antoinette Emch-Dériaz, *Tissot: Physician of the Enlightenment* (New York: Peter Lang, 1992).

43. Tissot, *Onanism*, vi: 'This work has nothing in common with the English *Onania* but the subject, except a quotation of two pages and a half, which I have taken from thence: such a rhapsody could afford me no assistance. Those who read the two works will I hope be sensible of the total difference there is between them: those who read this alone may be misled by the affinity of the titles, and inclined to think there is a great similitude between the two books: but happily there is none.'

44. *Ibid.*, iv. Quoting Tissot with approval, M. D. T. de Bienville in his *Nymphomania, or, a Dissertation Concerning the Furor Uterinus* (London: J. Bew, 1775), vi, argued: 'Can that book be considered as dangerous, the sole design of which is to prevent illicit pleasure; to intimidate those young persons who may be subject to this unhappy madness; and to restrain the vicious transports of the constitution, by striking lessons, and by principles, and consequence drawn from nature which must persuade?' Nymphomania (also known as *furor uterinus*) was often said to follow from onanism.

45. Jordanova, 'Popularisation of Medicine'.

46. Tissot, *Onanism*, xi.

47. *Ibid.*, vi.

48. *Ibid.*, 2.

49. See Roy Porter, *Doctor of Society: Thomas Beddoes and the Sick Trade in Late Enlightenment England* (London: Routledge, 1991), especially ch. 3 for Beddoes's political views.

50. Was this to do with personal factors? From around his fortieth year, Beddoes felt himself in decline. We know little about his sexual life and habits, beyond that he married in his mid-thirties and that within a few years his marriage was failing – his wife temporarily left him, which flung him upon his best friend, Davies Giddy. Whether Beddoes looked to some sexual vice in himself to explain his own decline cannot be ascertained, but there may be one clue. In a last letter to Humphry Davy just before his death, Beddoes described himself in failure as 'like one who has scattered abroad the Avena fatua of knowledge from which neither brand, nor blossom nor fruit has resulted'. The image strikingly echoes the sin of Onan, scattering his seed fruitlessly upon the ground. See Dorothy A. Stansfield, *Thomas Beddoes M.D., 1760–1808, Chemist, Physician, Democrat* (Dordrecht: Reidel, 1984), 249.

51. Thomas Beddoes, *Hygëia: or Essays Moral and Medical, on the Causes Affecting the Personal State of our Middling and Affluent Classes*, 3 vols (Bristol: J. Mills, 1802), Vol. I, essay iii, p. 77.

52. *Ibid.*, Vol. III, ix, 184–90. Far the most illuminating discussion of Swift and masturbation is Hugh Ormsby-Lennon, 'Swift's Spirit Reconjured: Das Dong-An-Sich', *Swift Studies*, iii (1988), 9–78.

53. Thomas Beddoes, *Manual of Health: or, the Invalid Conducted Safely through the Seasons* (London: Johnson, 1806), 79.

54. Beddoes, *Hygëia*, Vol. III, ix, 41. Whom is Beddoes trying to protect – women, or children?

55. *Ibid.*, Vol. III, ix, 157.

56. *Ibid.*, Vol. II, viii, 89.

57. *Ibid.*, Vol. III, ix, 194. This seems a splendid instance of the pot calling the kettle black.

58. For Sterne's smutty strategies, see M. New, 'At the Backside of the Door of Purgatory', in V. Grosvenor-Myer (ed.), *Lawrence Sterne: Riddles and Mysteries* (London: Vision, 1984), 15–23.

59. R. Darnton, 'The High Enlightenment and the Low-Life of Literature in Pre-revolutionary France', *Past and Present*, li (1971), 81–115; reprinted in his *The Literary Underground of the Old Regime* (Cambridge, Mass.: Harvard University Press, 1982), 1–40; *idem, The Great Cat Massacre and other Episodes in French Cultural History* (New York: Basic Books, 1984; Harmondsworth: Pen-

guin, 1985); *idem* and Daniel Roche (eds), *Revolution in Print: The Press in France 1775–1800* (Berkeley: University of California Press, 1989); Isabel Rivers (ed.), *Books and their Readers in Eighteenth Century England* (Leicester: Leicester University Press, 1982).

60. See Mary Fissell, 'Readers, Texts and Contexts: Vernacular Medical Works in Early Modern England', in Roy Porter (ed.), *The Popularization of Medicine, 1650–1850* (London and New York: Routledge, 1992), 72–96 and the items referred to in the footnotes.

61. Other erotica also claimed to be useful – for instance by providing ammunition against the evils of Popery or by reinforcing political radicalism against *ancien régime* monarchy and aristocracy: I. D. McCalman, *Radical Underworld: Prophets, Revolutionaries and Pornographers in London, 1795–1840* (Cambridge: Cambridge University Press, 1988); Peter Wagner, *Eros Revived: Erotica of the Enlightenment in England and America* (London: Secker and Warburg, 1988).

62. See Peter Wagner: 'The Pornographer in the Courtroom: Trial Reports about Cases of Sexual Crimes and Delinquencies as a Genre of Eighteenth Century Erotica', in P.-G. Boucé (ed.), *Sexuality in Eighteenth Century Britain* (Manchester: Manchester University Press, 1982), 120–40; *idem*, 'Researching the Taboo: Sexuality and Eighteenth-Century Erotica', *Eighteenth-Century Life*, iii (1983), 108–15; *idem*, 'Veil of Science and Mortality'; *idem*, *Eros Revived; idem*, 'The Discourse on Sex – or Sex as Discourse: Eighteenth Century Medical and Paramedical Erotica', in G. S. Rousseau and Roy Porter (eds), *Sexual Underworlds of the Enlightenment* (Manchester: Manchester University Press, 1987), 46–68.

63. Angus McLaren, *Reproductive Rituals: The Perception of Fertility in England from the Sixteenth to the Nineteenth Century* (London and New York: Methuen, 1984), 71ff.

64. Roy Porter, '"The Whole Secret of Health": Mind, Body and Medicine in *Tristram Shandy*', in John Christie and Sally Shuttleworth (eds), *Nature Transfigured* (Manchester: Manchester University Press, 1989), 61–84; Roy Porter, 'Against the Spleen', in Valerie Grosvenor Myer (ed.), *Laurence Sterne: Riddles and Mysteries* (London and New York: Vision, 1984), 84–99.

65. David Vincent, 'Love and Death and the Nineteenth Century Working Class', *Social History*, v (1980), 223–47.

66. Peter Burke (ed.), *New Perspectives on Historical Writing* (Cambridge: Polity Press, 1991).

5   Quackery and Erotica

1. Roy Porter and G. S. Rousseau (eds), *Sexual Underworlds of the Enlightenment* (Manchester: Manchester University Press, 1987), 'Introduction'; Rictor Norton, *Mother Clap's Molly House: The Gay Subculture in England 1700–1830* (London: Gay Men's Press, 1992); David F. Greenberg, *The Construction of Homosexuality* (Chicago: University of Chicago Press, 1988); Richard Davenport-Hines, *Sex, Death and Punishment: Attitudes to Sex and Sexuality in Britain since the Renaissance* (London: Collins, 1990).

2. Peter Wagner, *Eros Revived: Erotica of the Enlightenment in England and America* (London: Secker and Warburg, 1988).

3. Roy Porter, '"The Secrets of Generation Display'd": *Aristotle's Master-piece* in Eighteenth-Century England', in R. P. Maccubbin (ed.), *Unauthorized Sexual Behaviour during the Enlightenment* (special issue of *Eighteenth Century Life*), Vol. IX, ns 3 (May 1985), 1–21; Janet Blackman, 'Popular Theories of Generation: The Evolution of *Aristotle's Works*: The Study of an Anachronism', in John Woodward and David Richards (eds), *Health Care and Popular Medicine in Nineteenth-Century England: Essays in the Social History of Medicine* (London: Croom Helm, 1977), 56–88.

4. Roy Porter, 'Making Faces: Physiognomy and Fashion in Eighteenth-Century England', *Etudes Anglaises*, xxxviii (Oct.–Dec. 1985), 385–96.

5. Virginia S. Smith, 'Cleanliness: the Development of an Idea and Practice in Britain 1770–1850' (PhD thesis, University of London, 1985); N. Williams, *Powder and Paint* (London: Longmans, 1957).

6. Karl M. Figlio, 'Chlorosis and

Chronic Disease in Nineteenth-Century Britain: The Social Constitution of Somatic Illness in a Capitalist Society', *Social History*, iii (1978), 167–97; I. S. L. Loudon, 'Chlorosis, Anaemia and Anorexia Nervosa', *British Medical Journal*, cclxxxi, 2nd part (1980), 1–19.

7. Samuel Solomon, *An Account of that Most Excellent Medicine, The Cordial Balm of Gilead* (Stockport: Clarke, *c.* 1801), 55.

8. For women and child-bearing, see Barbara Duden, *The Woman Beneath the Skin: A Doctor's Patients in Eighteenth-Century Germany*, trans. Thomas Dunlap (Cambridge, Mass. and London: Harvard University Press, 1991); Patricia Crawford, 'Attitudes to Pregnancy from a Woman's Spiritual Diary, 1687–88', *Local Population Studies*, xxi (1978), 43–5; *idem*, 'Attitudes to Menstruation in Seventeenth Century England', *Past and Present*, xci (1981), 47–73.

9. *A Collection of 231 Advertisements*, 551.a. 32, 85.

10. See also W. F. Bynum, 'Treating the Wages of Sin: Venereal Disease and Specialism in Eighteenth-Century Britain', in W. F. Bynum and R. Porter (eds), *Medical Fringe and Medical Orthodoxy, 1750–1850* (London: Croom Helm, 1987), 5–28; H. MacGregor, 'Eighteenth-Century V.D. Publicity', *British Journal of Venereal Disease*, xxxi (1955), 117–18.

11. *A Collection of 185 Advertisements*, C112. f.9, 93.

12. *Ibid.*, f.9, 103.

13. *Ibid.*, f.9, 166.

14. *Ibid.*, f.9, 116.

15. Bynum, 'Treating the Wages of Sin'.

16. John Marten, *A Treatise of all the Degrees and Symptoms of the Venereal Disease in Both Sexes*, 6th edn (London: S. Crouch, 1708); John Spinke, *Quackery Unmasked* (London: D. Brown, 1709); R. Straus, *The Unspeakable Dr Curll* (New York: Kelley, 1970). Francis Doherty, *A Study in Eighteenth-Century Advertising Methods: The Anodyne Necklace* (Lewiston/Queenston/Lampeter: Edwin Mellen Press, 1992), 155ff., discusses the advertising of anti-onanistic products in a publication, *Eronania*, whose title mimicked *Onania*.

17. Jean H. Hagstrum, *Sex and Sensibility. Ideal and Erotic Love from Milton to Mozart* (Chicago and London: University of Chicago Press, 1980).

18. Roy Porter, 'Libertinism and Promiscuity', in J. Miller (ed.), *The Don Giovanni Book: Myths of Seduction and Betrayal* (London: Faber and Faber, 1990), 1–19; *idem*, 'The Rise of Physical Examination', in W. F. Bynum and Roy Porter (eds), *Medicine and the Five Senses* (Cambridge: Cambridge University Press, 1992), 179–97.

19. See William L. Whitwell, 'James Graham, Master Quack', *Eighteenth-Century Life*, iv (1977), 43–9.

20. James Graham, *Proposals for the Establishment of a New and True Christian Church* (Bath: Cruttwell, 1788), 4, terming himself 'formerly a physician but now a Christian philosopher'.

21. James Graham, *A Sketch, or Short Description of Dr Graham's Medical Apparatus* (London: Almon, 1780), 151.

22. *Ibid.*

23. James Graham, *Lecture on the Generation, Increase and Improvement of the Human Species* (London: M. Smith, 1780), 40. Electrification would also prolong sexual pleasures, turning the 'critical moment' into 'the critical hour' (47).

24. Quoted from a newspaper advertisement for the Temple of Health, in F. Grose, *A Guide to Health, Beauty, Riches and Honour* (London: Hooper and Wigstead, 1796), 25.

25. Though one of his sisters married Thomas Arnold, the Leicester mad-house keeper, and though he recommended Arnold's asylum to disturbed patients, Graham showed little interest in mental illness, or the use of electricity for treating melancholia or mania. Very few of his case histories deal with the mentally disturbed. Graham hardly fits into the tradition of psycho-healers from the Reformation exorcists through to the nineteenth-century pioneers of abnormal psychology.

26. Graham, *Lecture on the Generation*, 3.

27. *Ibid.*, 28.

28. A phrase he used in advertisements for his pamphlet, entitled 'DR GRAHAM's *Private Advice* (sealed up, price one guinea) to those ladies and gentlemen

who wish to have children, or to become snowy pillars of health and beauty, studded as it were with roses, and streaked with celestial blue, may now be had at only half-a-guinea; his other curious and eccentric works, containing full descriptions of his travels, discoveries, improvements, principles, cures, electrical apparatus, &c. &c. formerly 3s. 6d. now 1s. and 9d. and Vestina, The Rosy Goddess's warm lecture, price 2s. 6d'. Graham claimed to be able to extend life to about 150 years: 'I do myself expect . . . to live in perfect health, till I shall be at least an hundred and fifty years old, and to be, when an hundred years of age, as robust, healthy, fresh, active, and younglike as men in general are, in these degenerate and luxurious times, at fifty' (*Lecture on the Generation*, 42). Graham died at the age of 49. Marie Stopes shared similar illusions.

29. *Ibid.*, 7.
30. *Ibid.*, 22.
31. *Ibid.*, 4.
32. T. R. Malthus, *An Essay on the Principle of Population* (London: Johnson, 1798); Kenneth Smith, *The Malthusian Controversy* (London: Routledge and Paul, 1951).
33. Graham, *Lecture on . . . Generation*, 4.
34. 'Gentlemen, I do not conceive that any apology is necessary for this political digression, when it is remembered, that the *propagation* of the human species is the subject of our attention. Whatever the number of inhabitants of this country may be at present, certain it is, that by proper care and attention it may be doubled. Where the parents are healthy and in full bloom, were they to receive a small premium on the birth of every child, it would be a strong inducement to fertility, poor men would be comforted in their old age; their children would rise up and call them blessed. We can hardly form an idea to what extent the inhabitants of this country might be increased; instead of remitting such vast sums to America for the destructive purpose of carrying on this war, were it to be applied in the way I just mentioned, taxes, already overgrown, would be lessened, and men more happy than they are at present. From

ambition, luxury, they reduce one half to extreme poverty, and to gratify their pride, must send the other half to captivity' (*Lecture on the Generation*, 7).
35. *Ibid.*, 5. *Cf.*: 'Gentlemen, there is no maxim so clear as this, that men will propagate in proportion as matrimony is encouraged. Men must fly to other methods of indulging their passions; but we all know, that the children begotten out of wedlock, are but few in comparison, and these feeble.' Graham argued that the tax system should be changed to reward matrimony.
36. Graham, *The General State of Medical and Chirurgical Practice Exhibited* (London, Almon, 1779), 42.
37. Graham, *Lecture on the Generation*, 26. On aphrodisiacs, see Angus McLaren, *Reproductive Rituals: The Perception of Fertility in England from the Sixteenth to the Nineteenth Century* (London and New York: Methuen, 1984), 36ff.
38. Writing within the 'country' and 'commonwealth' moral-political tradition, Graham lambasts decadence, corruption and luxury. Sometimes his attacks are fixed on targets in the body politic (e.g. the medical monopoly of university professors – 'stupid blockheads'), but generally they are more biomedically focused on the body natural. For professional reasons, however, Graham sycophantically traded on the favour of the great, toadying to the Duchess of Devonshire, Catherine the Great of Russia, etc. He fawned on George III as 'very amiable and very much beloved' (quoted in Ida Macalpine and Richard Hunter, *George III and the Mad Business*, London: Allen Lane, 1969, 105). Though once a supporter of the American Revolution, by the 1790s he viewed the Birmingham riots against Priestley as a kind of nemesis for Priestley's Socinianism.
39. Graham, *Lecture on the Generation*, 4.
40. *Ibid.*
41. James Graham, *A Discourse Delivered August 17, 1783 in Edinburgh* (Hull: Briggs, 1787).
42. Graham, *Lecture on the Generation*, 27.
43. 'Fine, clean, shewy dresses, sweet smells, affected attentions, pretended affection, and PERFECT AND CONTINUAL personal sweetness and cleanness; – for all those who under-

stand perfectly their *trade*, are at all times, from the top of their head, to the end of the most distant toe, – sweet and pure, and firm, like the purest virgin wax candle, or like the most brilliant paste that glitters in the cap of folly' (*ibid.*, 34).

44. Graham argued 'that next to abstaining totally from animal food and strong liquors, from frequent venery, from warm meat and drink of any kind, and from close rooms and feather beds, BATHING THEIR PRIVATE PARTS WITH COLD WATER THOROUGHLY AND FOR A LONG WHILE, EVERY NIGHT AND MORNING, FROM THE FIRST MONTH OF THEIR LIFE TO THE LAST HOUR OF THEIR EXISTENCE [is] of the highest importance to the preservation of their health and strength, beauty, and brilliancy, bodily and intellectual, of any thing that can be recommended or observed' (*ibid.*, 30).

45. *Ibid.*, 25.

46. 'Early venery . . . steals *irrecoverably*, both from the thickness and the length of the wick, and from the quantity and quality of the oil of human life, – making our lamp for ever after, burn with a dim, tremulous and feeble flame, – and often incapacitates it from giving light, life, and vitality to embryo generations' (James Graham, *A New and Curious Treatise of the Nature and Effects of Simple Earth, Water and Air*, London and Bath: Cruttwell, 1780), 27.

47. Such beliefs were not unique to Graham. The emphasis on moderation and self-control was of course traditional and universal, operating within the framework of the 'nonnaturals'. What was perhaps special in Graham was his emphasis on restraint not primarily for the moral-religious goal of controlling the passions *per se*, but rather with a view to maximizing sexual effectiveness. Purity and sexuality were not at loggerheads but in league. In some ways Graham resembles one of Comfort's 'anxiety makers': those whose advice creates more problems than it resolves. Unlike some of Comfort's 'anxiety makers', however, Graham did not want to minimize sex because he fundamen-

tally distrusted it; he wanted self-control in order to enhance it: Alex Comfort, *The Anxiety Makers: Some Curious Preoccupations of the Medical Profession* (London: Nelson, 1967).

48. Graham, *Lecture on the Generation*, 23.

49. For another contemporary tirade on masturbation, see Ebenezer Sibly: 'A youth, apparently under age, applied to me for the cure of a disorder, which, he said, had deprived him of the power of erection, and all sensation in the privities. In so young a subject I could not suppose this want of tone arose from a general debility of the nervous system, particularly as no other symptoms warranted the conclusion. I had a strong suspicion it was the effect of Onanism, or secret venery, which usually ends in this species of absolute impotency. . . . After half an hour's close examination, I brought him to confess what I above suspected, that he had so much addicted himself to this shameful and destructive vice' (E. Sibly, *The Medical Mirror; or, Treatise on the Impregnation of the Human Female. Shewing the Origin of Diseases, and the Principles of Life and Death*, London: 1794, 145). One of the few medical men who mistrusted the attack on masturbation was John Hunter. See E. H. Hare, 'Masturbatory Insanity: The History of an Idea', *Journal of Mental Science*, cviii (1962), 1–25; Robert H. MacDonald, 'The Frightful Consequences of Onanism: Notes on the History of a Delusion', *Journal of the History of Ideas*, xxviii (1967), 423–31; Comfort, *The Anxiety Makers*. For Sibly, see Allen G. Debus, 'Scientific Truth and Occult Tradition: The Medical World of Ebenezer Sibly (1751–1799)', *Medical History*, xxvi (1982), 259–78.

50. Graham, *Lecture on the Generation*, 12; idem, *A New and Curious Treatise*, 27; 'Appendix, Containing Aphorisms, or Cautions to Youth and Advice to Old Age, against the Use of Venereal Pleasure'. For the same views, see S. A. A. D. Tissot, *Onanism or a Treatise upon the Disorders Produced by Masturbation: or, the Dangerous Effects of Secret and Excessive Venery*, trans. A. Hume (London: for Varenne, 1761), 58ff.

51. Graham, *A New and Curious Treatise*, 28.

An earlier tradition, by contrast, had thought that it was excessive *retention* of semen that caused ill-health. See N. Robinson, *The Theory of Physick* (London: Betteworth, 1729), 78.

52. Graham, *A New and Curious Treatise*, 28.

53. Graham, *A New and Curious Treatise*, 29; *cf. Lecture on the Generation*, 18: 'The early and ardent votary of either Bacchus or Venus, especially of the latter, and if he is an inhabitant of a great City, must be very careful, and very fortunate moreover, if he escapes diseases, and such diseases as will disqualify him from being the father of a stout, numerous and healthy offspring.'

54. For contemporary theories of the power of semen see G. J. Barker-Benfield, *The Horrors of the Half-Known Life: Male Attitudes toward Women and Sexuality in Nineteenth-Century America* (New York: Harper and Row, 1976); McLaren, *Reproductive Rituals*. For the role of semen in the development of mainstream embryology see Joseph Needham, *A History of Embryology*, 2nd edn (Cambridge: Cambridge University Press, 1959); P. G. Ritterbush, *Overtures to Biology* (New Haven: Yale University Press, 1964); Elizabeth Gasking, *Investigations into Generation, 1651–1828* (London: Hutchinson, 1967); Shirley A. Roe, *Matter, Life and Generation: Eighteenth-Century Embryology and the Haller–Wolff Debate* (Cambridge: Cambridge University Press, 1981); for broad discussion of the natural philosophy of superfine fluids see G. N. Cantor and M. J. S. Hodge (eds), *Conceptions of Ether* (Cambridge: Cambridge University Press, 1982).

55. Graham, *Lecture on the Generation*, 19.

56. *Ibid.*, 8. He also had some 'how to get and keep your man' advice for women: have 'a sweet attentive temper', 'read and study, and be continually washing, sponging, syringing and shifting' (*ibid.*, 35).

57. James Graham, *A Short Treatise on the All-Cleansing Earth* (Newcastle and Hall, 1790). For the idea of 'viriculture' see Brian Easlea, *Science and Sexual Oppression: Patriarchy's Confrontation with Women and Nature* (London: Weidenfeld and Nicolson, 1981). On alternative male and female visions of nature see also Carolyn Merchant, *The Death of Nature: Women, Ecology and the Scientific Revolution* (New York: Harper and Row, 1980; London: Wildwood House, 1982).

58. See for example S. Moravia, 'The Enlightenment and the Sciences of Man', *History of Science*, xviii (1980), 247–68; idem, *Il Pensiero degli Idéologues: Scienza e filosofia in Francia 1780–1815* (Firenze: La Nuova Italia, 1974); W. Coleman, 'Health and Hygiene in the *Encyclopédie*: A Medical Doctrine for the Bourgeoisie', *Journal of the History of Medicine and Allied Sciences*, xxix (1974), 399–421; Ludmilla Jordanova, 'Natural Facts: A Historical Perspective on Science and Sexuality', in C. MacCormack and M. Strathern (eds), *Nature, Culture and Gender* (Cambridge: Cambridge University Press, 1980), 42–69.

59. MacDonald, 'Frightful Consequences of Onanism'; J. Stengers and A. van Neck, *Histoire d'une grande peur: La Masturbation* (Brussels: University of Brussels Press, 1984).

60. Graham, *A New and Curious Treatise*, 28.

61. Graham, *Lecture on the Generation*, 20.

62. Tissot, *Onanism*; Ludmilla Jordanova, 'The Popularisation of Medicine: Tissot on Onanism', *Textual Practice*, i (1987), 68–80; Peter Wagner, 'The Veil of Science and Mortality: Some Pornographic Aspects of the ONANIA', *British Journal for Eighteenth Century Studies*, iv (1983), 179–84.

63. T. Beddoes, *Hygëia*, 3 vols (Bristol: Phillips, 1802–3), Vol. I, 40.

64. Lawrence Stone, *The Family, Sex and Marriage in England 1500–1800* (London: Weidenfeld and Nicolson, 1977).

65. Debus, 'Scientific Truth and Occult Tradition'.

66. W. Brodum, *A Guide to Old Age or a Cure for the Indiscretions of Youth. Nervous and Consumptive Complaints, Scurvy, Leprosy and Scrofula, and on A Certain Disease and Sexual Debility, in which is added An Address to Boys, Young Men, Parents, Tutors, and Guardians of Youth* (London: J. W. Myers, 1795); Samuel Solomon, *A Guide to Health, or, Advice to Both Sexes*, 2nd edn (Stockport: the author, *c.* 1800).

67. Debus, 'Scientific Truth and Occult

Tradition'; Comfort, *The Anxiety Makers*, 69ff.
68. Brodum, *A Guide to Old Age*.
69. Solomon, *A Guide to Health*.
70. *Ibid.*, 49.
71. *Ibid.*, 217.
72. *Ibid.*, 46.
73. *Ibid.*, 218.
74. *Ibid.*, 213.
75. *Ibid.*, 211.
76. *Ibid.*, 209.
77. *Ibid.*, 203. For Tissot, see Tissot, *Onanism*, 39ff.
78. Solomon, *A Guide to Health*, 198.
79. *Ibid.*, 195.
80. *Ibid.*, xi.

Introduction: Towards Victoria

1. Angus McLaren, 'The Pleasures of Procreation', in W. F. Bynum and Roy Porter (eds), *William Hunter and the Eighteenth Century Medical World* (Cambridge: Cambridge University Press, 1985), 323–420; *idem, Reproductive Rituals: The Perception of Fertility in England from the Sixteenth to the Nineteenth Century* (London and New York: Methuen, 1984).
2. Randolph Trumbach, 'London's Sodomites: Homosexual Behavior and Western Culture in the Eighteenth Century', *Journal of Social History*, xi (1977), 1–33; *idem,* 'Sodomitical Subcultures, Sodomitical Roles, and the Gender Revolution of the Eighteenth Century: The Recent Historiography', in R. P. Maccubbin (ed.), *Unauthorized Sexual Behavior during the Enlightenment* (Williamsburg, Va.: College of William and Mary, 1985), *Eighteenth-Century Life*, ix (1978), 109–21; *idem,* 'Sex, Gender and identity in Modern Cultures: Male Sodomy and Female Prostitution in 18th Century London', in Ad van der Woude (ed.), *The Role of the State and Public Opinion in Sexual Attitudes and Demographic Behaviour* (Paris: International Commission of Historical Demography, 1990), 271–374; Rictor Norton, *Mother Clap's Molly House: The Gay Subculture in England 1700–1830* (London: Gay Men's Press, 1992).
3. One feature apparent from a close reading of Michael Mason, *The Making of Victorian Sexuality* (Oxford: Oxford University Press, 1994), John Maynard, *Victorian Discourses on Sexuality and Religion* (Cambridge: Cambridge University Press, 1993) and Peter Gay, *The Bourgeois Experience: Victoria to Freud*, Vol. II: *The Tender Passion* (Oxford and New York: Oxford University Press, 1986), our best modern scholarly guides to Victorian sexuality, is the absence of any new kind of sexual Bible, the equivalent of *Aristotle's Master-Piece* a century earlier or the writings of Marie Stopes or perhaps Havelock Ellis around 1920.

Henry Thomas Kitchener, *Letters on Marriage, on the Causes of Matrimonial Infidelity, and on the Reciprocal Relations of the Sexes*, 2 vols (London: Chapple, 1812): this volume represents the nearest approximation to an early nineteenth-century successor to *Aristotle's Master-Piece* or to Venette, though there in no indication that it enjoyed any substantial influence. Cast in epistolary form, it relies extremely heavily upon extensive quotation from eighteenth-century works, ranging from *Onania* to the writings of Tissot, Rousseau, Mary Wollstonecraft, Maria Edgeworth, John Armstrong and Thomas Beddoes, with plenty of literary references to sources like Montaigne. It seems transitional between the sexual advice works of the Georgian age and the exhortations to marriage of the Victorian era. It would repay further study.
4. See Gordon Rattray Taylor, *The Angel-Makers: A Study in the Psychological Origins of Historical Change* (London: Heinemann, 1958; New York: E. P. Dutton, 1974).
5. Louis Crompton, *Byron and Greek Love: Homophobia in Nineteenth Century England* (Berkeley: University of California Press, 1985).
6. M. Jaeger, *Before Victoria* (London: Chatto and Windus, 1956); Boyd Hilton, *The Age of Atonement: the Influence of Evangelicalism on Social and Economic Thought, 1750–1865* (Oxford: Clarendon Press; New York: Oxford University Press, 1988); K. Brown, Ford, *Fathers of the Victorians: The Age of Wilberforce* (Cambridge: Cambridge

University Press, 1961).

7. N. Perrin, *Dr Bowdler's Legacy – A History of Expurgated Books in England and America* (New York: Atheneum, 1969; London: Macmillan, 1970).

8. M. Thale (ed.), *The Autobiography of Francis Place* (Cambridge: Cambridge University Press, 1972).

9. Mikhail M. Bakhtin, *Rabelais and his World*, trans. H. Iswolsky (Cambridge, Mass.: MIT Press, 1968); P. Stallybrass and A. White, *The Politics and Poetics of Transgression* (Ithaca, NY: Cornell University Press, 1986); Ronald Paulson, *Representations of Revolution 1789–1820* (New Haven: Yale University Press, 1983); Peter Wagner, *Eros Revived; Erotica of the Enlightenment in England and America* (London: Secker and Warburg, 1988); I. D. McCalman, *Radical Underworld: Prophets, Revolutionaries and Pornographers in London, 1795–1840* (Cambridge: Cambridge University Press, 1988).

10. T. R. Malthus, *An Essay on the Principle of Population* (London: Johnson, 1798); Kenneth Smith, *The Malthusian Controversy* (London: 1951); Gertrude Himmelfarb, *The Idea of Poverty: England in the Early Industrial Age* (London: Faber and Faber; New York: Knopf, 1984); D. C. Coleman and R. S. Schofield, *The State of Population Theory: Forward from Malthus* (Oxford: Basil Blackwell, 1986); Catherine Gallagher, 'The Body Versus the Social Body in the Works of Thomas Malthus and Henry Mayhew', in Catherine Gallagher and Thomas Laqueur (eds), *The Making of the Modern Body: Sexuality and Society in the Nineteenth Century* (Berkeley and Los Angeles: University of California Press, 1987), 83–106; Patricia James, *Population Malthus: His Life and Times* (London: Routledge and Kegan Paul, 1979).

11. There is an attack upon radical neo-Malthusian birth controllers in Michael Ryan, *The Philosophy of Marriage in its Social, Moral and Physical Relations* (London: Ballière, 1843), 15. Characteristically of its age, Ryan's book combines a moral paean to matrimony with an account of the medical and moral evils of pre- and extramarital sexual intercourse. The amatory discussions characteristic of eighteenth-century texts are almost wholly lacking.

See also Peter Fryer, *The Birth Controllers* (London: Secker and Warburg, 1965); Angus McLaren, *A History of Contraception from Antiquity to the Present Day* (Oxford: Basil Blackwell, 1991). Contraception and condoms had of course been discussed in the eighteenth century. See McLaren, *Reproductive Rituals*, 82ff.; Jeannette Parisot, *Johnny Come Lately: A Short History of the Condom*, trans. and enlarged by Bill McCann (London: Journeyman Press, 1987).

12. Mason, *Making of Victorian Sexuality*.

13. For example: John Power, *Essays on the Female Economy* (London: 1821); Thomas J. Graham, *The Diseases Peculiar to Females* (London: Simkin and Marshall, 1834); James Blundell, *Observations on Some of the More Important Diseases of Women* (London: Cox, 1837); see also Ornella Moscucci, *the Science of Woman: Gynaecology and Gender in England, 1800–1929* (Cambridge: Cambridge University Press, 1990); Carroll Smith-Rosenberg, 'The Hysterical Woman: Sex Roles and Conflict in Nineteenth-Century America', *Social Research*, xxxix (1972), 652–78; Carroll Smith-Rosenberg and Charles Rosenberg, 'The Female Animal: Medical and Biological Views of Woman and Her Role in Nineteenth-Century America', *Journal of American History*, lx (1973), 332–56; Moscucci, *Science of Woman*. There is a parallel but smaller genre of works on male sexual disorders. See for instance R. Dawson, *An Essay on Marriage, Being a Microscopic Investigation into its Physiological and Physical Relations, with Observations on the Nature, Causes and Treatment of Spermatorrhoea* (London: Hughes, 1845), and, for discussion, G. J. Barker-Benfield, 'The Spermatic Economy: A Nineteenth-Century View of Sexuality', *Feminist Studies*, i (1972), 45–74.

14. This fourth version will be quoted from *The Works of the Famous Philosopher Aristotle, Containing His Complete Master-Piece and Family Physician, His Experienced Midwife, His Book of Problems and Remarks on Physiognomy. To the Original Work is Added, Essay on Marriage;*

its Duties and Enjoyments (London, printed for the booksellers, no date, but clearly Victorian); it claims to be the 'original edition unabridged'. Here p. 13. An undated but late Victorian edition of this version carries an 'Advertisement' reassuring the reader that 'The odium in which the book has been held by the moral and the virtuous, does not apply to the present edition. That which was good and useful has been retained, and that only; the omission being supplied by new matter of an interesting and valuable character. . . . To supply a good and moral edition of a work hitherto accounted the reverse of either, is he [the publisher] believes, both important and useful.' For the admonitions, see ch. III. 'Words of Warning', 13–18.

15. *Ibid.*, 18.
16. *Ibid.*, 15.
17. *Ibid.*
18. *Ibid.*, 43.
19. *Ibid.*, 18, 43. The reader is warned not merely of the horrors of illicit sexuality but even of the pitfalls of unwise marriage. See ch. 5: 'Some of the errors of Marriage. Age – inequality of age'; ch. 6: 'Some of the errors of Marriage. Inadequate means of support – want of Reciprocity in Taste, &c'; ch. 7: 'Some of the errors in Marriage. Incompatibility of Temper – want of Candour'.
20. *Ibid.*, 9.
21. *Ibid.*, 15:

> Poor Traviata, with no splendour round her, no devoted admirer to rush in at the last, coughs her way through life and sinks into an early grave – a watery grave, sometimes, made by a leap from a bridge into the dark sullen river that chafes on the stone abutments, and sings under the shadow of the arch a syren song to the despairing.

22. *Ibid.*, 8. The text approvingly cites the pro-marriage writings of Martin Tupper. It argues that

> Celibacy, like the fly in the heart of an apple, dwells in perpetual sweetness, but sits alone, and dies in singularity; while marriage, like the useful bee, builds a house,

and gathers sweetness from every flower, and labours and unites into societies and republics, and sends out colonies, and obeys kings, and keeps order, and exercises many virtues, and promotes the interests of mankind. (*ibid.*, 12)

23. *Ibid.*, 43.
24. *Ibid.* Chapter 10 is entitled: 'Family Affection'.

> The eager pursuit of sensual gratification disqualifies for the exercise of the loftier powers. Experience proves that abstinence and moderation are caterers to the palate, while the wretched epicure who gluttons away the organs of taste, becomes impotent of the sweets that are crowded on his table. The libertine destroys at once animal power and intellectual faculty. But the temperate enjoyments of mind and of person give a durability of rapture to wedlock, which joined to the pleasures of rearing, training, and maturing the fruits of hallowed love, sets man on the summit of terrestrial bliss. There is nothing debasing in connubial love. It is blessed of heaven. Free to make friendship with the senses, man must have dominion over the passions, or forgo all the superior privileges of humanity. Our first parents participated of both mental and bodily enjoyments, with their Maker's benign smile upon them, everything was hallowed, and for the pleasure of the senses they offered to the Great Father the incense of adoration.

25. *Ibid.*, 36.
26. *Ibid.*, ch. 10.
27. Mason, *Making of Victorian Sexuality* and Maynard, *Victorian Discourses* are excellent recent discussions.

6   *The Victorian Polyphony, 1850–85*

1. Some important and/or recent works are: J. A. Banks, *Prosperity and Parenthood: A Study of Family Planning among*

the Victorian Middle Classes (London: Routledge and Kegan Paul, 1954); idem, Victorian Values: Secularism and the Size of Families (London and Boston: Routledge and Kegan Paul, 1981); Françoise Barret-Ducrocq, L'Amour sous Victoria (Paris: Plon, 1989), trans. John Howe, as Love in the Time of Victoria: Sexuality, Class and Gender in Nineteenth Century London (London and New York: Verso, 1991); Peter T. Cominos, 'Late Victorian Respectability and the Social System', International Review of Social History, viii (1963), 18–48, 216–50; Frances Finnegan, Poverty and Prostitution: A study of Victorian Prostitutes in York (Cambridge and New York: Cambridge University Press, 1979); Peter Gay, The Bourgeois Experience – Victoria to Freud, Vol. I: Education of the Senses (Oxford and New York: Oxford University Press, 1984); Brian Harrison, 'Underneath the Victorians', Victorian Studies, x (1967), 239–62; Pat Jalland, Women, Marriage, and Politics, 1860–1914 (Oxford: Oxford University Press, 1986); Paul McHugh, Prostitution and Victorian Social Reform (London: Croom Helm, 1980); Angus McLaren, Birth Control in Nineteenth Century England (London: Croom Helm, 1978); Linda Mahood, The Magdalenes: Prostitution in the Nineteenth Century (London and New York: Routledge, 1990); Steven Marcus, The Other Victorians: A Study of Sexuality and Pornography in Mid-Nineteenth Century England (London: Weidenfeld and Nicolson, 1966); Lynda Nead, Myths of Sexuality: Representations of Women in Victorian Britain (Oxford: Basil Blackwell, 1988); Mary Poovey, Uneven Developments: The Ideological Work of Gender in Mid-Victorian England (London: Virago, 1989); Cynthia Eagle Russett, Sexual Science: The Victorian Construction of Womanhood (London and Cambridge, Mass.: Harvard University Press, 1989); Mary Lyndon Shanley, Feminism, Marriage, and the Law in Victorian England, 1850–1895 (Princeton, NJ: Princeton University Press, 1989); Carol Z. Stearns and Peter N. Stearns, 'Victorian Sexuality: Can Historians Do It Better?', Journal of Social History, xviii (iv) (1985), 625–

34; Martha Vicinus (ed.), A Widening Sphere: Changing Roles of Victorian Women (Bloomington: Indiana University Press, 1977); Judith R. Walkowitz, Prostitution and Victorian Society: Women, Class and the State (Cambridge and New York: Cambridge University Press, 1980). Several studies of a wider chronological sweep nonetheless deal extensively with questions of 'Victorian values', for example Kenneth Ballhatchet, Race, Sex, and Class under the Raj: Imperial Attitudes and Policies and their Critics, 1793–1905 (London: Weidenfeld and Nicolson, 1980); J. Miriam Benn, The Predicaments of Love (London: Pluto Press, 1992); Alex Comfort, The Anxiety Makers: Some Curious Preoccupations of the Medical Profession (London: Nelson, 1967); Frank Mort, Dangerous Sexualities: Medico-Moral Politics in England since 1830 (London and New York: Routledge and Kegan Paul, 1987); and Ornella Moscucci, The Science of Woman: Gynaecology and Gender in England 1800–1929 (Cambridge: Cambridge University Press, 1990). Other studies not specifically about Victorian sexuality but which are illuminating about the omnipresence of sexual assumptions, include Mary S. Hartmann, Victorian Murderesses: A True History of Thirteen Respectable French and English Women Accused of Unspeakable Crimes (New York: Schocken Books; London: Robson Books, 1977) and Alex Owen, The Darkened Room: Women, Power and Spiritualism in Late Victorian England (London: Virago, 1989). Unfortunately Michael Mason's The Making of Victorian Sexuality (Oxford: Oxford University Press, 1994), came to hand too late for his insights fully to be engaged with.

2. A. James Hammerton, Cruelty and Companionship: Conflict in Nineteenth Century Married Life (London and New York: Routledge, 1992).

3. These issues are discussed in Shanley, Feminism, Marriage and the Law.

4. Cuttings found in 'Social Evil Abstracts' Part 3: 'The Preventive Reform Question', John Bull and Britannia, 15 Jan. 1859; Daily Telegraph 12 [?Jan.] 1859. These volumes of press cuttings and ephemera, now in the

Fawcett Library at London Guildhall University, appear to have been compiled by William Acton himself.

5. Social Evil Abstracts Part 3: 'The Argyll Rooms and their Votaries' [n. d.].

6. Thomas Boyle, *Black Swine in the Sewers of Hampstead: Beneath the Surface of Victorian Sensationalism* (New York: Viking, 1988), 12–20, 103–16; Richard D. Altick, *Victorian Studies in Scarlet* (London: J. M. Dent and Sons, 1972), deals mainly with murder, but see pp. 59–63 more generally on the rise of sensationalism; Lawrence Stone, *The Road to Divorce: England, 1530–1987* (Oxford: Oxford University Press, 1992), 252, 294–5 on crim. con. and divorce case reporting.

7. Mayhew, Henry, *London Labour and the London Poor*, Vol. IV: *Those That Will Not Work, comprising Prostitutes, Thieves, Swindlers, and Beggars, by Several Contributors* (London: Griffin, Bohn, 1861–2; New York: Dover Publications, 1968): 'The Agencies at Present in Operation within the Metropolis for the Suppression of Vice and Crime' by the Rev. William Tuckniss, xi–xl; see also F. K. Prochaska, *Women and Philanthropy in Nineteenth Century England* (Oxford: Oxford University Press, 1980), ch. 6: 'In Streets and "Dens of Vice"', 182–221.

8. First letter 4 Feb. 1858, and subsequent letters, are in Social Evil Abstracts, Part 1.

9. Social Evil Abstracts, Part 1: 'Gracchus' in *Reynolds' News Letter*, 7 Feb. 1858, Leading article in the *Leader*, 18 Sept. 1858.

10. Social Evil Abstracts, Part 1: *The Standard*, Nov. 1858.

11. *Ibid., The Leader*, 18 Sept. 1858, and n. d.

12. *Ibid., The Morning Chronicle*, 21 June 1858.

13. *Ibid.*, 24 May 1859, unidentified periodical.

14. *Ibid., Bell's Life in London*, n. d., c. 1858.

15. *Ibid.*, 'Prostitution: Its Medical Aspects', *The Lancet*, 13 March 1858.

16. T. J. Wyke, 'Hospital Facilities for, and Diagnosis and Treatment of, Venereal Disease in England, 1800–1870', *British Journal of Venereal Diseases*, xlix (1973), 78–85, citing *Report of the Committee Appointed to Enquire into the Pathol-*

ogy and Treatment of Venereal Disease, with the View to Diminish its Injurious Effects on the Men of the Army and Navy . . ., Cd. 4031, 1868.

17. T. J. Wyke, 'The Manchester and Salford Lock Hospital, 1818–1917', *Medical History*, xix (1979), 73–86; L. W. Harrison, 'Those Were the Days! or Random Notes on Then and Now in VD', *Bulletin of the Institute of Technicians in Venereology*, Wellcome Institute Library Reprint Collection [n. d. ?1950s], 1–7.

18. Wyke, 'Hospital Facilities'; A. Fessler, 'Venereal Disease and Prostitution in the Reports of the Poor Law Commissioners, 1834–1850', *British Journal of Venereal Diseases*, xxvii (1951), 154–7.

19. Moscucci, *Science of Woman*, 112–27.

20. Wyke, 'Hospital Facilities'.

21. *Proceedings of the Royal Medical and Chirurgical Society of London*, viii (i) (1876), 74–6.

22. Marie Stopes papers in the Contemporary Medical Archives Centre, Wellcome Institute for the History of Medicine: CMAC: PP/MCS/A.1/25.

23. Harrison, 'Those Were the Days!'

24. M. Jeanne Peterson, *The Medical Profession in Mid-Victorian London* (Berkeley: University of California Press, 1978), 244–59, mentions a few cases, but largely in the context of older styles of medical entrepreneurship increasingly being replaced by a new model of professionalization which engaged in the market-place in a less overtly aggressive fashion.

25. Social Evil Abstracts, Part 1: Handbill of Messrs Sloan and Co., allegedly members of the Royal College of Surgeons, c. 1857.

26. Harrison, 'Those Were the Days!'

27. Wyke, 'Hospital Facilities'; Fessler 'Venereal Disease and Prostitution'; Social Evil Abstracts, Part 1: handbills, various.

28. Discussed in detail in Walkowitz, *Prostitution and Victorian Society*; McHugh, *Prostitution and Victorian Social Reform*; Mort, *Dangerous Sexualities*; Richard Davenport-Hines, *Sex, Death, and Punishment: Attitudes to Sex and Sexuality in Britain since the Renaissance* (London: Collins, 1990).

29. Wyke 'Hospital Facilities'.

30. *Ibid.*

31. Social Evil Abstracts Part 1: various reports to this effect, early 1858.

32. Walkowitz, *Prostitution and Victorian Society*, 74

33. McHugh, *Prostitution and Victorian Social Reform*, 37–8.

34. Walkowitz, *Prostitution and Victorian Society*, ch. 10: 'The Making of an Outcast Group: Prostitutes and Working Women in Plymouth and Southampton', 192–213.

35. *Ibid.*, ch. 5: 'The Repeal Campaign', 90–112; McHugh, *Prostitution and Victorian Social Reform*, ch. 3: 'The Attack on the Acts launched', 55–90.

36. Mort, *Dangerous Sexualities*, 90.

37. Cited in Keith Thomas, 'The Double Standard', *Journal of the History of Ideas*, xx (1959), 195–216.

38. Thus causing 'Class and gender conflict within the repeal movement': Walkowitz, *Prostitution and Victorian Society*, ch. 7, 137–47.

39. McHugh, *Prostitution and Victorian Social Reform*, 259–62.

40. For example *The Lancet*, i (1870), 880, 889; ii, 89–90; *British Medical Journal* [*BMJ*], i (1879), 823–4.

41. *The Lancet*, ii (1870), 89–90, 124–6, 159–60, 224–5.

42. Social Evil Abstracts, Part 1: handbill of Messrs Sloan and Co., *c.* 1857.

43. *Ibid.*: cutting of advertisement.

44. *Descriptive Catalogue of the Liverpool Museum of Anatomy*, *c.* 1877 (first published *c.* 1851). I am indebted to David Brady for drawing this item to my attention.

45. Social Evil Abstracts, Part 1: advertisements for Dr Kahn's Museum, handbill 'Beware of Waxwork Quacks!' (De Roos), *c.* 1857; Richard D. Altick, *The Shows of London* (Cambridge, Mass. and London: Belknap Press of Harvard University Press, 1978), 340–1, gives a brief account of Kahn's museum.

46. 'A Graduate', *A Lecture to Young Men on the Preservation of Health and Personal Purity of Life*, 7th edn (Pulvermacher's World Famed Galvanic Belt Co.) (London: H. Renshaw, 1892); numerous advertisements for electro-therapeutic devices in the 'Patent Medicines' section of the John Johnson Ephemera Collection in the Bodleian Library.

47. *The Lancet*, ii (1857), 537.

48. O. S. Fowler, *Creative and Sexual Science; or, Manhood, Womanhood and Their Mutual Interrelations; Love, its Laws, Power, etc.; Selection, or Mutual Adaptation; Courtship, Married Life and Perfect Children; Their Generation, Endowment, Paternity, Maternity, Bearing, Nursing and Rearing; together with Puberty, Boyhood, Girlhood, etc., Sexual Impairments Restored, Male Vigour and Female Health and Beauty Perpetuated and Augmented, etc., as Taught by Phrenology and Physiology* (New York: O. S. Fowler, 1870; 2nd edn *c.* 1900), 603, 620.

49. *Ibid.*, 801–4.

50. T. L. Nichols, *Esoteric Anthropology (The Mysteries of Man) A Comprehensive and Confidential Treatise on the Structure, Functions, Passional Attractions, and Perversions, True and False Physical and Social Conditions and the Most Intimate Relations of Men and Women. Anatomical, Physiological, Pathological, Therapeutical and Obstetrical. Hygienic and Hydropathic. From the American Stereotype Edition, Revised and Rewritten* (Hygienic Institute, Museum St, London WC: the author, n. d., *c.* 1873).

51. Cominos, 'Late Victorian Respectability'.

52. S. Nissenbaum, *Sex, Diet, and Debility in Jacksonian America: Sylvester Graham and Health Reform* (Westport, Conn. and London: Greenwood Press, 1980), 158–73, discusses Nichols and his wife Mary Gove Nichols in the context of health reform and free love movements in the USA, and explores the contradictions inherent in their 'free love' stance.

53. Havelock Ellis, review article in *Reynolds News*, 26 April 1936, in E. F. Griffith's press-cuttings scrapbook, Papers of Edward Fyfe Griffith, Wellcome Institute, CMAC, PP/EFG/A.41; similar opinion expressed in Havelock Ellis, *Eonism and Other Supplementary Studies, Studies in the Psychology of Sex Volume VII* (Philadelphia: F. A. Davis, 1928), 156.

54. Hartmann, *Victorian Murderesses*, 185, mentions this, and Adelaide Bartlett's consultation of Mary Gove Nichols (T. L.'s wife), p. 200. I am indebted to Heather Creaton of the Institute of Historical Research, London, for draw-

ing my attention to the Nicholses and *Esoteric Anthropology*'s connection with one of the most famous of Victorian murder cases.

55. Nichols, *Esoteric Anthropology*, 280–1.
56. Moscucci, *Science of Woman*; Poovey, *Uneven Developments*; Russett, *Sexual Science*; Susan Mendus and Jane Rendall (eds), *Sexuality and Subordination: Interdisciplinary Studies of Gender in the Nineteenth Century* (London: Routledge, 1989), to name but a few.
57. *The Lancet*, i (1854), 243–6, 269–70, 467–8, 595–6.
58. *The Lancet*, ii (1856), 215–17, 300–3, 482–4, 643–4; i (1857), 376–7.
59. *The Lancet*, ii (1856), 644.
60. Marris Wilson, *On Diseases of the Vesiculae Seminales and their Associated Organs, with Special Reference to the Morbid Secretions of the Prostatic and Urethral Mucous Membrane* (London: published for the author by Tallart and Allen, 1856); reviewed in *The Lancet*, i (1856), 289–90.
61. *The Lancet*, i (1857), 556–7.
62. Marcus, *The Other Victorians*, ch. 1: 'Mr Acton of Queen Anne Street, or, The Wisdom of our Ancestors', 1–33.
63. F. B. Smith, *The People's Health, 1830–1910* (London: Croom Helm, 1979) and 'Sexuality in Britain, 1800–1900: Some Suggested Revisions', in M. Vicinus, *A Widening Sphere*, 182–98; M. Jeanne Peterson, 'Dr Acton's Enemy: Medicine, Sex, and Society in Victorian England', *Victorian Studies*, xxix (iv) (1986), 569–90; *idem*, 'No Angels in the House: The Victorian Myth and the Paget Women', *American Historical Review*, lxxxix (iii) (1984), 677–708; *idem, Family, Love and Work in the Lives of Victorian Gentlewomen* (Bloomington and Indianapolis: Indiana University Press, 1989); Gay, *Education of the Senses*; an early critique of this revisionist school is to be found in Stearns and Stearns, 'Victorian Sexuality: Can Historians Do It Better?'
64. Smith, *The People's Health*, Section 4, Adults, Part 4, 'Venereal Diseases, Contraception and Sexuality', 294–315.
65. Peterson, 'Dr Acton's Enemy'; Paget's views and their influence are discussed below.
66. William Acton, *The Functions and Disorders of the Reproductive Organs in Youth,* *Adult, Age, and Advanced Life, considered in their Physiological, Social and Psychological Relations* (London: John Churchill, 1857; 3rd edn 1862), 101–2.
67. *Ibid.*, 98.
68. *Ibid.*, 92–5.
69. *Ibid.*, 130–1.
70. *Ibid.*, 138.
71. *Ibid.*, 140–1.
72. John L. Milton, 'On the Nature and Treatment of Spermatorrhoea', *The Lancet*, i (1854), 243–6, 269–70.
73. Smith, *The People's Health*, 295.
74. Cominos, 'Late Victorian Respectability'.
75. Acton, *Functions and Disorders*, 74.
76. *British Medical Journal*, ii (1881), 904.
77. James Copland, *A Dictionary of Practical Medicine: Comprising General Pathology, the Nature and Treatment of Diseases, Morbid Structures and the Disorders Especially Incident to Climates, to the Sex, and to the Different Epochs of Life*, 4 vols (London: Longmans, 1844–58), 'Pollutions', 441–8.
78. Peterson, 'Dr Acton's Enemy'.
79. Sir James Paget, 'Sexual Hypochondriasis', in his *Clinical Lectures and Essays* (London: Longmans Green, 1875; 2nd edn 1879), 275–98.
80. John Laws Milton, *On Spermatorrhoea: Its Results and Complications*, 9th edn (London: Robert Hardwicke, 1872; from original papers in *The Lancet*, 1852 and *The Medical Circular*, 1858).
81. *The Lancet*, ii (1870), 159.
82. Samuel La'mert, *Self-Preservation: A Medical Treatise on Nervous and Physical Debility, Spermatorrhoea, Impotence and Sterility, with Practical Observations on the Use of the Microscope in the Treatment of Diseases of the Generative System*, '64th edn' (London: 'Published by the Author and sold at all Booksellers', *c.* 1850s–60s) contains credentials pertaining to La'mert's career and qualifications. The registers of licentiates of the Society of Apothecaries in the Guildhall Library (Guildhall Mss 8241/6, 8241B/1) confirm his licence (1833) to practise as an apothecary, qualified through apprenticeship.
83. La'mert, *Self-Preservation*, Introduction, ix.
84. *BMJ*, i (1863), 567; ii, 586–7; *The Lancet*, ii (1863), 634–5.
85. *The Lancet*, i (1857), 556–7.

86. *The Lancet*, i (1862), 518–19.
87. La'mert, *Self-Preservation*, 23.
88. Discussed further in Lesley A. Hall '"The English Have Hot-Water Bottles': the Morganatic Marriage of Medicine and Sexology in Britain since William Acton', in Roy Porter and Mikuláš Teich (eds), *Sexual Knowledge, Sexual Science: The History of Attitudes to Sexuality* (Cambridge: Cambridge University Press, 1994), 350–66.
89. Peterson, 'Dr Acton's Enemy'.
90. See Peterson, *Medical Profession in Mid-Victorian London*.
91. For example *The Lancet*, i (1862), 518; and see 'Introduction' to the 3rd edition of Acton, *Functions and Disorders*, vii–viii.
92. *BMJ*, i (1866), 440. Isaac Baker Brown, *On the Curability of Certain Forms of Insanity, Epilepsy, Catalepsy, and Hysteria in Females* (London: R. Hardwicke, 1866).
93. *BMJ*, ii (1866), 665.
94. *The Lancet*, ii (1866), 566; *BMJ*, i (1867), 395–410; I am indebted to Ornella Moscucci for letting me see her (so far unpublished) paper on Baker Brown and the clitoridectomy debate; the case is also discussed in Ann Dally, *Women under the Knife: A History of Surgery* (London: Hutchinson Radius, 1991), 162–81.
95. George Drysdale, *Elements of Social Science: or Physical, Sexual, and Natural Religion, an Exposition of the True Cause and Only Cure of the Three Primary Social Evils: Poverty, Prostitution, and Celibacy, by a Doctor of Medicine* (London [anonymously], E. Truelove, 1854; London: G. Standring, 1905), 80–1.
96. *Ibid.*, 77–8, 87.
97. Phyllis Grosskurth, *Havelock Ellis: A Biography* (London: Allen Lane, 1980), 39.
98. Drysdale, *Elements of Social Science*, 78.
99. *Ibid.*, 88.
100. *Ibid.*, 125.
101. *Ibid.*, 163, 255–7.
102. *Ibid.*, 270.
103. Havelock Ellis, *Sex in Relation to Society, Studies in the Psychology of Sex Volume VI* (Philadelphia: F. A. Davis, 1910), 596.
104. Peter Agate, MD, *Sexual Economy as Taught by Charles Bradlaugh, M.P., with an addendum by Saladin* (London: W.

Stewart, n. d. ?1878).
105. See Benn, *Predicaments of Love*: a magnificently researched study of George Drysdale, his brother and sister-in-law, and nephew and niece, in their relations to the Malthusian movement.
106. C. Knowlton, *Fruits of Philosophy: An Essay on the Population Question*, new edn, with notes, ed, G. Drysdale, printed by Charles Bradlaugh and Annie Besant (London: Freethought Publishing, [1877]; first published USA, 1847) for an account of the trial of this work see S. Chandrasekhar, '*A Dirty Filthy Book*': *The writings of Charles Bradlaugh and Annie Besant on Reproductive Physiology and Birth Control, and an Account of the Bradlaugh-Besant Trial* (Berkeley: University of California Press, 1981).
107. H. A. Allbutt, *The Wife's Handbook: How a Woman Should Order Herself during Pregnancy, in the Lying-In Room, and After Delivery. With Hints on the Management of the Baby, and Other Matters of Importance Necessary to be Known by Married Women* (London: W. J. Ramsay, 1886); for an account of the trial see *BMJ*, i (1889), 270; ii, 1162–3, 1221–2. In spite, or perhaps because, of this notoriety, this work had gone into over 40 editions by the time of the First World War, and was still, according to Norman E. Himes, *The Medical History of Contraception* (Baltimore, Md.: Williams and Wilkins, 1936), 326n, widely available in the 1930s.
108. Donald Thomas, *A Long Time Burning: The History of Literary Censorship in England* (London: Routledge and Kegan Paul, 1969), 240–1.
109. McLaren, *Birth Control in Nineteenth Century England*, 116.
110. C. H. F. Routh, *On the Moral and Physical Evils likely to Follow if Practices Intended to Act as Checks to Population be not Strongly Discouraged and Condemned*, originally given as a paper before the Obstetrical section of the British Medical Association, and first published in the *Medical Press and Circular*, October 1878; repr. London, 1879.
111. *BMJ*, ii (1889), 88.
112. Social Evil Abstracts Part 1: *Man's Body, God's Temple: An Earnest Appeal to Young People, and All Who Wish Them*

Well by the Rev. Peter Lilly, MA, curate of Kegworth Leicestershire, (n. d. *c.* 1858); *An Address to Young Men*, (n. d., mid-19th century), John Johnson Ephemera Collection, Bodleian Library: 'Sex Population and Eugenics' I.

113. *BMJ*, ii (1881), 904.
114. Hon. E. Lyttelton, *The Causes and Prevention of Immorality in Schools* (London: Social Purity Alliance, printed for private circulation, 1887), 15.
115. Arthur T. Barnett, 'The Testimony of Medical Men', citing F. Le Gros Clark, in The White Cross League, *The Blanco Book* (London: White Cross League, 1913), reprinting League papers which had been in circulation for some decades, 223.
116. C. G. Wheelhouse, in Barnett, 'Testimony of Medical Men', 226.
117. Marcus, *The Other Victorians*, ch. 7: 'Conclusion: Pornotopia', 266–86; Coral Lansbury, *The Old Brown Dog: Women, Workers and Vivisection in Edwardian England* (Madison: University of Wisconsin Press, 1985), chs 6 and 7: 'Riding Masters and Young Mares', 'A Woman is Being Beaten', 96–129; Thomas, *A Long Time Burning*, 273–4.
118. Iain McCalman, *Radical Underworld: Prophets, Revolutionaries and Pornographers in London, 1795–1840* (Cambridge: Cambridge University Press, 1988), ch. 10: 'Grub Street Jacks: Obscene Populism and Pornography', 204–31; see also Richard D. Altick, *The English Common Reader: A Social History of the Mass Reading Public 1800–1900* (Chicago: University of Chicago Press, 1957), 292–3, 346, on the commercial motivation and acumen, and pornographic output, of 'pariah publishers'.
119. Thomas, *A Long Time Burning*, 193.
120. McCalman, *Radical Underworld*, 235.
121. Mayhew, *London Labour and the London Poor*, Vol IV, 267.
122. Social Evil Abstracts Part 1: Traffic in obscene literature; Mr Prichard of the Society for the Suppression of Vice: letter to Lord Campbell about obscene publications, (n. d. ?1858).
123. Social Evil Abstracts Part 1: Prosecution under Lord Campbell's Act, reported in *Morning News*, 19 March

[no year].
124. Cited in Thomas, *A Long Time Burning*, 272–3.
125. John Johnson Ephemera Collection, Bodleian Library: 'Sex Population and Eugenics' boxes, for all the above and a number of works on nuns and the confessional; lurid reporting about the Catholic menace also in Social Evil Abstracts.
126. *BMJ*, ii (1881), 904.
127. Acton, *Functions and Disorders*, 18–19.
128. See newspaper reports collected in Social Evil Abstracts cited above.
129. Mayhew, *London Labour and the London Poor*, Vol. IV, 27, definition of 'Cohabitant Prostitutes'.
130. *Man's Body, God's Temple* in Social Evil Abstracts Part 1; *An Address to Young Men*, John Johnson Ephemera Collection.
131. Judith R. Walkowitz, *City of Dreadful Delight: Narratives of Sexual Danger in Late-Victorian London* (London: Virago, 1992), chs 3 and 4: '"The Maiden Tribute of Modern Babylon"', '"The Maiden Tribute": cultural consequences', 81–134.

7   *From the Primeval Protozoa to the Laboratory: the Evolution of Sexual Science from 1889 to the 1930s*

1. Ornella Moscucci, *The Science of Woman: Gynaecology and Gender in England 1800–1929* (Cambridge: Cambridge University Press, 1990), 21–2; Cynthia Eagle Russett, *Sexual Science: The Victorian Construction of Womanhood* (Cambridge, Mass. and London: Harvard University Press, 1989), 40–43, and *passim*.
2. Phyllis Grosskurth, *Havelock Ellis: A Biography* (London: Allen Lane, 1980), 114–15.
3. Cited in Paddy Kitchen, *A Most Unsettling Person: An Introduction to the Ideas and Life of Patrick Geddes* (London: Gollancz, 1975), 96.
4. *Ibid.*, 299; quoting C. R. Ashbee.
5. Philip Boardman, *The Worlds of Patrick Geddes, Biologist, Town Planner, Reeducator, Peace-warrior* (London and

Boston: Routledge and Kegan Paul, 1978), 299.

6. Kitchen, *A Most Unsettling Person*, 76–9.

7. Prof. Patrick Geddes and J. Arthur Thomson, *The Evolution of Sex*, Contemporary Science Series, ed. Havelock Ellis (London: Walter Scott, 1889). Introduction to the 2nd edn, 1901, p. v (the first edition only said 'such unity as our present knowledge renders possible'). Subsequent citations are from the first edition.

8. *Ibid.*, 17.

9. *Ibid.*, 267.

10. *Ibid.*, 257–8.

11. *Ibid.*, 270–1.

12. Boardman, *The Worlds of Patrick Geddes*, 299.

13. Geddes and Thomson, *The Evolution of Sex*, 295.

14. *Ibid.*, 296.

15. *Ibid.*, 297.

16. *Ibid.*, 269.

17. Edward Carpenter to Havelock Ellis, 27 March 1890; Harry Ransom Humanities Research Center, University of Texas at Austin (HRC).

18. Kitchen, *A Most Unsettling Person*, 100, quoting letter of 1889 from Mrs J. Butt of Eastbourne.

19. Boardman, *The Worlds of Patrick Geddes*, 113.

20. *Ibid.*; Unfortunately, letters of comment survive only sporadically among the Geddes papers; although two large collections are to be found in both Edinburgh and at Strathclyde, there are what Paddy Kitchen describes as 'tantalizing gaps': *A Most Unsettling Person*, 25.

21. Boardman, *The Worlds of Patrick Geddes*, 112; reported by Geddes's daughter Norah.

22. Alfred R. Wallace to Patrick Geddes, 1 Dec. 1889; Sir Patrick Geddes papers in the University of Strathclyde Library (Geddes/Strathclyde), T–GED 9/42.

23. Merriley Borell, 'Organotherapy, British Physiology, and Discovery of the Internal Secretions', *Journal of the History of Biology*, ix (ii) (1976), 235–68; *idem*, 'Setting the Standards for a New Science: Edward Schäfer and Endocrinology', *Medical History*, xxii (1978), 282–90.

24. *British Medical Journal* [*BMJ*], i, (1893), 1325–6; Richard von Krafft-Ebing, *Psychopathia Sexualis: With Especial Reference to the Antipathetic Sexual Instinct. A Medico-Forensic Study* (Stuttgart: Erke, 1886; first English edition 1892, numerous subsequent editions).

25. Sheila Rowbotham and Jeffrey Weeks, *Socialism and the New Life: the Personal and Sexual Politics of Edward Carpenter and Havelock Ellis* (London: Pluto Press, 1977); Part 1: 'Edward Carpenter: Prophet of the New Life' by Sheila Rowbotham, 25–138; Jeffrey Weeks, *Coming Out: Homosexual Politics in Britain from the Nineteenth Century to the Present* (London: Quartet, 1977), ch. 6: 'Edward Carpenter and Friends', 68–83.

26. Edward Carpenter, *Love's Coming of Age. A Series of Papers on the Relation of the Sexes* (London: Allen and Unwin, 1896; 13th edn 1930): 'The Intermediate Sex', 130–48.

27. *Ibid.*, 'Love's Ultimate Meaning', 149–68.

28. Such as Edward Carpenter, *Iolaus: An Anthology of Friendship* (London, 1902); *The Intermediate Sex* (London: Swan Sonnerschein, 1908); and *Intermediate Types among Primitive Folk* (London, 1914), directed at, and extremely popular with, a more specific constituency.

29. Carpenter, *Love's Coming of Age*, 'The Intermediate Sex', 130–48.

30. Havelock Ellis, *Man and Woman: A Study of Human Secondary Sexual Characters*, Contemporary Science Series (London: Walter Scott, 1894).

31. Weeks, *Coming Out*, ch. 2: 'The Medical Model', 23–32; ch. 4: 'Speaking Out: John Addington Symonds', 47–56; *idem, Sex, Politics and Society: The Regulation of Sexuality since 1800*, Themes in British Social History (London: Longman, 1981), 111–12.

32. Havelock Ellis to Edward Carpenter, 17 Dec. 1892, Edward Carpenter papers in Sheffield City Archives (Carpenter/Sheffield), MSS 357/5.

33. Grosskurth, *Havelock Ellis*, 181–2.

34. *Ibid.*, ch. 13: 'The Bedborough Trial', 191–204; Weeks, *Coming Out*, ch. 5: 'Havelock Ellis and *Sexual Inversion*', 57–67; *idem, Sex, Politics and Society*, 180–1.

35. *The Lancet*, ii (1898), 1344–5: 'The Question of Indecent Literature'.

36. *BMJ*, ii (1898), 1466.

37. Grosskurth, *Havelock Ellis*, 196.

38. *Shafts: A Paper for Women and the Working Classes* ed. Margaret Shurmer Sibthorp, Nov. 1892; June 1895.

39. T. L. Nichols, *Esoteric Anthropology (The Mysteries of Man) A Comprehensive and Confidential Treatise on the Structure, Functions, Passional Attractions, and Perversions, True and False Physical and Social Conditions and the Most Intimate Relations of Men and Woman. Anatomical, Physiological, Pathological, Therapeutical and Obstetrical. Hygienic and Hydropathic. From the American Stereotype Edition, Revised and Rewritten* (Hygienic Institute, Museum St, London WC: the author, *c.* 1873), 109.

40. 'Ellis Ethelmer' [Mrs Wolstenholme Elmy], *Woman Free* (Congleton: Woman's Emancipation Union, 1893).

41. *Shafts*, July 1896.

42. *Shafts*, July 1895.

43. *BMJ*, i (1909), 1547.

44. Ellis to Carpenter, 8 April 1907, Carpenter/Sheffield, MSS 357/13.

45. *BMJ*, i (1902), 339–40.

46. *The Lancet*, i (1910), 1207.

47. *The Lancet*, ii (1908), 1373.

48. *BMJ*, i (1908), 102–3.

49. Dean Rapp, 'The Early Discovery of Freud by the British General Public', *Social History of Medicine*, iii (1990), 217–43.

50. J. A. Campbell to Geddes, 24 Jan. 1912, Geddes/Strathclyde, T–GED 9/1041.

51. Prof. Patrick Geddes and J. Arthur Thomson, *Sex*, Home University Library (London: Williams and Norgate, 1914), 118, 150; see also 138, 144.

52. *The Lancet*, i (1917), 912–14.

53. *BMJ*, i (1902), 339–40.

54. Otto Weininger, *Sex and Character*, authorized trans. from the 6th German edn (London: Heinemann, 1906).

55. Harold Hodge of the *Saturday Review* to Geddes, 27 Feb. 1906, Geddes Strathclyde T–GED 6/638.

56. Review of *Sex and Character*, *Saturday Review* 5 May 1906.

57. Grace French of Bedford to Carpenter, *c.* 1906, Carpenter/Sheffield MSS 386/141.

58. Carpenter to Ellis, 8 Oct. 1906, HRC.

59. Ellis to Carpenter, 12 Nov. 1916: Carpenter/Sheffield, MSS 357/28.

60. Carpenter, *Love's Coming of Age*, 162–3.

61. Carpenter to Ellis, 23 June 1914, HRC.

62. Frances Swiney, *The Cosmic Procession, or the Feminine Principle in Evolution: Essays of Illumination*, Higher Thought Series (London: Ernest Bell, 1906), 71n.

63. *Ibid.*, 'Introduction', x.

64. *Ibid.*, 158fn.

65. Ellis to Carpenter, 17 May 1907, Carpenter/Sheffield, MSS 357/14.

66. Iwan Bloch, *The Sexual Life of Our Time, in its Relations to Modern Civilisation*, trans. from the 6th German edn by M. Eden Paul (London: Rebman, 1909), v.

67. Ernest Jones, Toronto, to Ellis, 12 June 1910, Havelock Ellis papers in the Department of Manuscripts, British Library, BL Add. MS 70539.

68. Rebecca West, *The Young Rebecca: Writings of Rebecca West 1911–1917* selected and introduced by Jane Marcus (London: Macmillan, 1982), review of Ellis's *Essays in Wartime*, 332–5.

69. Havelock Ellis, *Studies in the Psychology of Sex*: Volume I: *The Evolution of Modesty: The Phenomena of Sexual Periodicity; Auto-Erotism, Studies in the Psychology of Sex* (Leipzig and Watford, 1899; Philadelphia: F. A. Davis 1901); Volume II: *Sexual Inversion* (with J. Addington Symonds), London, Wilson and Macmillan, 1897 (withdrawn), Philadelphia: F. A. Davis, 1901 (subsequent volumes all first published by F. A. Davis); Volume III: *The Analysis of the Sexual Impulse: Love and Pain: The Sexual Impulse in Women* (1903); Volume IV: *Sexual Selection in Man* (1905); Volume V: *Erotic Symbolism: The Mechanism of Detumescence: the Psychic State in Pregnancy* (1906); Volume VI: *Sex in Relation to Society* (1910); Volume VII: *Eonism and Other Supplementary Studies* (1928).

70. Ellis to E. Westermarck, 1902, BL Add. MS 70539.

71. Grosskurth, *Havelock Ellis*, 185.

72. See, for example, Jeffrey Weeks in *Sex Politics and Society*, 147–51, and his 'Havelock Ellis: The Politics of Sexual Reform', in Rowbotham and Weeks, *Socialism and the New Life*, 162, 168–71. For a swingeing, and rather unnuanced, attack on Ellis's view of

women see Sheila Jeffreys, *The Spinster and Her Enemies: Feminism and Sexuality 1800–1930* (London: Pandora Press, 1985); similar arguments are advanced by Margaret Jackson, 'Eroticizing Women's Oppression: Havelock Ellis and the Construction of the "Natural" ', in *idem, The Real Facts of Life: Feminism and the Politics of Sexuality c. 1850–1940* (London: Taylor and Francis, 1994), 106–28.

73. See, for example, the tribute paid him by F. W. Stella Browne in *The Sexual Variety and Variability among Women and their Bearing upon Social Reconstruction* (London: British Society for the Study of Sex Psychology, 1917).

74. Ellis, *Evolution of Modesty; The Phenomena of Sexual Periodicity; Auto-Erotism*, p. 98.

75. *Ibid.*, 166.

76. *Ibid.*, 261.

77. *Ibid.*, 263.

78. Ellis to Carpenter, 16 April 1910, 17 Feb. 1918, Carpenter, Sheffield, MSS 357/16 and 32.

79. Havelock Ellis, *Essays in War-Time: First Series* (London: Constable, 1916); *idem, The Philosophy of Conflict, and Other Essays in War-Time: Second Series* (London: Constable, 1919); *idem, Little Essays of Love and Virtue* (London: A. and C. Black, 1922); *idem, More Essays of Love and Virtue* (London: Constable, 1931).

80. A. Radcliffe Brown, Professor of Social Anthropology, Cape Town, to Ellis, 12 June 1922: BL Add. MS 70555.

81. *The Lancet*, ii (1939), 165.

82. Discussed in Chapter 9 on the marriage manual; see p. 211ff.

83. Ellis to Marie Stopes, 22 Nov. 1921, Stopes papers in the British Library Department of Manuscripts, BL Add. MS 58564.

84. Francis H. A. Marshall, *The Physiology of Reproduction*, with a Preface by Professor E. A. Schäfer and contributions by William Cramer and James Lochhead (London, New York, Bombay and Calcutta: Longmans Green, 1910), 'Introduction', 1.

85. See, for example, *ibid.*, 1, 71n, 654–7; W. Blair Bell, *The Sex Complex: A Study of the Relationships of the Internal Secretions to the Female Characteristics and Functions in Health and Disease* (London: Baillière, Tindall and Cox, 1916), 1–6, 18, 113–15.

86. The scientific discourse concerning sex hormones and their relation to social attitudes to sexuality have been discussed over the past twenty years in several very valuable articles: Diana Long Hall, 'Biology, Sex Hormones and Sexism in the 1920s', *Philosophical Quarterly*, v (1973–4), 81–96; Borell, 'Organotherapy, British Physiology, and Discovery of the Internal Secretions'; *idem*, 'Setting the Standards for a New Science'; *idem*, 'Organotherapy and the Emergence of Reproductive Technology', *Journal of the History of Biology*, xviii (i) (1985), 1–30, and *idem*, 'Biologists and the Promotion of Birth Control Research, 1918–1938', *Journal of the History of Biology*, xx (i) (1987), 51–88; Nelly Oudshoorn, 'On the Making of Sex Hormones: Research Materials and the Production of Knowledge', *Social Studies of Science*, xx (i) (1990), 5–33; *idem*, 'Endocrinologists and the Conceptualization of Sex, 1920–1940', *Journal of the History of Biology*, xxiii (ii) (1990), 163–86; and *idem*, 'On Measuring Sex Hormones: the Role of Biological Assays in Sexualizing Chemical Substances', *Bulletin of the History of Medicine*, lxiv (1990), 243–61. None of them, however, appears to consider the possibility that wider debates on sexuality at the time may have influenced conceptualizations and the course of investigations, and some rather naive assumptions are made about science, society, sex, the developing acceptability of birth control and the medical profession.

87. Marshall, *Physiology of Reproduction*, 1.

88. Sir Alan Parkes, 'Prospect and Retrospect in the Physiology of Reproduction', Inaugural Lecture of the Mary Marshall Chair of the Physiology of Reproduction, Cambridge, Nov. 1961, in *Sex, Science and Society: Addresses, Lectures and Articles* (Newcastle-upon-Tyne: Oriel Press, 1966), 37–53.

89. Marshall, *Physiology of Reproduction*, 1.

90. George W. Corner, 'The Early History of the Oestrogenic Hormones', The Sir Henry Dale Lecture for 1964, *Journal of Endocrinology*, xxxi (1965) iii–xvii.

91. Hall, 'Biology, Sex Hormones and Sexism'.
92. Marshall, *Physiology of Reproduction*, 111.
93. *Ibid.*, 635–6.
94. *Ibid.*, 640–7, 650–8.
95. *Ibid.*, 303.
96. *Ibid.*, 304, 307.
97. *Ibid.*, 349–50.
98. *Ibid.*, 308.
99. Corner, 'Early History of the Oestrogenic Hormones'.
100. See Lesley Hall, *Hidden Anxieties: Male Sexuality 1900–1950* (Cambridge: Polity Press, 1991) for further discussion of this.
101. Marshall, *Physiology of Reproduction*, 242.
102. *Ibid.*, 257.
103. *Ibid.*, 242.
104. *Ibid.*, 262.
105. Borell, 'Organotherapy and the Emergence of Reproductive Technology'.
106. Corner, 'Early History of the Oestrogenic Hormones'.
107. Walter Heape, *Sex Antagonism* (London: Constable, 1913), 49.
108. *Ibid.*, 203.
109. *Ibid.*, 49.
110. *Ibid.*, 16–17.
111. *Ibid.*, 51.
112. *Ibid.*, 203.
113. *Ibid.*, 214.
114. *Ibid.*, 205–8.
115. *Ibid.*, 213.
116. Bell, *The Sex Complex*, 120–1.
117. *Ibid.*, 13–14.
118. *Ibid.*, 'Introduction', 1–6.
119. *Ibid.*, 100–2.
120. *Ibid.*, 104–5.
121. *Ibid.*, 106–7.
122. *Ibid.*
123. *Ibid.*, 109–12.
124. *Ibid.*, 113–14.
125. *Ibid.*, 109–12.
126. *Ibid.*, 21–2.
127. *Ibid.*, 113–14.
128. *Ibid.*, 118–19.
129. *Ibid.*, 120–1.
130. *Ibid.*, 177.
131. *Ibid.*, 179.
132. *Ibid.*, 200.
133. *Ibid.*, 109.
134. *Ibid.*, 108.
135. Cited in Hall, 'Biology, Sex Hormones and Sexism'.
136. Borell, 'Biologists and the Promotion of Birth Control Research'.
137. Hall, 'Biology, Sex Hormones and Sexism'.
138. Sir Alan Parkes, 'The Rise of Reproductive Endocrinology, 1926–1940', The Sir Henry Dale Lecture of the Society for Endocrinology, May 1965, in Parkes (ed.), *Sex, Science and Society*, 14–36.
139. Hall, 'Biology, Sex Hormones and Sexism'.
140. Parkes, 'The Rise of Reproductive Endocrinology'.
141. Marie C. Stopes, *Enduring Passion: Further New Contributions to the Solution of Sex Difficulties, Being the Continuation of Married Love* (London: G. P. Putnam's Sons, 1928; 2nd edn 1929), 105.
142. Hall, 'Biology, Sex Hormones and Sexism'.
143. Stopes, *Enduring Passion*, 205.
144. Corner, 'Early History of the Oestrogenic Hormones'.
145. Hall, 'Biology, Sex Hormones and Sexism'.
146. Papers of R. A. McCance and Elsie M. Widdowson in the Contemporary Medical Archives Centre, Wellcome Institute for the History of Medicine: CMAC, GC/97/C: prefatory note to the completed forms of this study; R. A. McCance, M. C. Luff and E. E. Widdowson 'Physical and Emotional Periodicity in Women', *Journal of Hygiene*, xxxvii (1937), 571–611; Royal Society archives: Register of Papers, Series B 1936 – no mention of this paper in earlier years; Minutes of Sectional Committee on Physiology; further discussion in Chapter 8, pp. 191–2.
147. Borell 'Biologists and the Promotion of Birth Control Research, 1918–1938'.
148. R. A. Soloway, *Demography and Degeneration: Eugenics and the Declining Birthrate in Twentieth Century Britain* (Chapel Hill: University of North Carolina Press, 1990), 220–4.
149. Correspondence of J. R. Baker with C. P. Blacker of the Eugenics Society, 1925–1936, Eugenics Society archives in the Contemporary Medical Archives Centre at the Wellcome Institute for the History of Medicine: CMAC, SA/EUG/C.10–11.

8   The Authority of Individual Experience and the Opinions of Experts: Sex as a Social Science

1. Letter from Olive Schreiner to Karl Pearson, 14 July 1885, cited in Ruth First and Anne Scott, *Olive Schreiner* (London: André Deutsch, 1980), 148.

2. Judith R Walkowitz, *City of Dreadful Delight: Narratives of Sexual Danger in Late-Victorian London* (London: Virago, 1992), ch. 5: 'The Men and Women's Club', 135–70; Lucy Bland, 'Marriage Laid Bare: Middle-Class Women and Marital Sex c. 1880–1914', in Jane Lewis (ed.), *Labour and Love: Women's Experience of Home and Family, 1850–1940* (Oxford: Basil Blackwell, 1986), 122–46; Carol Dyhouse, *Feminism and the Family in England 1880–1939* (Oxford: Basil Blackwell, 1989), 157–66; Phyllis Grosskurth, *Havelock Ellis: A Biography* (London: Allen Lane, 1980); First and Scott, *Olive Schreiner*; Ruth Brandon, *The New Women and the Old Men: Love, Sex and the Woman Question* (London: Secker and Warburg, 1990). These latter three deal with the club from a biographical perspective.

3. Havelock Ellis, *Analysis of the Sexual Impulse; Love and Pain; The Sexual Impulse in Women. Studies in the Psychology of Sex Volume III* (Philadelphia: F. A. Davis, 1903; New York: Random House omnibus edition, Vol. I, 1937), Appendix B: 'The Development of the Sexual Instinct', 277–8; Harry Oosterhuis's recent work on Krafft-Ebing would tend to indicate that Krafft-Ebing too was the recipient of unsolicited, volunteered accounts of personal experience (presentation and discussion at the Triennial European History of Psychiatry Conference, London, July 1993).

4. Havelock Ellis, *The Evolution of Modesty; The Phenomena of Sexual Periodicity; Auto-Erotism, Studies in the Psychology of Sex Volume I* (Philadelphia: F. A. Davis, 1901; 3rd edn 1910; New York: Random House omnibus edn, Vol. I, 1937), Appendix B: 'Sexual Periodicity in Man' by F. H. Perrycoste, 297–309. This had been published earlier, in 1898, and a 'preliminary communication' on the subject in *Nature* in 1891.

5. Michel Foucault, *The History of Sexuality Volume I: An Introduction* (first published as *La Volonté de savoir*, Paris: Gallimard, 1976) trans. Robert Hurley (London: Allen Lane, 1979; Harmondsworth: Penguin, 1981), 61–70.

6. 'The Confessional in Belgravia: Astounding Disclosures', *Morning Advertiser*, 12 June 1858, Social Evil Abstracts Vol. I Fawcett Library, London Guildhall University; National Vigilance Association archives, Fawcett Library, subcommittee minutes, Sept. 1889, anti-Catholic pamphlets deemed to be obscene; pamphlets in the John Johnson Ephemera Collection, Bodleian Library: Sex Population and Eugenics: *Police News Edition: The Extraordinary Disclosures of a Nunnery. Action by a Sister of Mercy (Saurin v. Starr and Kennedy) Life of the Plaintiff. Mysteries of Convent Life. Examination of the Witnesses. Summing Up and Verdict, The Poor Nun: or the Trap of Beelzebub* by Thomas Godfrey Jack (prurient account of prurience of the confessional, sadism/masochism in convents, etc.), *The Thrilling Story of Six Months in a Convent!* by Maria Theresa Reed . . . Published by the United States Protestant Association, *The Betrayed Maiden; or, the Confession of a Priest by Mahallah* (London: National Union Publishing Company).

7. E.g. letter to *The Lancet*, ii (1897), 684, from L. A. Parry deprecating suggestions in article by M. C. Hime, 'Immorality among Schoolboys' (*The Lancet*, ii, 1897, 614–17) as 'approximating too closely to the French system'; evidence of A. H. Evans of Winchester, to the National Birth-rate Commission (1920–3) published in *Youth and the Race: The Development and Education of Young Citizens for Worthy Parenthood, Being the Fourth Report of and the Chief Evidence Taken*, ed. Sir James Marchant, secretary (London: Kegan Paul/Trench Trubner, 1923), 52–63, struck a similar note.

8. See ch. 5, pp. 120–22.

9. Marion Shaw, ' "To Tell the Truth of Sex": Confession and Abjection in Late Victorian Writing', in Linda M. Shires (ed.), *Rewriting the Victorians: Theory, History and the Politics of Gender*

(London: Routledge, 1992), 86–100.

10. *Ibid.*, 90–1.

11. Ellis, *Analysis of the Sexual Impulse [etc.]*, 189.

12. Discussed in Lesley A. Hall, *Hidden Anxieties: Male Sexuality, 1900–1950* (Cambridge: Polity Press, 1991), especially 'Introduction: Deconstructing the Monolithic Phallus', 1–7.

13. Carolyn Steedman, *Childhood, Culture and Class in Britain: Margaret McMillan, 1860–1931* (London: Virago, 1990), 122–3; see also Dyhouse, *Feminism and the Family*, 165–6 for some other groups.

14. *The Freewoman*, March–Oct. 1912. V. Glendinning, *Rebecca West: A Life* (London: Weidenfeld and Nicolson, 1987), 37–9, mentions West as a 'lively presence' at these groups, which she herself described as 'too like being in church'; see also Jane Lidderdale and Mary Nicholson, *Dear Miss Weaver: Harriet Shaw Weaver 1876–1961* (London: Faber and Faber, 1970), 48–9, 56.

15. F. W. Stella Browne, 'A New Psychological Society', *International Journal of Ethics*, xxviii (1917–18), 266–9; for a more detailed discussion of this society, see L. A. Hall, '"Disinterested Enthusiasm for Sexual Misconduct": the British Society for the Study of Sex Psychology 1913–1947' (article forthcoming in *Journal of Contemporary History*).

16. Publication No. 1 of the British Society for the Study of Sexual Psychology [Laurence Housman], *Policy and Principles: General Aims* (London: 1914; 2nd revised edition 1929).

17. Browne, 'A New Psychological Society'; Hall, '"Disinterested Enthusiasm for Sexual Misconduct"'.

18. Virginia Woolf, *The Diary of Virginia Woolf*, Vol. I *1915–19*, ed. Anne Olivier Bell (London: Penguin, 1979), entry for 21 Jan. 1918, 110; W. David Wills, *Homer Lane: A Biography* (London: Allen and Unwin, 1964), 200–1.

19. Archives of the British Sexology Society (BSS) at the Harry Ransom Humanities Research Center (HRC), University of Texas at Austin: 'Misc.': Stella Browne to Janet Carson, 27 March 1919, 28 April 1920; Minutes Vol. II, 71st meeting 16 April 1920.

20. BSS archives 'Misc.': Attendance Books 1925–31, 1931–40; Members' Roll 1913–21 also has some lists of attendance at meetings in the 1930s; 'Lecture Lists'.

21. BSS archives 'Misc.': Study Group III, (Heterosexuality), Minutes 1919–[?1923]; Minutes of Joint Meeting between members of Education, Heterosexual and Psycho-Analytic Study Groups, 16 March 1921.

22. E.g. BSS 'Misc.': Minutes of 55th meeting 15 Jan. 1919, re suggestion of a Mr Ernest Crawford.

23. BSS archives 'Misc.': Committee Minutes, 1920, and Minutes of the Heterosexuality Group.

24. Martin Bulmer, 'The Development of Sociology and of Empirical Social Research in Britain', and Raymond Kent 'The Emergence of the Sociological Survey, 1887–1939', in M. Bulmer (ed.), *Essays on the History of Sociological Research* (Cambridge: Cambridge University Press, 1985), 3–36, 52–69.

25. R. A. Soloway, *Birth Control and the Population Question in England, 1877–1930* (Chapel Hill and London: University of North Carolina Press, 1982), 34.

26. Sidney Webb, *The Decline in the Birth-Rate*, Fabian Tract no. 131 (London: Fabian Society, 1907), 9–10 [cost one penny].

27. Soloway, *Birth Control and the Population Question*, 34.

28. Webb, *Decline in the Birth-Rate*, 13.

29. Ethel M. Elderton, *Report on the English Birthrate Part I. England, North of the Humber* Eugenics Laboratory Memoirs nos 19 and 20 (London: University of London, 1914).

30. *The Declining Birth-Rate: its Causes and Effects, Being the Report of and the Chief Evidence Taken by the National Birth-Rate Commission, Instituted, with Official Recognition, by the National Council of Public Morals – for the Promotion of Race Regeneration – Spiritual, Moral and Physical*, ed. James Marchant, secretary to the Commission and the Council (London: Chapman and Hall, 1916), vi, ix–x.

31. *Problems of Population and Parenthood, Being the Second Report of and the Chief Evidence Taken by the National Birth-Rate Commission, 1918–1920* (London:

Chapman and Hall, 1920), xi.

32. *Youth and the Race*, xi.

33. Enid Charles, *The Practice of Birth Control: An Analysis of the Birth-Control Experiences of Nine Hundred Women* (London: Williams and Norgate, 1932), 85.

34. *The State and Sexual Morality* (London: Allen and Unwin, 1920).

35. Archives of the Association for Moral and Social Hygiene at the Fawcett Library at London Guildhall University (AMSH): Box 49: Committee of Enquiry into Sexual Morality 1918–19; Notes of preliminary meeting 14 Oct. 1918.

36. *Ibid.*, Box 49: Minutes of 3rd meeting, 5 Nov. 1918.

37. *Ibid.*: Minutes of 11th meeting, 24 March 1919.

38. *Ibid.*: Minutes of 6th meeting, 13 Jan. 1919.

39. *Ibid.*: list of names 'For Co-option And As Witnesses: Suggested names for Consideration', [n. d.]; and minutes of evidence from witnesses called.

40. *Ibid.*: evidence of W. Clarke Hall, Police Magistrate, 19 May 1919.

41. *Ibid.*: Evidence of Archibald Allen, barrister, of the London Council for the Promotion of Public Morality and the National Vigilance Association, 30 June 1919; Miss Costin, formerly of the Police Service, 27 Jan. 1919; Dr Mary Gordon, Medical Inspector of Women's Prisons, 13 Jan. 1919; Inspector Harburn of Women's Police Service, 10 March 1919.

42. *Ibid.*: Evidence of W. J. H. Brodrick, 1 Dec. 1919.

43. *Ibid.*: Evidence of Rev. A. Herbert Gray, 24 March 1919.

44. BSS 'Misc': Minute Book [1] 1913–19; Ernest Jones in Toronto to Havelock Ellis 12 June 1910, Ellis papers in British Library Department of Manuscripts: BL Add. MS 70539.

45. Jeffrey Weeks, *Sex, Politics and Society: The Regulation of Sexuality since 1800* (London: Longman, 1981), 152–6.

46. *The Lancet*, i (1917), 912–14.

47. Unpublished autobiography of Professor Vernon Henry Mottram, Physiological Society deposited papers of individuals in the Contemporary Medical Archives Centre at the Wellcome Institute for the History of Medicine, CMAC, GC/151/7; I am indebted to my colleague Isobel Hunter for drawing my attention to this document.

48. Such as Katherine B. Davis, *Factors in the Sex Life of Twenty-two Hundred Women* (New York: Harper and Bros, 1929); G. V. T. Hamilton, *A Research in Marriage* (New York: A. & C. Boni, 1929); Robert L. Dickinson and Lura Beam, *A Thousand Marriages* (Baltimore Md.: Williams and Wilkins, 1932); L. Terman, *Psychological Factors in Marital Happiness* (New York: McGraw-Hill, 1939).

49. Martin Bulmer, Kevin Bales and Kathryn Kish Sklar, 'The Social Survey in Historical Perspective 1880–1940', in *idem* (eds), *The Social Survey in Historical Perspective 1880–1940* (Oxford: Oxford University Press, 1991), 1–48; Catherine Marsh, *The Survey Method: the Contribution of Surveys to Sociological Explanation* (London: Allen and Unwin, 1982), 10.

50. M. Leonora Eyles, *The Woman in the Little House* (London: Grant Richards, 1922), ch. 7: 'The Sex Problem', 129; for more on Eyles see Chapter 11, n. 110.

51. Marie C. Stopes, *Enduring Passion. Further New Contributions to the Solution of Sex Difficulties, Being the continuation of 'Married Love'* (London: G. P. Putnam's Sons, 1928; 2nd edn 1929), 76.

52. Stopes papers in the Department of Manuscripts, British Library, BL Add. MS 58569.

53. *Ibid.*, Add. MS 58562.

54. *Ibid.*, Add. MS 58550.

55. Margaret Llewellyn Davies (ed.), *Maternity: Letters from Working Women collected by the Women's Co-operative Guild* (London: G. Bell and Sons, 1915; London: Virago, 1978); *idem* (ed.), *Life as We Have Known It, by Co-operative Working Women* (London: Hogarth, 1931; London: Virago, 1977).

56. R. A. McCance, M. C. Luff and E. E. Widdowson, 'Physical and Emotional Periodicity in Women', *Journal of Hygiene*, xxxvii (1937), 571–611; the detailed records of this study are in the Contemporary Medical Archives Centre at the Wellcome Institute for the History of Medicine: CMAC,

GC/97/C.

57. Royal Society archives: Reader's Reports 1936; Minutes of the Sectional Committee on Physiology.

58. CMAC, GC/97/C, prefatory note to records of study.

59. Charles, *Practice of Birth Control*, 17, 25.

60. *Ibid.*, Part III, 107–21; Part IV, 125–50.

61. *Ibid.*, 13–14.

62. *Ibid.*, 25.

63. *Ibid.*, 15–16.

64. McCance *et al.*, 'Physical and Emotional Periodicity in Women'; CMAC: GC/97/C.1.

65. Charles, *Practice of Birth Control*, 26.

66. *Ibid.*, 16, 50.

67. See chs 4–6 of Hall, *Hidden Anxieties*.

68. BSS 'Misc.': Minutes Vol. [V], 198th meeting of committee, 9 April 1931.

69. *Ibid.*: Minutes [V]; Aims and Policy of the Society, 1932.

70. *Ibid.*: Harold Clare Booth (National Physical Laboratory, Molesey) to E. Lonsdale Deighton, 10 Nov. 1931.

71. *Ibid.*: George Ives, 'A Commentary upon the Role and Purpose of the Order' 2252 [1914]; see also Jeffrey Weeks, *Coming Out: Homosexual Politics in Britain, from the Nineteenth Century to the Present* (London: Quartet, 1977), 122–7.

72. BSS 'Misc.': Minutes Vol. [IV], 154th meeting 3 March 1927; 'Letters received': Dora F. Kerr to Deighton, 25 Sept. 1929, 16 May 1931, 26 Feb. 1932; also H. C. Booth to Deighton, 20 Jan. 1932; Kerr's earlier career in Canada is discussed in Angus McLaren, 'Sex Radicalism in the Canadian Pacific Northwest, 1890–1920', *Journal of the History of Sexuality*, ii (iv) (1992), 527–46.

73. Mentioned in passing in Paul Delany, *The Neo-Pagans: Friendship and Love in the Rupert Brooke Circle* (London: Macmillan, 1987), 13.

74. Virginia Woolf, *The Diary of Virginia Woolf*, Volume IV: *1931–1935* (London: Hogarth Press, 1982), 223.

75. Brighton branch: BSS 'Misc.': Minutes Vol. II: 110th meeting 12 April 1923; Vol [III]: 127th and 128th meetings 6 Nov. 1924, 4 Dec. 1924; 'Letters Received', Mary Ryder, [n. d., ?1923]. Other branches (or queries as to whether they exist) 'Letters Received', R. C. Klavehn, 17 May 1936 re a Scot-tish branch; 'Misc.' 'Letters of enquiry' file – inquiry re Glasgow branch [W. Young, n. d.].

76. For a brief account of Mass Observation and its work, see Tom Harrisson, *Britain Revisited* (London: Gollancz, 1961); also Angus Calder and Dorothy Sheridan (eds), *Speak for Yourself: A Mass Observation Anthology 1937–1949* (Oxford: Oxford University Press, 1985), and A. Calder, 'Mass Observation 1937–1949', in Bulmer (ed.) *Essays on the History of Sociological Research*, 121–36. There is a useful short discussion of the organization in Samuel Hynes, *The Auden Generation: Literature and Politics in England in the 1930s* (London: Bodley Head, 1976; Pimlico Press, 1992), 279–87.

77. Marsh, *The Survey Method*, 32–3, has a brief discussion of Mass Observation in the broader context of the development of survey methods; see also comments in Bulmer, 'The Development of Sociology and of Empirical Social Research'.

78. Calder and Sheridan, *Speak for Yourself*, 48–62.

79. See 'Selection from M-O Reports File, 1939–1959', Appendix to Harrisson, *Britain Revisited*, 271–4, Calder and Sheridan, *Speak for Yourself*, 8–15 for a 'Day Report' and 18–19 for observations in a pub.

80. Tom Harrisson – Mass Observation Archives at the University of Sussex (MO): 'Sex Survey 1929–1950' A.9; Box 1 Venereal Disease Survey 1942–1943, 1/C, 1/F.

81. MO VD Survey, A.9, 1/A.

82. *Ibid.*, A.9, 1/E.

83. *Ibid.*, A.9, 1/B.

84. *Ibid.*, A.9, 1/E, 1/B.

85. *Ibid.*, A.9, 1/G Feb.–March 1943, F30G.

86. 'Report on an Enquiry into Family Limitation and its Influence on Human Fertility during the past fifty years by E. Lewis-Faning, B.Sc, Ph.D, conducted at the request of the Royal Commission on Population'; held in the Royal College of Obstetricians and Gynaecologists. Published by HMSO in 1949, as *Papers from the Royal Commission on Population*, Vol. I.

87. Eliot Slater and Moya Woodside, *Patterns of Marriage: A Study of Marriage*

Relationships in the Urban Working Classes (London: Cassell, 1951), 21.

88. Ibid., 'Introduction', 7–30.
89. Ibid., 112–13.
90. Ibid., 120.
91. Ibid., 149.
92. Ibid., ch. 10: 'Sex Life in Marriage', 165–76.
93. Ibid., ch. 12: 'Contraception', 194–213.
94 'Sexual Behaviour 1929–1950', A.9 'Sex Survey 1949'; file 5/D, 'Organisational Material'.
95. Liz Stanley of Manchester University is currently editing the 'Little Kinsey' for publication.
96. MO 'Sex Survey', A.9, 3/B 'Report on Sex: Chapter One: Sex Surveyed'.
97. Ibid., A.9, 3/C 'Report on Sex: Chapter Two: Discovering Sex'.
98. Eustace Chesser, Joan Maizels, Leonard Jones and Brian Emmett, The Sexual, Marital and Family Relationships of the English Woman (with the assistance of an Advisory Committee comprising Professor F. A. E. Crew, Professor Alexander Kennedy, Kenneth Walker, Doris Odlum and Canon Hugh Walker), (London: Hutchinson's Medical Publications, 1956).
99. Ibid., ch. 1: 'Aims and Scope', 3–9.
100. Ibid., ch. 2: 'The Method of Enquiry', 10–29.
101. Ibid., ch. 12: 'The Authority in the Home', 144–54.
102. Ibid., ch. 14: 'Trends in Sex Education', 160–9.
103. BSS 'Misc.': Aims and Policy of the Society, 1932, in Minutes, Vol. [V].
104. Chesser et al., Sexual, Marital and Family Relationships of the English Woman, paras 7–11, 4–5.
105. The two volumes of this survey published so far are A. Johnson et al., Sexual Attitudes and Lifestyles (Oxford: Blackwell Scientific Publications, 1994) and Kaye Wellings et al., Sexual Behaviour in Britain (Harmondsworth: Penguin, 1994).

9   'Good Sex': the New Rhetoric of Conjugal Relations

1. T. L. Nichols, Esoteric Anthropology (The Mysteries of Man) A Comprehensive and Confidential Treatise on the Structure, Functions, Passional Attractions, and Perversions, True and False Physical and Social Conditions and the Most Intimate Relations of Men and Women. Anatomical, Physiological, Pathological, Therapeutical and Obstetrical. Hygienic and Hydropathic. From the American Stereotype Edition, Revised and Rewritten (Hygienic Institute, Museum St, London WC: the author, n. d. c. 1873); O. S. Fowler, Creative and Sexual Science; or, Manhood, Womanhood and Their Mutual Interrelations; Love, its Laws, Power, etc.; Selection, or Mutual Adaptation; Courtship, Married Life and Perfect Children; Their Generation, Endowment, Paternity, Maternity, Bearing, Nursing and Rearing; together with Puberty, Boyhood, Girlhood, etc., Sexual Impairments Restored, Male Vigour and Female Health and Beauty Perpetuated and Augmented, etc., as Taught by Phrenology and Physiology (New York: O. S. Fowler, 1870); Havelock Ellis on the clandestine popularity of Esoteric Anthropology, review article in Reynolds News, 26 April 1936 in E. F. Griffith's press-cuttings scrapbook, Griffith papers in the Contemporary Medical Archives Centre at the Wellcome Institute for the History of Medicine (CMAC), PP/EFG/A.41; similar opinion expressed in Havelock Ellis, Eonism and Other Supplementary Studies, Studies in the Psychology of Sex Volume VII (Philadelphia: F. A. Davis, 1928), 156.
2. S. Nissenbaum, Sex, Diet and Debility in Jacksonian America: Sylvester Graham and Health Reform (Westport, Conn. and London: Greenwood Press, 1980), 158–73, discusses Nichols and his wife Mary Gove Nichols in the context of health reform and free-love movements in the USA, and explores the contradictions inherent in their free-love stance.
3. Nichols, Esoteric Anthropology, 100–1.
4. Ibid., 120.
5. Ibid., 119.
6. R. T. Trall, Sexual Physiology and Hygiene: An Exposition Practical, Scientific, Moral, and Popular of Some of the Fundamental Problems in Sociology (1st edn USA, c. 1888; Glasgow: T. D. Morison, and London: Simpkin, Marshall, Hamilton and Kent, 1908).
7. Lyman Beecher Sperry, Confidential

Talks with Husband and Wife: A Book of Information and Advice for the Married and the Marriageable (London and Edinburgh: Oliphant Anderson and Ferrier, 1900).

8. *Ibid.*, 105–6.
9. *Ibid.*, 119.
10. Trall, *Sexual Physiology*, 226.
11. Sperry, *Confidential Talks*, 113.
12. Trall, *Sexual Physiology*, 222.
13. Sperry, *Confidential Talks*, 119.
14. Trall, *Sexual Physiology*, 232.
15. *Ibid.*, 234.
16. Sperry, *Confidential Talks*, 110.
17. E.g. Sperry, *Confidential Talks*, 117–20; Trall, *Sexual Physiology*, 226.
18. [Anon.] *Nature's Revelations for the Married Only*, printed for private circulation only, Electric Life Invigorator Co. (Gloucester: G. W. Ventnor, The Limes, Painswick Rd, ?1904).
19. Aristotle [pseud.] *The Works of Aristotle the Famous Philosopher, Containing his Complete Masterpiece, and Family Physician; His Experienced Midwife, His Book of Problems, and His Remarks on Physiognomy*, complete edn, with engravings (High Holborn, London: J. Smith, n. d.); Part I: 'The Masterpiece'; ch. 13: 'Of the External and Internal Organs of Generation in Women'; ch. 15: 'A Description of the Use and Action of the Several Generative Parts in Women'; ch. 17: 'A Word of Advice to Both Sexes, consisting of several Directions with regard to Copulation'. For the *Master-piece* during the eighteenth and early nineteenth centuries, see Chapter 2; it was clearly in circulation at least as late as the beginning of the Second World War but who bought it and how it was read remain open and intriguing questions.
20. Edward Carpenter, *Love's Coming of Age. A Series of Papers on the Relation of the Sexes* (London: Allen and Unwin, 1896; 13th edn 1930), 'Marriage: A Retrospect', 93–109.
21. *Ibid.*, 'Marriage: A Forecast', 110–29.
22. E.g., *ibid.*, 'The Sex Passion', 11–31; 'Remarks and Notes: On Preventive Checks to Population', 202–5.
23. Discussed in detail in Mary Lyndon Shanley, *Feminism, Marriage, and the Law in Victorian England, 1850–1895* (Princeton, NJ: Princeton University Press, 1989).

24. E.g. Geoffrey Mortimer on 'Enforced Maternity', *Shafts: A Paper for Women and the Working Classes*, 14 Jan. 1893.
25. *Shafts*, 18 Feb. 1893.
26. *Shafts*, July 1893: 'What the Editor Means'.
27. Havelock Ellis, *Sex in Relation to Society, Studies in the Psychology of Sex Volume VI* (Philadelphia: F. A. Davis, 1910), ch. 11: 'The Art of Love', 508.
28. *Ibid.*, 510.
29. *Ibid.*, 518.
30. *Ibid.*, 520–7.
31. *Ibid.*, 535–8.
32. *Ibid.*, 544–51.
33. *Ibid.*, 528–9.
34. *The Lancet*, i (1910), 1207.
35. Ellis, *Sex in Relation to Society*, 554–8.
36. See Chapter 10, p. 238.
37. Most recently June Rose, *Marie Stopes and the Sexual Revolution* (London: Faber and Faber, 1992); see also Lesley A. Hall, 'Uniting Science and Sensibility: Marie Stopes and the Narratives of Marriage in the 1920s', in A. Ingram and D. Patai (eds), *Rediscovering Forgotten Radicals: British Women Writers, 1880–1939* (Chapel Hill: University of North Carolina Press, 1993), 118–36, for a more detailed discussion of Stopes and the marriage advice genre; also Lesley A. Hall, *Hidden Anxieties. Male Sexuality, 1900–1950* (Cambridge: Polity Press, 1991), ch. 3: ' "Most Men Act in Ignorance": the Marriage Manual and Changing Concepts of Marriage', 63–88.
38. Laurie Taylor, 'The Unfinished Sexual Revolution', First Marie Stopes Memorial Lecture, 12 March 1971, *Journal of Biosocial Science*, iii (1971), 473–92.
39. Marie Stopes, *Married Love. A New Contribution to the Solution of Sex Difficulties. With a Preface by Dr Jessie Murray, and Letters from Professor E. H. Starling FRS, and Father Stanislaus St John, SJ* (London: A. C. Fifield, 1918; later edns by G. P. Putnam's Sons) 4th edn, 1918, Author's Preface, xiii.
40. Peter Eaton and Marilyn Warnick, *Marie Stopes: A Checklist of Her Writings* (London: Croom Helm, 1977); Billie Melman, *Woman and the Popular Imagination in the 1920s: Flappers and Nymphs* (London: Macmillan, 1988), 3.
41. Marie Stopes papers in the Contemporary Medical Archives Centre,

Wellcome Institute for the History of Medicine CMAC, PP/MCS/A.169 MCS to Mr RDM, 1919.

42. Naomi Mitchison, *You May Well Ask: A Memoir 1920–1940* (London: Gollancz, 1979; Flamingo paperback edn, 1986), 69–70.

43. *The Lancet*, ii (1918), 886.

44. *British Medical Journal* [*BMJ*], i (1918), 510.

45. Lesley A. Hall, '"Somehow Very Distasteful": Doctors, Men and Sexual Problems between the Wars', *Journal of Contemporary History*, xx (iv) (1985), 553–74; also *idem, Hidden Anxieties*, especially ch. 6: '"I Shouldn't Care to Face the Experience Again": Male Sexual Problems in the Consulting Room', 139–69.

46. CMAC, PP/MCS/A.265.

47. Norman Haire, *Hymen, or the Future of Marriage* (New York: E. P. Dutton, 1928), 80.

48. Marie Stopes papers in the Department of Manuscripts, British Library, 'Physicians: British Isles', BL Add. MS 58570.

49. Hall, *Hidden Anxieties*, 157–9.

50. *BMJ*, i (1932), *passim.*

51. As discussed in Lesley A. Hall, '"The English Have Hot-Water Bottles": The Morganatic Marriage of Medicine and Sexology in Britain since William Acton', in Roy Porter and Mikuláš Teich (eds), *Sexual Knowledge, Sexual Science: The History of Attitudes to Sexuality* (Cambridge: Cambridge University Press, 1994), 350–66.

52. 'Dr' G. Courtenay Beale, *Wise Wedlock: The Whole Truth: A Book of Counsel and Instruction for All Who Seek for Happiness in Marriage*, 2nd edn (London: Health Promotion, *c.* 1922).

53. CMAC, PP/MCS/A.22 includes correspondence 'Re Dr Courtenay Beale' in which Stopes voiced her suspicions as to 'Beale's' bona fides in the light of the fact that she had been unable to track him down in order to serve upon him a writ for plagiarism.

54. Ellis, *Eonism and Other Supplementary Studies*, IV, 'The Menstrual Curve of Sexual Impulse', 213–36.

55. *BMJ*, i (1918), 510; *The Lancet*, ii (1918), 886.

56. Rev. A. Herbert Gray, *Men, Women, and God. A Discussion of Sex Questions from the Christian Point of View* (London: Student Christian Movement, 1923); republished in 1987 as 'a modern Christian classic' with a new extended introduction by David R. Mace (Worthing: Churchman, 1987).

57. Isabel Elmslie Hutton, *The Hygiene of Marriage* (London: Heinemann Medical Books, 1923; 4th edn 1933).

58. Isabel Elmslie Hutton, *Memories of a Doctor in War and Peace* (London: Heinemann, 1960), 214–15.

59. Th. H. Van de Velde, *Ideal Marriage: Its Physiology and Technique*, trans. F. W. Stella Browne (Holland, 1926; London: Heinemann Medical Books, 1928).

60. Eustace Chesser, *Sexual Behaviour: Normal and Abnormal* (London: London Medical Publications, 1949), 16–17.

61. Eustace Chesser, *Love without Fear: A Plain Guide to Sex Technique for Every Married Adult* (London: Rich and Cowan Medical Publications, 1941; 2nd edn July 1942), 67.

62. Chesser, *Sexual Behaviour: Normal and Abnormal*, 17.

63. Gray, *Men, Women, and God*, 145.

64. Stopes, *Married Love*, 27.

65. Hutton, *Hygiene of Marriage*, 31.

66. Beale, *Wise Wedlock*, 49.

67. Hutton, *Hygiene of Marriage*, 64.

68. Beale, *Wise Wedlock*, 51–2.

69. Gray, *Men, Women, and God*, 146.

70. Honoré de Balzac, *The Physiology of Marriage* (Paris 1826; London: translation, privately printed, 1904), 56–8: 'comparing the majority of husbands to this orang-outang trying to play the violin'.

71. Beale, *Wise Wedlock*, 87.

72. Hutton, *Hygiene of Marriage*, 68.

73. Stopes, *Married Love*, 22.

74. Beale, *Wise Wedlock*, 69.

75. Hutton, *Hygiene of Marriage*, 49.

76. *Ibid.*, 49–50.

77. Stopes, *Married Love*, 39.

78. Beale, *Wise Wedlock*, 75.

79. Gray, *Men, Women, and God*, 144.

80. Hutton, *Hygiene of Marriage*, 54.

81. Marie Stopes, *Enduring Passion: Further New Contributions to the Solution of Sex Difficulties, Being the Continuation of 'Married Love'* (London: G. P. Putnam's Sons, 1928), ch. 4: 'Undersexed Husbands'; ch. 5: 'Premature Ejaculation' (of 'wide prevalence').

82. Van de Velde, *Ideal Marriage*, 238.
83. *Ibid.*, 165.
84. *Ibid.*, 6.
85. Beale, *Wise Wedlock*, 83.
86. Hutton, *Hygiene of Marriage*, 64.
87. *Ibid.*, 65-6.
88. Stopes, *Enduring Passion*, 57-62.
89. Van de Velde, *Ideal Marriage*, 240.
90. Stopes, *Married Love*, 42-5.
91. Hutton, *Hygiene of Marriage*, 69-70.
92. Stopes, *Enduring Passion*, 83.
93. Beale, *Wise Wedlock*, 83.
94. Stopes, *Married Love*, 204.
95. Gray, *Men, Women, and God*, 146-8.
96. Hutton, *Hygiene of Marriage*, 62.
97. Stopes, *Married Love*, 68.
98. Edward F. Griffith, *Modern Marriage and Birth Control* (London: Gollancz, 1935), 117.
99. Eustace Chesser, *Love without Fear*, July 1942 edn (slightly expurgated, following the obscenity trial discussed in Chapter 13), 26.
100. Leslie D. Weatherhead, (assisted by Dr Marion Greaves), *The Mastery of Sex through Psychology and Religion* (London: Student Christian Movement Press, 1931), 40-1.
101. Griffith, *Modern Marriage*, 69.
102. *Ibid.*, 151.
103. Sheila Jeffreys, 'Sex Reform and Anti-Feminism in the 1920s', in London Feminist History Group, *The Sexual Dynamics of History: Men's Power, Women's Resistance* (London: Pluto Press, 1983), 177-202, and *idem, The Spinster and Her Enemies: Feminism and Sexuality 1880-1930* (London: Pandora Press, 1985) has put forward this view. It is also mentioned in Frank Mort, *Dangerous Sexualities: Medico-moral Politics in England since 1830* (London and New York: Routledge and Kegan Paul, 1987), and Johanna Alberti, *Beyond Suffrage: Feminists in War and Peace, 1914-1928* (London: Macmillan, 1989), largely on the basis of Jeffreys's arguments. Similar arguments are advanced in M. Jackson, *The Real Facts of Life: Feminism and the Politics of Sexuality c. 1850-1940* (London: Taylor and Francis, 1994).
104. Lesley A. Hall, 'A New Man in the 1920s? Questions of Social/Sexual Change' (unpublished paper circulated at conference 'Sexual Cultures in Europe', Amsterdam, 24-26 June 1992, papers Group C: Sexual Codes and Practices, 51-61.)
105. Hall, *Hidden Anxieties*, 108-10.
106. Van de Velde, *Ideal Marriage*, 158.
107. Hutton, *Hygiene of Marriage*, 67.
108. Stopes, *Enduring Passion*, 90-1.
109. 'Medica' [Joan Malleson], *Any Wife or Any Husband: A Book for Couples who have met sexual difficulties and for doctors* (London: Heinemann Medical Books, 1950), 58-64.
110. Chesser, *Love without Fear*, 85, 98.
111. CMAC, PP/MCS/A.36 MCS to Mr PJB, 1924.
112. Alec Craig, *Above All Liberties* (London: Allen and Unwin, 1942), 103.
113. Stopes, *Enduring Passion*, 40-2.
114. Weatherhead, *Mastery of Sex*, 151-3.
115. Chesser, *Love without Fear*, 111-14.
116. 'Medica', *Any Wife or Any Husband*, 123-34.
117. E.g. CMAC, PP/MCS/A.88 F, A.134 CGH, A.205 Lt Col RMP, RMC, A.129 FH.
118. Jay Mechling, 'Advice to Historians on Advice to Mothers', *Journal of Social History*, ix (1975-6), 44-57.
119. See Chapter 11, p. 257.
120. Hutton, *Memories of a Doctor*, 217.
121. CMAC, PP/MCS/A.150 CK.
122. *Ibid.*, PP/MCS/A.134 CGH.
123. *Ibid.*, PP/MCS/A.235 WT.
124. *Ibid.*, PP/MCS/A.94 EGF, A.194 EP, A.135 Capt. BH, Indian Army.
125. *Ibid.*, PP/MCS/A.173 AJM, A.250 JHW, A.246 RHW.
126. *Ibid.*, PP/MCS/A.114 ACH, A.165 HL.
127. *Ibid.*, PP/MCS/A.246 HPW, A.197 EWP, A. 165 HL.
128. *Ibid.*, PP/MCS/A.239 Mrs AEW.
129. *Ibid.*, PP/MCS/A.117 GPH.
130. *Ibid.*, PP/MCS/A.254 HJY.
131. E.g. *ibid.*, PP/MCS/A.188 F, A.109 Major JG, A.112 Pte WG, A.124 SJH, A.128 FJH, A.174 Cpl HM (RAF), A.185 AGM, A.202 WJP, A.182 CKM, A.160 SL, A.136 Capt. LDAH (RGA), A.129 FH.
132. Michael Gordon, 'From an Unfortunate Necessity to a Cult of Mutual Orgasm: Sex in American Marital Education Literature 1830-1940', in J. Henslin (ed.), *Studies in the Sociology of Sex* (New York: Appleton-Century Crofts, 1975), 53-77.
133. Edward M. Brecher, *The Sex Researchers* (London: André Deutsch, 1970), 102.

134. E. L. Packer, 'Aspects of Working Class Marriage', *Pilot Papers: Social Essays and Documents*, ii (i) (March 1947), 92–104. Packer was a probation officer. This shortlived journal was edited by Charles Madge, who was also involved with Mass Observation.

135. Randolph Trumbach, 'Review Essay: Is There a Modern Sexual Culture in the West; or, Did England Never Change between 1500 and 1900?', *Journal of the History of Sexuality*, i (ii) (Oct. 1990), 296–309.

136. E.g. Naomi Mitchison, *All Change Here: Girlhood and Marriage* (London: Bodley Head, 1975), and *idem, You May Well Ask*; Lady Cynthia Asquith, *Diaries 1915–1918* (London: Hutchinson, 1968), 477, describes a 'fairly obscene hair-combing arising from a discussion of Dr Stopes' *Married Love*' with Lady Diana Manners, later Cooper, 'quite a missionary' about the book (I am indebted to Heather Creaton for this citation). A letter from Harold Nicolson to his wife, Vita Sackville-West, about Stopes's revelations is cited in Victoria Glendinning, *Vita* (Harmondsworth: Penguin, 1985), 99. Charlotte Mackenzie has drawn my attention to Virginia Woolf's awareness of the circulation among the 'younger generation' of the works and ideas of 'Mary [*sic*] Stopes', mentioned in a letter to Molly Macarthy, 19 Jan. 1923.

137. CMAC, PP/MCS/A.108 EWG.

138. *Ibid.*, PP/MCS/A.148 FCK.

139. *Ibid.*, PP/MCS/A.233 DLLT.

140. *Ibid.*, PP/MCS/A.66 C.

141. *Ibid.*, PP/MCS/A.244 Miss LW, A.118 Mr LH.

142. *Ibid.*, PP/MCS/A.32 JJB.

143. *Ibid.*, PP/MCS/A.118 Miss KH.

144. *Ibid.*, PP/MCS/A.254 NHY.

145. *Ibid.*, PP/MCS/A.233 DLLT.

146. *Ibid.*, PP/MCS/A.92 F.

147. *Ibid.*, PP/MCS/A.1/70 anonymous correspondent.

148. Tom Harrisson – Mass Observation Archive at the University of Sussex: A.9 Sex Survey, Box 14, 'Leaders of Opinion'.

149. Kenneth M. Walker, *Marriage: A Book for the Married and About to be Married* (London: Secker and Warburg for the British Social Hygiene Council,

1951), 1.

150. Stopes, *Enduring Passion*, 76.

151. Stopes, *Married Love*, 12th edn, 1923, 92: this passage does not appear in the 1918 edition and may well have been inserted following the many revelations of sexual ignorance Stopes received: e.g., CMAC, PP/MCS/A.196 EP, A.197 AHP, A.121 JH, A.132 HPH.

152. Alan Rusbridger, *A Concise History of the Sex Manual, 1886–1986* (London and Boston: Faber and Faber, 1986), 11–12.

10 Public Faces in Private Places: Sex, Law, Politics and Pressure Groups

1. Linda Mahood, *The Magdalenes: Prostitution in the Nineteenth Century* (London and New York: Routledge, 1990), 119–22; Frank Mort, *Dangerous Sexualities: Medico-moral Politics in England since 1830* (London and New York: Routledge and Kegan Paul, 1987), 134–5, also 'Purity, Feminism and the State: Sexuality and Moral Politics, 1880–1914', in M. Langdon and B. Schwarz (eds), *Crises in the British State 1880–1930* (London: Hutchinson, 1985), 209–25; Judith Walkowitz, *Prostitution and Victorian Society: Women, Class and the State* (Cambridge and New York: Cambridge University Press, 1980), 250–2.

2. Richard Davenport-Hines, *Sex, Death and Punishment: Attitudes to Sex and Sexuality in Britain since the Renaissance* (London: Collins, 1990), 130–6; see also Jeffrey Weeks, *Coming Out: Homosexual Politics in Britain from the Nineteenth Century to the Present* (London: Quartet, 1977), 14–16.

3. Jeffrey Weeks, *Against Nature: Essays in History, Sexuality and Identity* (London: Rivers Oram Press, 1991), 19; Elaine Showalter, *Sexual Anarchy: Gender and Culture at the 'Fin de Siècle'* (New York: Viking Penguin, 1990; London: Bloomsbury, 1991).

4. Weeks, *Coming Out*, especially Part Four: 'Approaches to Reform', 113–82; Davenport-Hines, *Sex, Death, and Punishment*; Kevin Porter and Jeffrey Weeks (eds), *Between the Acts: Lives of*

Homosexual Men 1885–1967 (London: Routledge, 1991); Stephen Jeffrey-Poulter, *Peers, Queers and Commons: The Struggle for Gay Law Reform from 1950 to the Present* (London: Routledge, 1991).

5. Edward J. Bristow, *Vice and Vigilance: Purity Movements in Britain since 1700* (Dublin: Gill and Macmillan, 1977), ch. 7: 'Social Purity and Prostitution', 154–74.

6. Mort, *Dangerous Sexualities*, 135.

7. See National Vigilance Association Archives in Fawcett Library, London Guildhall University (NVA), Committee Minutes 1887, 1888, 1889, 1890.

8. L. W. Harrison, 'Those Were the Days! Or Random Notes on Then and Now in VD', *Bulletin of the Institute of Technicians in Venereology*, Wellcome Institute Library Reprint Collection (n. d. ?1950s), 1–7; Michael Adler, 'The Terrible Peril: a Historical Perspective on the Venereal Diseases', *British Medical Journal*, ii (1980), 202–11.

9. T. J. Wyke, 'Hospital Facilities for, and Diagnosis and Treatment of, Venereal Disease in England, 1800–1870', *British Journal of Venereal Diseases*, xlix (1973), 78–85; *Departmental Committee on Sickness Benefit Claims under the National Insurance Act*, Cd 7687, 1914, paras 134–41; Local Government Board, *Report as to the Practice of Medicine and Surgery by Unqualified Persons in the United Kingdom*, Cd 5422, 1910; *Royal Commission on Venereal Diseases [RC on VD]: Final Report*, Cd 8189, 1916, paras 188, 133.

10. *RC on VD, First Report: Appendix: Minutes of Evidence (1913–1914)*, Cd 7475, 1914, para. 2822.

11. E. B. Turner, 'The History of the Fight against Venereal Disease', *Science Progress*, xi (1916–17), 83–8.

12. This is discussed more fully in terms of imperial concerns and pervasive themes within the British administration in India, in Kenneth Ballhatchet, *Race, Sex, and Class under the Raj: Imperial Attitudes and Policies and their Critics, 1793–1905* (London: Weidenfeld and Nicolson, 1980).

13. Published in *Shafts: A Paper for Women and the Working Classes*, ed. Margaret Shurmer Sibthorp, July–Aug. 1897 issue.

14. Turner, 'History of the Fight against Venereal Disease'.

15. Bristow, *Vice and Vigilance*, 94–140.

16. *British Medical Journal [BMJ]*, ii (1885), 303–4.

17. *The Lancet*, ii (1885), 350–1.

18. Arthur T. Barnett, 'The Testimony of Medical Men', in The White Cross League, *The Blanco Book* (London: White Cross League, 1913), 217–48.

19. Bristow, *Vice and Vigilance*, 139–40.

20. Quoted in *BMJ*, i (1894), 1266–7.

21. Edith MacDuff to Edward Carpenter, 7 April 1894, Carpenter papers in Sheffield City Archives MSS 271/51.

22. 'Ellis Ethelmer' [Mrs Wolstenholme Elmy], *The Human Flower, Baby Buds* (Congleton: Mrs Wolstenholme Elmy, 1894, 1895).

23. *Shafts*, April, June 1894, letter from 'ETH of Dawlish', April 1895.

24. *Ibid.*, Jan.–Feb. 1896, 'What the Editor Means'.

25. *BMJ*, ii (1889), 88.

26. National Vigilance Association [NVA], Executive Committee Minutes, 1887.

27. Press cutting in John Johnson Ephemera Collection at the Bodleian Library: 'Sex Population and Eugenics', Box I.

28. Edith A. MacDuff to Edward Carpenter, 16 April 1894, Carpenter/Sheffield MSS 271/52.

29. *Shafts*, July 1893.

30. Cited in Paddy Kitchen, *A Most Unsettling Person: An Introduction to the Ideas and Life of Patrick Geddes* (London: Gollancz, 1975), 99–100; for more detailed discussions of debates around birth control at this period see Angus McLaren, *Birth Control in Nineteenth Century England* (London: Croom Helm, 1978); R. A. Soloway, *Birth Control and the Population Question in England, 1870–1930* (Chapel Hill and London: University of North Carolina Press, 1982); Carol Dyhouse, *Feminism and the Family in England 1880–1939* (Oxford: Basil Blackwell, 1989).

31. As discussed in detail in R. A. Soloway, *Demography and Degeneration: Eugenics and the Declining Birthrate in Twentieth Century Britain* (Chapel Hill: University of North Carolina Press, 1990).

32. Lesley A. Hall, 'Illustrations from the Wellcome Institute Library: the Eugenics Society Archive in the Contemporary Medical Archives Centre',

Medical History, xxxiv (1990), 327–33; for the BSSSP see discussion in Chapter 8; see also Soloway, *Demography and Degeneration*.

33. Lord Baden-Powell, *Rovering to Success: A Book of Life-Sport for Young Men* (London: Herbert Jenkins, 1922), 111; Norah March, *Toward Racial Health. A Handbook for Parents, Teachers and Social Workers on the Training of Boys and Girls*, with a foreword by J. Arthur Thomson (London: George Routledge and Sons, 1915; 4th revised edn 1920).

34. Marie Stopes papers in the Contemporary Medical Archives Centre (CMAC), Wellcome Institute for the History of Medicine: 'Statement Issued by the C.B.C. Executive Committee on the Racial Contraceptives of the C.B.C.' [n. d., c. 1924/5?]: PP/MCS/C.45.

35. Turner, 'History of the Fight Against Venereal Disease'.

36. A. C. A. Magian, *Handbook of Venereal Diseases, Being an Outline of These Affections and of Their History and Treatment* (Manchester and London: John Heywood, 1909), ch. 6.

37. Local Government Board, *Report on Venereal Diseases by Dr R. W. Johnstone* [Cd.7029], HMSO, 1913; 'occasional or clandestine' prostitutes in many cases strictly speaking may not have been prostitutes at all.

38. Samuel Hynes, *The Edwardian Turn of Mind* (Princeton: Princeton University Press, 1968; London, Pimlico Press, 1991), 192–4, 208–9; O. M. McGregor, *Divorce in England: A Centenary History* (London: Heinemann, 1957), 25–9.

39. Rebecca West, 'The Divorce Commission: A Report that Will Not Become Law', first published in *The Clarion*, 29 Nov. 1912, in *The Young Rebecca: Writings of Rebecca West 1911–1917*, selected and introduced by Jane Marcus (London: Macmillan, 1982), 124–7.

40. Paul Ferris, *Sex and the British: A Twentieth Century History* (London: Michael Joseph, 1993), 34–41; Bristow, *Vice and Vigilance*, 191–2.

41. Weeks, *Against Nature*, 19.

42. Association for Moral and Social Hygiene archives (AMSH) at the Fawcett Library, London Guildhall University: Enquiry into Sexual Morality, Box 49: evidence of Mr W. Clarke Hall, Police Magistrate, 19 May 1919.

43. G. W. Johnson, 'The Injustice of the Solicitation Laws'; 'Woman, Where Are Thine Accusers?', *The Shield: The Journal of the Association of Moral and Social Hygiene*, 3rd series, iii (1920–2), 267–9, 307–9.

44. AMSH, Box 49: evidence of Dr Mary Gordon, HM Inspector of Women's Prisons, 13 Jan. 1919; Inspector Harburn, of the Women's Police Service, 10 March 1919; Miss Shaw, formerly in preventive and rescue work in Southsea and Portsmouth, 2 June 1919.

45. Ferris, *Sex and the British*, 27; *The Pelican: A Journal of Today*, 1910 and 1900; AMSH archives: Box 49: Enquiry into Sexual Morality, evidence of Mr W. J. H. Brodrick, 1 Dec. 1919.

46. March, *Toward Racial Health*, 4th edn revised, 1920, 24.

47. Mary Scharlieb and F. A. Sibly, *Youth and Sex: Dangers and Safeguards for Girls and Boys* (London: T. C. and E. C. Jack, 1913), 48.

48. Dr A. R. Schofield, and Dr P. Vaughan-Jackson, *What a Boy Should Know* (London: Cassell, 1913), 27–8.

49. March, *Toward Racial Health*, Appendix I, 262.

50. Bristow, *Vice and Vigilance*, 140–6; and see account of the Dronfield case in Mort, *Dangerous Sexualities*, 153–63, 183–5.

51. L. W. Harrison, 'Some Lessons Learnt in Fifty Years' Practice in Venereology', *British Journal of Venereal Diseases* [*BJVD*], xxx (1954), 184–90.

52. Local Government Board, *Report on Venereal Diseases*, Introduction by the Medical Officer to the Board (Arthur Newsholme), iii.

53. Turner, 'History of the Fight Against Venereal Disease'.

54. Christabel Pankhurst, *The Great Scourge and How to End It* (London: E. Pankhurst, 1913).

55. *RC on VD: Final Report*, paras 10–11.

56. *Ibid.*, paras 127–32, 136.

57. *Ibid.*, para. 143.

58. *Ibid.*, para. 144.

59. 'Venereal Diseases: State Provision for their Diagnosis and Treatment', *BMJ*, ii (1916), 111; 'Medical Notes in Parliament: The Venereal Diseases Bill', *BMJ*, i (1917), 557.

60. B. Towers, 'Health Education Policy, 1916–1926: Venereal Disease and the Prophylaxis Dilemma', *Medical History*, xxiv (1980), 70–87.

61. *History of the Great War Based on Official Documents: Medical Services: Diseases of the War Volume II* (London: HMSO, 1923), 74.

62. *Ibid.*, 72.

63. *Ibid.*, 78; Brig.-Gen. F. D. Crozier, *A Brass Hat in No-Man's Land: A Personal Record of the European War* (London: Jonathan Cape, 1930), 64–7.

64. The leaflet is cited in Ferris, *Sex and the British*, 67; A subtle and nuanced study by Mark Harrison on the politics of venereal disease control in the British Army, 1914–18, will appear shortly in *Medical History.*

65. AMSH, Box 49: evidence of Rev. Herbert Gray, 24 March 1919.

66. CMAC, PP/MCS/A.60 – a 2nd lieutenant in the RAF, so presumably fairly intelligent and educated.

67. Towers, 'Health Education Policy, 1916–1926'.

68. Crozier, *A Brass Hat in No-Man's Land*, 66–7.

69. See the debate in *The Nineteenth Century* between Sir Bryan Donkin and Sir Francis Champneys: Donkin, 'The Fight against Venereal Infection', lxxxii (Sept. 1917), 580–95; Champneys, 'The Fight against Venereal Infection: A Reply to Sir Bryan Donkin', lxxxii (Nov. 1917), 1044–54; Donkin, 'The Fight against Venereal Infection: A Rejoinder', lxxxiii (Jan. 1918), 184–90; Champneys, 'The Fight against Venereal Infection: A Further Reply to Sir Bryan Donkin', lxxxiii (March 1918), 611–18. There was also considerable correspondence on this topic in the *BMJ* during 1919 and 1920.

70. AMSH, Box 49: evidence of Dr R. A. Lyster of the SPVD, 15 Dec. 1919.

71. *BMJ*, ii (1919), 832; i (1920), 61.

72. A. Neilans, 'The Protection of Soldiers', *The Shield*, 3rd series, i (1916–17), 216–23, citing press controversies including contributions by Sir Arthur Conan Doyle and Rev. F. B. Meyer.

73. M. H. Mason, 'Public Morality: Some Constructive Suggestions', *The Nineteenth Century*, lxxxii (1917), 185–94.

74. *History of the Great War,* 121.

75. Mason, 'Public Morality'.

76. *History of the Great War*, 121.

77. AMSH, Box 49: evidence of Dr R. A. Lyster, 15 Dec. 1919.

78. *BMJ*, i (1920), 273.

79. Towers, 'Health Education Policy'; Cate Haste, *Rules of Desire: Sex in Britain, World War I to the Present* (London: Chatto and Windus, 1992), 32–8; Ferris, *Sex and the British*, 57–62.

80. AMSH, Box 49: evidence of Dr Mary Gordon, HM Medical Inspector of Women's Prisons, 13 Jan. 1919.

81. *Ibid.*, evidence of Miss Shaw, of Cope Hall Training Colony and formerly in preventive and rescue work in Southsea and Portsmouth, 2 June 1919.

82. Ferris, *Sex and the British*, 57–71; Haste, *Rules of Desire*, 33–8; Martin Pugh, *Women and the Women's Movement in Britain 1914–1959* (London: Macmillan, 1992), 32–4.

83. Paul Langford Adams, 'Health of the State: British and American Public Health Policies in the Depression and World War II' (unpublished dissertation for the Doctorate of Social Welfare, University of California Berkeley, 1979), ch. 7: 'Reforming Morals and Making Fornication Safe: Venereal Disease Control in Wartime', 326–67; Harrison, 'Those Were the Days!'; Ambrose King, 'The First Harrison Lecture, 1974: The Life and Times of Colonel Harrison', *BJVD*, l (1974), 391–403.

84. Editorial: 'Criminal Law Amendment and Sexual Offences Bills', *The Shield*, 3rd series, ii (1918–20), 5.

85. L. W. Harrison, 'The Public Health Services and Venereal Diseases', *BJVD*, i (1925), 12–22.

86. W. Metcalfe Chambers, 'Prostitution and Venereal Disease', *BJVD*, ii (v) (1926), 68–75.

87. Towers, 'Health Education Policy, 1916–1926'.

88. Ministry of Health Circular 202, 31 May 1921, 'Prevention and Treatment of Venereal Diseases'; Norah March to Alison Neilans of the Association of Moral and Social Hygiene, 21 Dec. 1921: both in AMSH, Venereal Diseases, 311/2.

89. National Birth-Rate Commission, *The*

Declining Birth-Rate: its Causes and Effects, Being the Report of and the Chief Evidence Taken by the National Birth-Rate Commission, Instituted, with Official Recognition, by the National Council of Public Morals – for the Promotion of Race Regeneration – Spiritual, Moral and Physical, ed. James Marchant, Secretary to the Commission and the Council (London: Chapman and Hall, for the National Birth-Rate Commission, 1916), v–viii.

90. Soloway, *Birth Control and the Population Question*, 236–8.
91. *Ibid.*, 215–16.
92. Audrey Leathard, *The Fight for Family Planning* (London: Macmillan, 1980), 15–16.
93. Ruth Hall, *Marie Stopes: A Biography* [*Passionate Crusader: The Life of Marie Stopes* in the USA] (London: André Deutsch, 1977), 237–42.
94. Soloway, *Birth Control and the Population Question*, 241–2; Lord Dawson to Marie Stopes, 1922, in Stopes papers in the Department of Manuscripts, British Library, Add. MS 59567.
95. Soloway, *Birth Control and the Population Question*, 190–2; and see *The Practitioner*, Birth Control issue, July 1923.
96. Stopes papers, BL Add. MS 58569.
97. A very large proportion of the correspondence to be found in both the Stopes Collection in the Contemporary Medical Archives Centre, in the section 'ML–DRS', CMAC, PP/MCS/A.256–96, and among the Stopes papers in the British Library Department of Manuscripts, Add. MS 58568–71, 'Physicians, British Isles, General', consists of routine requests of this nature.
98. Marie Stopes 'ML–DRS': CMAC, PP/MCS/A.274 J, A.283 M, A.287 R.
99. CMAC, PP/MCS/A.278 RML.
100. *Ibid.*, PP/MCS/A.64 A.
101. Soloway, *Birth Control and the Population Question*, 229.
102. *Ibid.*, 281–2.
103. *Ibid.*, 283–6.
104. Bristow, *Vice and Vigilance*, 198; George Ryley Scott, *A History of Prostitution from Antiquity to the Present Day*, revised and illustrated limited edn (London: Torchstream Books, 1954), 249.
105. Pugh, *Women and the Women's Movement*, 247–8.

106. Gladys M. Hall, *Prostitution: a Survey and a Challenge* (London: Williams and Norgate, 1933), 34–5; C. H. Rolph (ed.), *Women of the Streets: A Sociological Study of the Common Prostitute* (London: Secker and Warburg for and on behalf of the British Social Biology Council, 1955), 38–9; frequently mentioned in evidence to the Enquiry on Sexual Morality of the Association of Moral and Social Hygiene, see Chapter 8.
107. See Chapter 11, p. 264.
108. Lesley A. Hall, *Hidden Anxieties: Male Sexuality 1900–1950* (Cambridge: Polity Press, 1991), 52–3.
109. McGregor, *Divorce in England*, 29.
110. Ferris, *Sex and the British*, 94; Lawrence Stone, *The Road to Divorce: England 1530–1987* (Oxford: Oxford University Press, 1992), 295.
111. National Vigilance Association [NVA]: Box 104 S46 A Assaults, *Vigilance Record*, Comments, Dec. 1923.
112. *Woman's World: The Favourite Paper of a Million Homes* (weekly 2d), 17 Jan. 1925.
113. See Chapter 9.
114. Meyrick Booth, *Youth and Sex: A Psychological Study* (London: Allen and Unwin, 1932), 102n, citing Dr Stanford Read, *The Struggles of Male Adolescence*; Marie Stopes, *Enduring Passion: Further New Contributions to the Solutions of Sex Difficulties, Being the Continuation of 'Married Love'* (London: G. P. Putnam's Sons, 1928, 2nd edn 1929), 62–3.
115. A. Herbert Gray, *Sex Teaching* (London: National Sunday School Union [n. d. 1929]), ch. 4: 'To Teachers of Boys', 50–7; [Margaret] Leonora Eyles, *Commonsense about Sex* (London: Gollancz, 1933), ch. 2: 'Masturbation', 34–41.
116. Gray, *Sex Teaching*, 53.
117. Soloway, *Birth Control and the Population Question*, 287–302.
118. *Ibid.*, 308–12; Leathard, *Fight for Family Planning*, 44–50; British Sexology Society (BSS) archives at the Harry Ransom Humanities Research Center, University of Texas at Austin (HRC), 'Misc.': Minutes Vol. [V] 198th meeting 9 April 1931, 'Letters out', to Arthur Greenwood, Minister of Health, 27 March 1931.
119. Soloway, *Demography and Degeneration*, 208–9.

120. Bristow, *Vice and Vigilance*, 153.
121. Davenport-Hines, *Sex, Death and Punishment*, 261.
122. 'Free Treatment for Venereal Patients': Letters from H. Wansey Bayly and M. Browdy, *The Lancet*, i (1932), 1229, 1279.
123. Langford Adams, 'Health of the State', 327.
124. Contribution by L. W. Harrison to discussion of Sir Weldon Dalrymple-Champneys, 'The Epidemiological Control of Venereal Disease', *BJVD*, xxiii (1947), 101–8; J. A. Burgess, 'Is There a New Deal in the Control of Venereal Disease?', in the same issue of *BJVD*, p. 24, pointed out the great regional variations in routine testing of pregnant women for latent syphilis.
125. C. Mills, 'Collaboration between the Venereal Disease and Other Departments', *BJVD*, x (1934), 233–48.
126. Ambrose King, 'The Life and Times of Colonel Harrison', mentions that Harrison, in spite of his national and international reputation, was 'not particularly popular' with other consultants at St Thomas's.
127. Ambrose King, 'These Dying Diseases: Venereology in Decline?', *The Lancet*, i (1958), 651–7.
128. Dalrymple-Champneys, 'Epidemiological Control of Venereal Disease'.
129. 'Scotland versus VD', *The Lancet*, i (1944), 668.
130. Dalrymple-Champneys, 'Epidemiological Control of Venereal Diseases'; Robert Lees, 'Venereal Diseases in the Armed Forces Overseas (1)', *BJVD*, xxii (1946), 149–58; D. J. Campbell, 'Venereal Diseases in the Armed Forces Overseas (2)', *BJVD*, xxii (1946), 158–68; *History of the Second World War: United Kingdom Medical Series; The Army Medical Services: Administration II*, ed. F. A. E. Crew (London: HMSO, 1955), 236.
131. John Macnicol, 'Eugenics and the Campaign for Voluntary Sterilization in Britain Between the Wars', *Social History of Medicine*, ii (1989), 147–69; *idem*, 'The Voluntary Sterilization Campaign in Britain, 1918–1939', in John C. Fout (ed.), *Forbidden History: The State, Society and the Regulation of Sexuality in Modern Europe: Essays from*

'The Journal of the History of Sexuality' (Chicago: University of Chicago Press, 1992), 317–33.
132. Barbara Brookes, *Abortion in England, 1900–1967* (London: Croom Helm, 1988) is an overview of this subject.
133. 'Notes of the Quarter: "Dangers to Men"', *The Shield*, 5th series, v (iii) (1937), 99.
134. 'Notes of the Quarter', *The Shield*, 5th series, ix (ii) (1942), 3–7.
135. McGregor, *Divorce in England*, 29–34; Stone, *Road to Divorce*, 401.
136. *Army Medical Services: Administration II*, 231–2.
137. Lees, 'Venereal Diseases in the Armed Forces Overseas'.
138. *Army Medical Services: Administration II*, 234.
139. Campbell, 'Venereal Diseases in the Armed Forces Overseas (2)'.
140. *Army Medical Services: Administration II*, 238.
141. *The Lancet*, ii (1942), 577.
142. *The Lancet*, i (1943), 276.
143. Tom Harrisson – Mass Observation archive at the University of Sussex (MO): 'Sex Survey' A.9, Box 1 Venereal Disease Survey 1942–1943; discussed further in Chapter 8.
144. *The Lancet*, ii (1942), 18.
145. *The Shield*, 5th series, lx (ii) (1942), 58.
146. *The Lancet*, i (1944), 167.
147. I. N. Orpwood Price and J. A. Burgess, 'Is a New Deal in the Control of Venereal Disease Necessary?' (two papers and discussion), *BJVD*, xx (1944), 19–30.
148. 'The Social Aspect of the Venereal Diseases': Hilda M. Johns, 'Contact Tracing' and Margaret A. Wailes, 'Contact Tracing and the Prostitute', *BJVD*, xxi (1945), 15–17, 17–21; Col. J. E. Gordon, 'The Control of Venereal Disease: An Epidemiological Approach', *The Lancet*, ii (1944), 711–15.
149. E.g. A. D. Frazer, 'The Problem of the Defaulter', *BJVD*, viii (1932), 56–8, and in 1935, Vol. xi, a series of papers on particular classes of defaulter.
150. Major G. O. Watts and Major R. A. Wilson, 'A Study of Personality Factors among Venereal Disease Patients', *Canadian Medical Association Journal*, liii (1945), 119–22.
151. E. D. Wittkower, 'The Psychological Aspects of Venereal Disease', *BJVD*,

xxiv (1948), 59–67.

152. E.g. Alec Craig, *Above All Liberties* (London: Allen and Unwin, 1942), citing 'Sheila Cousins', *To Beg I Am Ashamed: The Autobiography of a London Prostitute* (Paris: Obelisk Press, 1938), 119.

153. Cyril Bibby, *Sex Education: A Guide for Parents, Teachers and Youth Leaders* (London: Macmillan, 1946), 109.

154. Eustace Chesser, *Grow Up – and Live* (Harmondsworth: Penguin, 1949), 237; idem, *Love without Fear: A Plain Guide to Sex Technique for Every Married Adult*, 2nd edn (London: Rich and Cowan, Medical Publications, 1942), 91–100.

155. Chesser, *Grow Up – and Live*, 247.

156. Bibby, *Sex Education*, 130–1.

157. Lesley A. Hall, ' "The Cinderella of Medicine": Sexually-Transmitted Diseases in Britain in the Nineteenth and Twentieth Centuries', *Genitourinary Medicine*, lxix (1993), 314–19.

158. Leathard, *The Fight for Family Planning*, 78–85; Jane Lewis, David Clark and David Morgan, *Whom God Hath Joined Together: The Work of Marriage Guidance* (London: Routledge, 1992), 74–85.

159. Leathard, *Fight for Family Planning*, 201–4.

160. BSS 'Letters out', to G. Gardiner; 'Misc.' Gardiner's comments on whether Rockstro's *A Plain Talk on Sex Difficulties* is liable to prosecution; transcript of Gardiner's chairman's introduction to paper by Margaret Lowenfeld and comments on it, 16 Feb. 1933. The biography by his second wife, Muriel Box, *Rebel Advocate: a Biography of Gerald Gardiner* (London: Gollancz, 1983) does not mention this facet of his career.

161. Haste, *Rules of Desire*, 174.

162. Davenport-Hines, *Sex, Death and Punishment*, 151–3; Haste, *Rules of Desire*, 85; Ferris, *Sex and the British*, 107.

163. A much severer attitude towards divorce was noticeable in returns from Scotland of the Mass Observation 'Sex Survey' of 1947–9, MO A.9, 9/A.

164. Hynes, *The Edwardian Turn of Mind*, 296–306; Ferris, *Sex and the British*, 20–3; Haste, *Rules of Desire*, 74–7; Donald Thomas, *A Long Time Burning: The History of Literary Censorship in England* (London: Routledge and Kegan Paul,

1969), 302–5; the effects of censorship are further discussed in Chapter 11, p. 257.

165. Ferris, *Sex and the British*, 103–4; Haste, *Rules of Desire*, 77–8.

166. Bristow, *Vice and Vigilance*, ch. 9: 'The Pursuit of the Obscene', 200–28.

167. Brookes, *Abortion in England*.

168. See Porter and Weeks, *Between the Acts*, 63, 148 for mentions of this.

169. Even in the 1950s: see Rolph (ed.), *Women of the Streets*, 18–23.

170. Kaye Wellings, Julia Field, Anne Johnson and Jane Wadsworth, with Sally Bradshaw, *Sexual Behaviour in Britain: The National Survey of Sexual Attitudes and Lifestyles* (Harmondsworth: Penguin, 1994), p. 236.

11 Silent Stares, Smut, Censorship and Surgical Stores: the Makings of Popular Sexual Knowledges

1. Steve Humphries, *A Secret World of Sex: Forbidden Fruit, the British Experience 1900–1950* (London: Sidgwick and Jackson, 1988), 'Introduction: Taboo Talk', 9–13.

2. Marie Stopes 'ML–Gen' correspondence in the Contemporary Medical Archives Centre at the Wellcome Institute for the History of Medicine: CMAC, PP/MCS/A.220 WS, A.146 BJ.

3. *Ibid.*, CMAC, PP/MCS/A.115 HPH, A.244 WPW.

4. Humphries, *Secret World of Sex*, 36–40.

5. National Vigilance Association archives in the Fawcett Library, London Guildhall University (NVA): Box 104, file S.46 Assaults Departmental Committee; undated [c. 1926] cutting from *Vigilance Record*.

6. Humphries, *Secret World of Sex*, 35.

7. Maureen Sutton, '*We Didn't Know Aught': A Study of Sexuality, Superstition and Death in Women's Lives in Lincolnshire during the 1930s, '40s and '50s* (Stanford: Paul Watkins, 1992), 8–9.

8. Tom Harrisson – Mass Observation Archive at the University of Sussex (MO), 'Sex Survey' A.9 5/E, Fulham male, aged 54.

9. Stephen Graham, *A Private in the*

Guards (1919), cited in a review in *The Shield: The Journal of the Association for Moral and Social Hygiene*, 3rd series, ii (1919–20), 228.

10. Inquiry into *The Army and Religion*, reviewed *ibid.*, 231.

11. Association for Moral and Social Hygiene archives at the Fawcett Library, London Guildhall University (AMSH): Box 49, Committee of Enquiry into Sexual Morality 1918–19, evidence of Reverend Herbert Gray, 24 March 1919.

12. Brig.-Gen. F. D. Crozier, *A Brass Hat in No-Man's Land: A Personal Record of the European War* (London: Jonathan Cape, 1930), 66–7.

13. *Ibid.*, 90.

14. AMSH, Box 49: Evidence of Rev. Herbert Gray.

15. *The Shield*, 3rd series, ii (1919–20), 231.

16. 'British Troops in France: Provision of Tolerated Brothels', *The Shield*, 3rd series, i (1916–17), 393–7; 'The Maisons Tolerées', *The Shield*, 3rd series, ii (1918–20), 53–64.

17. Crozier, *A Brass Hat in No-Man's Land*, 143.

18. CMAC, PP/MCS/A.211 MR, A.168 Capt. McK, A.118 Capt. WPH, A.120 HHK, A.135 Capt. BH.

19. *Ibid.*, PP/MCS/A.32 HMB 1921, A.57 JC 1918, A.135 WH 1919.

20. *Ibid.*, PP/MCS/A.220 WS; A.67 GHG 1929 S. Africa; A.205 HWP in Bengal; and see also Lesley A. Hall, *Hidden Anxieties: Male Sexuality 1900–1950* (Cambridge: Polity Press, 1991), 51–2.

21. CMAC, PP/MCS/A.193 RP.

22. *Ibid.*, PP/MCS/A.129 FH, 1921 age 48.

23. *Ibid.*, PP/MCS/A.88.

24. *Ibid.*, PP/MCS/A.114 Miss HH (Australia), A.215 Miss BR, A.115 Miss MH.

25. *Ibid.*, PP/MCS/A.6 Miss EMA, A.245 Mrs AW, DMW, A.248 Mrs AW, A.167 Mrs MMcD.

26. Virginia Woolf, *The Diary of Virginia Woolf*, Vol. I: *1915–1919*, ed. Anne Olivier Bell (Harmondsworth: Penguin, 1979), entry for Thursday 18 April 1918, 141.

27. CMAC, PP/MCS/A.118 Miss MH, A.114 Miss HH.

28. Sutton, *'We Didn't Know Aught'*, 48.

29. Elsa Lanchester, *Elsa Lanchester Herself* (London: Michael Joseph, 1983), 35.

30. Sutton, *'We Didn't Know Aught'*, 50, 43.

31. CMAC, PP/MCS/A.114 Mrs EH, A.118 Miss MH.

32. Naomi Mitchison, *All Change Here: Girlhood and Marriage* (London: Bodley Head, 1975), 157; *idem, You May Well Ask: A Memoir 1920–1940* (London: Gollancz, 1979), 69–70.

33. Sutton, *'We Didn't Know Aught'*, 2, 90–3, 59.

34. Nicky Leap and Billie Hunter, *The Midwife's Tale: an Oral History from Handywoman to Professional Midwife* (London: Scarlet Press, 1993), 78–9; the whole of the chapters on 'Women's Knowledge about the "Facts of Life"' and 'Birth Control', 72–82, 83–91, are illuminating on this topic.

35. CMAC, PP/MCS/A.242 Miss TCW, A.74 Miss FD, A.68 Mr C, 1923.

36. *Ibid.*, PP/MCS/A.168 Miss REM, A.167 Mr RMcD, A.115 Miss MH, A.3 Miss A.

37. *Ibid.*, PP/MCS/A.246 Mrs W, A.247 Mrs DW.

38. Sutton, *'We Didn't Know Aught'*, 54–5, 92.

39. *Ibid.*, 56–7; 'Ask the Family Doctor', *Lucky Star: The New Home Story Paper*, 22 March, 28 June 1941.

40. *Woman's Weekly* [2d], Jan.–April 1925.

41. Leap and Hunter, *The Midwife's Tale*, xi.

42. Lesley A. Hall, 'Forbidden by God, Despised by Men: Masturbation, Medical Warnings, Moral Panic and Manhood in Great Britain, 1850–1950', *Journal of the History of Sexuality*, ii (iii) (1992), 365–87.

43. CMAC, PP/MCS/A.252 AEW, 1932, A.222, JAS, soldier, Egypt, 1937, A.183 JM India 1936, A.157, FJL, 1933.

44. *Ibid.*, PP/MCS/A.222 PDS, 1941, A.185 AGM, 1940.

45. MO, A.9 'Sex Survey' 1947–9 5/C: completed questionnaire, 50-year-old male 'in insurance'.

46. *Ibid.*, 4/G 'Report on Sex: Miscellaneous and Unsorted Draft Material'.

47. *Ibid.*, 3/C 'Report on Sex: Chapter Two: Discovering Sex'.

48. *Ibid.*, 5/F completed questionnaires.

49. *Ibid.*, 5/E 1949 Fulham.

50. *Ibid.*, 10/C.

51. *Ibid.*, 10/A, 10/B.

52. *Ibid.*, 5/E 1949 Fulham.

53. *Ibid.*, 5/H 65-year-old policeman's widow, 9/A (Scotland), daily house-

keeper, aged 41, 45-year-old dock labourer's wife.

54. Eliot Slater and Moya Woodside, *Patterns of Marriage: A Study of Marriage Relationships in the Urban Working Classes* (London: Cassell, 1951), 173.

55. Eustace Chesser, Joan Maizels, Leonard Jones and Brian Emmett, *The Sexual, Marital and Family Relationships of the English Woman* (with the assistance of an Advisory Committee comprising Professor F. A. E. Crew, Professor Alexander Kennedy, Kenneth Walker, Doris Odlum and Canon Hugh Walker), (London: Hutchinson's Medical Publications, 1956), ch. 14, paras 21–3, p. 177.

56. MO, A.9, 3/C: 'Report on Sex: Chapter Two: Discovering Sex'.

57. *Ibid.*, 4/G: 'Report on Sex: Miscellaneous and Unsorted Draft Material'; 16/G: 'Advertising and Publications: Proprietary Medicines and Tonics'.

58. *Ibid.*, 16/A: 'Advertising and Publications: Published Material on Sex'; one correspondent wrote to Marie Stopes: 'if the claims made for the Energiser are borne out in practice, it would be an immense boon to millions of men' (CMAC, PP/MCS/A.243 GWW 1934); Blakoe still in business, July 1993.

59. CMAC, PP/MCS/A.216 Lt. LS 1919, see also A.184 JFM 1924.

60. NVA Box 116, Case files No. 24: Indecent window displays – Victoria Docks area; Sempkins of NVA to Scotland Yard, 24 Jan. 1928.

61. Humphries, *Secret World of Sex*, 60.

62. *The Lancet*, Annotation on 'Birth Control', ii (1917), 207–8.

63. Parliamentary Papers: *Select Committee on Patent Medicines* (1914) (414), para. 4693.

64. Marie Stopes papers in the Department of Manuscripts at the British Library: Sir W. Arbuthnot Lane to Stopes, 1922, BL Add. MS 58566.

65. CMAC, PP/MCS/A.204 KAP.

66. *Ibid.*, PP/MCS/A.266 FE.

67. See advertisements reproduced in *Report as to the Practice of Medicine and Surgery by Unqualified Persons in the United Kingdom* (1910), Cd 5422; literature produced by and relating to J. Greevz Fisher of Leeds, supplier of Domestic and Surgical Specialities, during the 1890s, also a member of the National Secular Society and the Legitimation League, and a protester against medical monopoly, in John Johnson Ephemera Collection, the Bodleian Library: 'Sex Population and Eugenics', Box I; Frank Poller, *Holmes of Hanney*, Hanney History Group, Occasional Paper, no. 1 (E. Hanney, Oxon: Hanney History Group, 1993), on J. R. Holmes, an active Malthusian in this small Oxfordshire village.

68. NVA, Box 104 S46 Assaults Departmental Committee; offences against young persons *c.* 1926.

69. *Ibid.*, Box 107 Objectionable Literature 88E, 1925.

70. *Ibid.*, Objectionable Literature S88, Deputation from London Public Morality Council to Joynson Hicks, 1929, report in *Vigilance Record*.

71. British Sexology Society (BSS) archives in the Harry Ransom Humanities Research Center, University of Texas at Austin (HRC), 'Misc.': H. C. Booth to E. L. Deighton, 10 Nov. 1931.

72. Alec Craig, 'Recent Developments in the Law of Obscene Libel', in Dr A Pillay and Albert Ellis (eds), *Sex, Society and the Individual: Selected Papers, Revised and Brought up to Date, from 'Marriage Hygiene' (1934–1937) and 'International Journal of Sexology' (1947–1952)* (Bombay: International Journal of Sexology, 1953), 302–27.

73. CMAC, PP/MCS/A.223 MWS *c.* 1930s.

74. *British Medical Journal*, ii (1934), 95.

75. Information supplied by librarian friends.

76. Francis Jekyll to Edward Carpenter, 8 June 1912; Carpenter papers in Sheffield City Archives, MSS 386/199.

77. BSS 'Letters out': to Sir F. G. Kenyon, British Museum, 22 Jan., 6 March 1920; 'Misc.': Minutes Vol. II, 77th meeting, 24 Sept. 1920.

78. E.g. Iwan Bloch, *The Sexual Life of Our Time, in its Relations to Modern Civilisation*, trans. from the 6th German edn by M. Eden Paul (London: Rebman, 1909), 'Publisher's Note to the English Edition': '... The publishers have, after very serious and careful consideration, come to the conclusion that the sale of the English translation of this book shall be limited to members of the legal and medical profession'; Wilhelm Stekel, *Impotence in the Male:*

The Psychic Disorders of Sexual Function in the Male, 2 vols, authorized English version by Oswald H. Boltz (Germany, 1927; New York: Liveright, 1927): 'The sale of this work, because of its scientific character, is positively restricted to physicians, lawyers, ministers and educators'; Dr Magnus Hirschfeld, *Sexual Anomalies and Perversions: Physical and Psychological Development and Treatment. A Summary of the Works of the Late Professor Dr Magnus Hirschfeld, Compiled as a Humble Memorial by His Pupils* (London: Torch Publishing *c.* 1936), 'A Textbook for Students, Psychologists, Criminologists, Probation Officers, Judges and Educationists'; George Ryley Scott, *Scott's Encyclopaedia of Sex: A Practical Encyclopaedia Arranged in Alphabetical Order, Explanatory of Everything Pertaining to Sexual Physiology, Psychology and Pathology* (London: T. Werner Laurie, 1939): 'The sale of this book is restricted to members of the Medical and Legal Professions, Scientists, Anthropologists, Psychologists, Sociologists, Criminologists and Social Workers.'

79. The Viscountess Rhondda, *This Was My World* (London: Macmillan, 1933), 126–7.

80. Walter Gallichan, *The Poison of Prudery; An Historical Survey* (London: T. Werner Laurie, 1929), 147.

81. CMAC, PP/MCS/A.158 JL, 1923.

82. Oral communication to L. H., Sydney, Oct. 1988.

83. Marie Stopes correspondence with A. C. Fifield Ltd, BL Add. MS 58524.

84. Isabel Elmslie Hutton, *Memories of a Doctor in War and Peace* (London: Heinemann, 1960), 216–17.

85. E.g. Mrs S Herbert, *Sex-Lore: A Primer on Courtship, Marriage and Parenthood* (London: A. & C. Black, 1918); A. J. Cokkinis, *The Reproduction of Life: a Handbook of the Science of Reproduction in Nature and Man* (London: Baillière, 1926).

86. CMAC, PP/MCS/A.169 MCS to Mr RDM.

87. *The Lancet*, i (1933), 1349.

88. Lesley A. Hall, ' "Somehow Very Distasteful": Doctors, Men and Sexual Problems between the Wars', *Journal of Contemporary History*, xx (iv) (1985), 553–74; *idem, Hidden Anxieties*, in particular ch. 6: ' "I Shouldn't Care to Face the Experience Again": Male Sexual Problems in the Consulting Room', 139–69.

89. Eustace Chesser, *Love without Fear: A Plain Guide to Sex Technique for Every Married Adult* (London: Rich and Cowan Medical Publications, 1941; revised edn, July 1942), inside dustjacket.

90. Craig, 'Recent Developments in the Law of Obscene Libel'.

91. Chesser, *Love without Fear*, revised edn July 1942, 26; ch. 11 'Byways of Sex', and ch. 12 'Painful Pleasures', 105–24.

92. Craig, 'Recent Developments in the Law of Obscene Libel'.

93. MO, A.9, 16/A: 'Advertising and Publications: Published Material on Sex'; similar catalogues produced by the 'Economy Educator Service', *c.* 1930s–40s (with a particularly strong leaning towards nudism, theoretical and pictorial) in NVA archives: 'Objectionable Literature' S885, Box 107.

94. Bernarr A. MacFadden, *The Virile Powers of Superb Manhood: How Developed, How Lost, How Regained* (New York: Physical Culture Publishing, 1900); M. Huhner, *A Practical Treatise on Disorders of the Sexual Function in the Male and Female* (Philadelphia: F. A. Davis, 1916; 3rd edn 1929); A. K. Gardner, *The Conjugal Relationship as Regards Personal Health and Hereditary Well-Being Practically Treated* (New York: G. J. Moutton, 1892; Glasgow: T. D. Morison, 1892; London: Simpkin, Marshall, Hamilton and Kent, 1894); R. T. Trall, *Sexual Physiology and Hygiene: An Exposition Practical, Scientific, Moral, and Popular of Some of the Fundamental Problems in Sociology* (1st edn USA *c.* 1888; Glasgow: T. D. Morison; London: Simpkin, Marshall, Hamilton and Kent, 1908 edn); Prof. W. H. Walling, *Sexology* (Philadelphia: Puritan Publishing Co., 1902).

95. Cyril Bibby, *Sex Education: A Guide for Parents, Teachers and Youth Leaders* (London: Macmillan, 1946), 128.

96. Thomas Boyle, *Black Swine in the Sewers of Hampstead: Beneath the Surface of Victorian Sensationalism* (New York: Viking, 1988; Harmondsworth: Penguin, 1989); Richard Davenport-Hines, *Sex, Death, and Punishment:*

Attitudes to Sex and Sexuality in Britain since the Renaissance (London: Collins, 1990).

97. Keith Soothill and Sylvia Walby, *Sex Crime in the News* (London: Routledge, 1991), for example, is a useful study of the reporting of rape and other crimes of sexual violence from the 1950s to the 1980s, emphasizing the distortions created by sensationalist press construction of selected cases into a particular narrative of rape.

98. HRC, Havelock Ellis from Radclyffe Hall, 23 and 28 Aug. 1929; Rebecca O'Rourke, *Reflecting on 'The Well of Loneliness'*, 'Heroines?' series (London: Routledge, 1989), 92, states that 'the initial impact' of the *Sunday Express*'s attack on Hall and her book 'was to increase interest and sales'; HRC, Morris Ernst papers, uncatalogued bundles 383–4, English legal papers re *The Well of Loneliness*.

99. NVA, Box 110, S109, S127: traffic cases.

100. CMAC, PP/MCS/A.169, A.166 Mrs C. McC, A.168 Mrs McI, 1922.

101. Claire Davey, 'Birth Control in Britain during the Inter-War Years: Evidence from the Stopes Correspondence', *Journal of Family History*, xiii (iii) (1988), 329–45.

102. CMAC, PP/MCS/A.248 Mrs AW.

103. Most works which have analysed women's magazines have done so in order to elaborate their implication in wider issues of constructing ideologies of womanhood rather than considering more specific messages about female sexuality: Cynthia L. White, *Women's Magazines 1693–1968* (London: Michael Joseph, 1970); Marjorie Ferguson, *Forever Feminine: Women's Magazines and the Cult of Femininity* (London: Heinemann, 1983); Bridget Fowler, 'True to Me Always: An Analysis of Women's Magazine Fiction', in Christopher Pawling (ed.), *Popular Fiction and Social Change* (London: Macmillan, 1984); Billie Melman, *Woman and the Popular Imagination in the 1920s; Flappers and Nymphs* (London: Macmillan, 1988): 'Part Three: Realistic Fantasies: The World of the Story Papers', 107–44.

104. *Woman's World: The Favourite Paper of a Million Homes* [weekly 2d], 21 March,

25 April, 21 Feb. 1925.

105. *Ibid.*, 10 Jan., 4 April 1925.

106. *Ibid.*, 28 Feb., 21 March, 25 April 1925.

107. *Ibid.*, *Woman's Weekly* [2d], Jan.–April 1925.

108. R. A. McCance, M. C. Luff and E. E. Widdowson, 'Physical and Emotional Periodicity in Women', *Journal of Hygiene*, xxxvii (1937), 571–611; more detailed discussion in Chapters 7 and 8.

109. E.g. in *Woman's World*, 1935, 1945; *Silver Star*, 1940; *Lucky Star*, 1941.

110. For more on Eyles see Maroula Joannou, '"The Woman in the Little House": Leonora Eyles and Socialist Feminism', in A. Ingram and D. Patai (eds), *Rediscovering Forgotten Radicals: British Women Writers 1880–1939* (Chapel Hill: University of North Carolina Press, 1993), 75–89.

111. *Modern Woman (incorporating Leach's Newest Fashions)* [6d monthly], Sept., Aug., Oct., Dec., 1925.

112. Melman, *Woman and the Popular Imagination*, 'Part Three: Realistic Fantasies: The World of the Story Papers', 107–44; see also Fowler, 'True to Me Always'.

113. Joseph McAleer, *Popular Reading and Publishing in Britain 1914–1950* (Oxford: Clarendon Press, 1992).

114. Morris Ernst papers (HRC) bundles 383–4: English legal papers re *Well of Loneliness*; proofs of witnesses – Julian Huxley.

115. Lillian Fadermann, *Surpassing the Love of Men: Romantic Friendship and Love between Women from the Renaissance to the Present* (London: Junction Books, 1982), 'Fiction as a Weapon', 341–56.

116. AMSH, Box 49: evidence of J. B. Fagan, 3 Nov. 1919.

117. Marie Stopes, *A Banned Play and a Preface on the Censorship* (London: John Bale, Sons and Danielsson, 1926), Preface, 1–50.

118. Rebecca West, 'The Tosh Horse', in *The Strange Necessity: Essays and Reviews* (London: Jonathan Cape, 1928), 319–25.

119. The 'desert romance' in particular is discussed in ch. 6 '1919–28: "The Sheik of Araby" – Freedom in Captivity in the Desert Romance', in Melman, *Woman and the Popular Imagination*, 89–104, as part of her wider discussion of

' "Furtive Excitement": The Discourse in Best-sellers'; see also McAleer, *Popular Reading and Publishing*.

120. Claud Cockburn, *Bestseller: The Books that Everyone Read, 1900–1939* (London: Sidgwick and Jackson, 1972); Melman, *Woman and the Popular Imagination*, McAleer, *Popular Reading and Publishing*.

121. Eileen Arnot Robertson, *Cullum* (1928), *Three Came Unarmed* (1929), *Four Frightened People* (1931), *Ordinary Families* (1933).

122. All to be found in *Gay Life* (1933), but also in other novels of Delafield's.

123. Mitchison, *You May Well Ask*, 'A Note on the Literary Decencies', 171–9.

124. René J. A. Weiss, *Criminal Justice: The True Story of Edith Thompson* (London: Hamish Hamilton, 1988).

125. Stopes, *A Banned Play*, 112–14.

126. Fowler, 'True to Me Always'; Tania Modleski, *Loving with a Vengeance: Mass-Produced Fantasies for Women* (London: Methuen, 1984), ch. 2: 'The Disappearing Act: Harlequin Romances', 35–58.

127. MO, A.9, file 3/B: 'Report on Sex: Chapter One: Sex Surveyed', and VD surveys of 1942–3, files 1/A–G.

128. Davenport-Hines, *Sex, Death, and Punishment*, 297; Paul Ferris, *Sex and the British: A Twentieth Century History* (London: Michael Joseph, 1993), 60.

129. Craig, 'Recent Developments in the Law of Obscene Libel'; C. H. Rolph (ed.), *The Trial of Lady Chatterley: Regina v. Penguin Books Limited* (Harmondsworth: Penguin, 1961).

130. Alex Comfort, 'Sex Education in the Medical Curriculum', *International Journal of Sexology*, iii (iii) (1950), 175–7.

Conclusion

1. See, for example, R. Davenport-Hines, *Sex, Death, and Punishment: Attitudes to Sex and Sexuality in Britain since the Renaissance* (London: Collins, 1990), 326–9, and ch. 9: 'Hating Others: AIDS', 330–83.

2. Barbara Brookes, *Abortion in England, 1900–1967* (London: Croom Helm, 1988), 96–7; Paul Ferris, *Sex and the British: A Twentieth Century History* (London: Michael Joseph, 1993), 293–5.

3. Department of Health Circular EL(90) MB115 to Regional General Managers 6 June 1990; Family Planning Association, *What Is Happening to NHS Family Planning Clinics*, Nov. 1990; David Brindle, 'District Cuts NHS-Funded Abortions', *The Guardian*, 15 Nov. 1991; Celia Hall, 'Closure of Family Planning Clinics Proposed', *The Independent*, 13 Aug. 1992; Jane Roe, 'Abortion on Request or Quest for Abortion: the Law in Practice', *Breaking Chains*, lvii (Autumn 1992), 6. I am indebted to Margaret Chekri of the Family Planning Association for providing me with these and other supporting references.

4. See, for example, David Fernbach, 'Xq28 Marks the Spot', *New Statesman and Society*, 30 July 1993, 29–30.

5. Kaye Wellings, Julia Field, Anne Johnson and Jane Wadsworth, *Sexual Behaviour in Britain: The National Survey of Sexual Attitudes and Lifestyles* (Harmondsworth: Penguin, 1994), Preface, ix.

6. *British Medical Journal*, ii (1989), 701, 1065–6; Wellings *et al.*, *Sexual Behaviour in Britain*, Foreword by Sir Donald Acheson, vii.

7. J. Laurance, 'Bedroom Survey "Can't Be Trusted"', *The Times*, 24 Jan. 1994.

8. Peter Lennon, 'Why Mary, Mary Was Really Quite Contrary', *The Guardian*, 27 Nov. 1993.

9. Carol Lee, *Friday's Child: The Threat to Moral Education* (Wellingborough: Thorsons, 1988); Ferris, *Sex and the British*, 239–43, 292–3; Isobel Allen, *Education on the Sex and Personal Relationships* (London: Policy Studies Institute, 1987) – this indicates that most parents want some kind of sex education in schools; 'The Wonder Years', *Guardian Weekend*, 18 Dec. 1993, 6–12.

10. *The Guardian*, 24 March 1994, 2; Leader Comment, 25.

11. Jane Lewis, David Clark and David Morgan, *Whom God Hath Joined Together: The Work of Marriage Guidance* (London: Routledge, 1992).

12. On sex education see note 9 above; on AIDS prevention, see, for example, V. Berridge, 'The Early Years of AIDS in the United Kingdom 1981–6: Historical Perspectives', in T. Ranger and P. Slack (eds), *Epidemics and Ideas* (Cambridge: Cambridge University Press, 1992); Eric T. Juengst and Barbara A. Koenig (eds), *The Meaning of AIDS: Implication for Medical Science, Clinical Practice and Public Health Policy* (New York: Praeger, 1989); V. Berridge and P. Strong (eds), *AIDS and Contemporary History* (Cambridge: Cambridge University Press, 1993).

13. Prudence Tunnadine, *The Making of Love* (London: Unwin Paperbacks, 1985); Dr Tunnadine is Director of Training in the Institute of Psychosexual Medicine.

14. Wellings *et al.*, *Sexual Behaviour in Britain*, 244–52.

15. *Ibid.*, 265–9.

16. Wellings *et al.*, *Sexual Behaviour in Britain*, 264.

17. Ferris, *Sex and the British*, 262–3; Donald Thomas, *A Long Time Burning: The History of Literary Censorship in England* (London: Routledge and Kegan Paul, 1969), 272–3.

18. Some discussion of these may be found in Davenport-Hines, *Sex, Death, and Punishment*, Ferris, *Sex and the British*, and Cate Haste, *Rules of Desire. Sex in Britain: World War I to the Present* (London: Chatto and Windus, 1992), in the context of wider overviews; two recent studies of the 'sexual revolution' of the 1960s in particular are Linda Grant, *Sexing the Millennium: A Political History of the Sexual Revolution* (London: HarperCollins, 1993), and Jonathan Green, *It: Sex since the Sixties* (London: Secker and Warburg, 1993).

19. P. Robinson, *The Modernization of Sex: Havelock Ellis, Alfred Kinsey, William Masters and Virginia Johnson* (London and New York: Harper and Row, 1976); besides its somewhat Whiggish narrative, like Brecher's *The Sex Researchers* (London: André Deutsch, 1970) its narrative structure follows the model of 'Great Men [*sic*] of Science' and their Onward Progress to The Truth, which one might also wish to critique.

20. See, for example, Ann Snitow, Christine Stansell and Sharon Thompson (eds), *Desire: The Politics of Sexuality* (London: Virago, 1984); Carole S. Vance (ed.), *Pleasure and Danger: Exploring Female Sexuality* (Boston and London: Routledge and Kegan Paul, 1984); Feminist Review, *Sexuality; A Reader* (London: Virago, 1987).

21. Barbara Ehrenreich, Elizabeth Hess and Gloria Jacobs, *Remaking Love: The Feminization of Sex* (Garden City, NY: Anchor Press/Doubleday, 1986; London: Fontana, 1987).

22. Jonathan Goldberg, *Sodometries: Renaissance Texts, Modern Sexualities* (Stanford, Calif.: Stanford University Press, 1992); cf. John Donne, 'Elegy 16 On His Mistress':

'Th' indifferent Italian. . . well
    content to think thee Page
Will hunt thee with such lust, and
    hideous rage,
As Lots fair guests were vext.

This was first published in 1635, but presumably written in Donne's reprobate youth some thirty or more years previously.

23. Joseph McAleer, *Popular Reading and Publishing in Britain 1914–1950* (Oxford: Clarendon Press, 1992), 126–7.

24. *Ibid.*, 166, 185.

25. Tom Harrisson – Mass Observation archive at the University of Sussex (MO), A.9, Sex Survey, 4/C: 'Report on Sex: Chapter Nine: The Psychology of Sex'.

26. *Ibid.*, 4/F: 'Report on Sex: Early draft chapters, discarded: Chapter Fifteen: Vanguards and Resistance Movements'; 4/B: 'Report on Sex: Chapter Eight: Prostitution'.

27. *Ibid.*, Sex Survey, 3/B: 'Report on Sex: Sex Surveyed'.

28. See Lesley A. Hall, ' "The English Have Hot-Water Bottles": the Morganatic Marriage of Medicine and Sexology in Britain since William Acton', in Roy Porter and Mikuláš Teich (eds), *Sexual Knowledge, Sexual Science: The History of Attitudes to Sexuality* (Cambridge: Cambridge University Press, 1994) 349–65; and ' "The Cinderella of Medicine": Sexually Transmitted

Diseases in Britain in the Nineteenth and Twentieth Centuries', *Genitourinary Medicine*, lxix (1993), 314–19.

29. Brecher, *Sex Researchers*, 86; Wellings *et al.*, *Sexual Behaviour in Britain*, 12.

30. Janice M. Irvine, *Disorders of Desire: Sex and Gender in Modern American Sexology* (Philadelphia: Temple University Press, 1990), 64–6.

31. Wellings *et al.*, *Sexual Behaviour in Britain*, 12–13.

32. See, for example, Irvine, *Disorders of Desire* on sexology in the USA in the twentieth century; Angus McLaren and Arlene Tiger McLaren, *The Bedroom and the State: the Changing Practices and Politics of Contraception and Abortion in Canada, 1880–1980* (Toronto: McLelland and Stewart, 1986); John C. Fout, 'Sexual Politics in Wilhelmine Germany: The Male Gender Crisis, Moral Purity, and Homophobia', and other essays in John C. Fout (ed.), *Forbidden History: The State, Society, and the Regulation of Sexuality in Modern Europe* (Chicago: University of Chicago Press, 1992); Laura Engelstein, *The Key to Happiness: Sex and the Search for Modernity in Fin de Siècle Russia* (Ithaca, NY: Cornell University Press, 1992); Cornelie Usborne, *The Politics of the Body in Weimar Germany: Women's Reproductive Rights and Duties* (Ann Arbor, Mich.: University of Michigan Press; London: Macmillan, 1992); Robert A. Nye, *Masculinity and Male Codes of Honor in Modern France* (Oxford: Oxford University Press, 1993).

33. Françoise Barret-Ducrocq, *Love in the Time of Victoria: Sexuality, Class and Gender in Nineteenth Century London*, trans. John Howe (first published as *L'Amour sous Victoria*, Paris: Plon, 1989; London and New York: Verso, 1991). As a closure of 150 years was reimposed on the Foundling Hospital records by the present governors following Barret-Ducrocq's research, it is not at present possible for researchers to go back to the original documents. 'Crim. con.' was a common Victorian euphemism for sexual intercourse, derived from 'criminal conversation', which actually meant acts of adultery for which a husband could claim damages from the seducer.

34. Alan Rusbridger, *A Concise History of the Sex Manual, 1886–1986* (London: Faber and Faber, 1986).

35. Angus McLaren, *A History of Contraception from Antiquity to the Present Day* (Oxford: Basil Blackwell, 1991).

36. E.g. P. Fryer, *The Birth Controllers* (London: Secker and Warburg, 1965).

37. Wally Seccombe, *Weathering the Storm: Working-Class Families from the Industrial Revolution to the Fertility Decline* (London and New York: Verso, 1993).

38. MO, A.9 VD Survey 1/A: 'Re Dec. 1942 Survey'.

39. *Ibid.*, 1/E Nov.–Dec. 1942 F55B.

40. *Ibid.*, 1/B Dec. 1942 London F45C.

41. *Ibid.*, 1/B Dec. 1942 London, F35C 'Indirect'.

42. *Ibid.*, 1/B, Dec. 1942 London, F30B 'Indirect'.

43. George Ives, entry for 8 May 1940, 'Notes and Various Writings no. CV 1940', Harry Ransom Humanities Research Center, University of Texas at Austin.

44. 'Correspondence: general', 1937–45 in the archives of the National Society for the Prevention of Venereal Disease in the Contemporary Medical Archives Centre at the Wellcome Institute for the History of Medicine, CMAC, SA/PVD/1, 3–9, 11–13; there may well have been earlier correspondence which has not survived.

45. Wellings *et al.*, *Sexual Behaviour in Britain*, 356–80.

46. Sheila Rowbotham and Jeffrey Weeks, *Socialism and the New Life: the Personal and Sexual Politics of Edward Carpenter and Havelock Ellis* (London: Pluto Press, 1977); Jeffrey Weeks, *Coming Out: Homosexual Politics in Britain, from the Nineteenth Century to the Present* (London: Quartet Books; Totowa, NJ: Barnes and Noble, 1977); Phyllis Grosskurth, *Havelock Ellis: A Biography* (London: Allen Lane, 1980).

47. For further details about Haire, see Weeks, *Coming Out*, 128–43, 151–5.

48. June Rose, *Marie Stopes and the Sexual Revolution* (London: Faber and Faber, 1992); Lesley A. Hall, 'Uniting Science and Sensibility: Marie Stopes and the Narratives of Marriage in the 1920s', in A. Ingram and D. Patai (eds), *Rediscovering Forgotten Radicals: British*

Women Writers, 1880–1939 (Chapel Hill: University of North Carolina Press, 1993), 118–36.

49. Isabel Elmslie Hutton, *Memories of a Doctor in War and Peace* (London: Heinemann, 1960).

50. Edward F. Griffith, *The Pioneer Spirit* (Upton Grey, Hants: Green Leaves Press, 1981).

51. Papers of Sir Alan Sterling Parkes, FRS in the Contemporary Medical Archives Centre at the Wellcome Institute for the History of Medicine, 'Screwball Letters', 1930–80, n. d.; CMAC, PP/ASP/A.21.

52. Jay Mechling, 'Advice to Historians on Advice to Mothers', *Journal of Social History*, ix (1975–6), 44–57.

Bibliography

Archives

Bodleian Library, Oxford
    John Johnson Ephemera Collection: sections 'Patent Medicines', and 'Sex Population and Eugenics'
British Library, Department of Manuscripts (BL):
    Papers of Havelock Ellis (Ellis)
    Correspondence of Elizabeth Wolstenholme Elmy with Mrs McIlquham
    Papers of Marie C. Stopes (Stopes)
Contemporary Medical Archives Centre, Wellcome Institute for the History of Medicine (CMAC):
    British Medical Association 'Groups' files (SA/BMA)
    Eugenics Society archives (SA/EUG)
    Family Planning Association archives (SA/FPA)
    Papers of Edward Fyfe Griffith (PP/EFG)
    Papers of James Randal Hutchinson (PP/MCS)
    Papers of R. A. McCance and Elsie M. Widdowson (GC/97)
    Unpublished autobiography of Professor Vernon Henry Mottram (GC/151/7)
    Papers of Sir Alan Sterling Parkes, FRS (PP/ASP)
    National Society for the Prevention of Venereal Disease archives (SA/PVD)
    Papers of Marie C. Stopes (PP/MCS)
Fawcett Library at London Guildhall University (Fawcett):
    'Social Evil' scrapbooks of William Acton
    Archives of the Association for Moral and Social Hygiene (AMSH)
    Archives of the National Vigilance Association (NVA)
Harry Ransom Humanities Research Center, University of Texas at Austin (HRC):
    Archives of the British Society for the Study of Sex Psychology (British Sexology Society) (BSS)
    George Ives: Uncatalogued papers
    Havelock Ellis: correspondence with Horatio Brown, Edward Carpenter and Radclyffe Hall
    Edward Carpenter: correspondence with George Ives, George Ives correspondence with Henry Salt

Morris Ernst: Uncatalogued papers, bundles 383–4 relating to prosecution
of *The Well of Loneliness*
London University:
Bentham Papers, University College
Royal College of Obstetricians and Gynaecologists (RCOG):
Records of Human Fertility Investigation Committee
Royal Society:
Registers of Papers, Series B
Referees' Reports, 1936
Sectional Committee on Physiology
Sheffield City Archives (Sheffield):
Edward Carpenter papers (Carpenter)
University of Strathclyde:
Papers of Sir Patrick Geddes (Geddes)
Tom Harrisson – Mass Observation Archive at the University of Sussex (MO):
A.9 'Sex Survey' 1929–1950; Venereal Disease Survey 1942–1943, 'Little
Kinsey' 1947–1949

Government Reports

Departmental Committee on Sickness Benefit Claims under the National Insurance Act,
Cd 7687, 1914
Local Government Board, *Report as to the Practice of Medicine and Surgery by
Unqualified Persons in the United Kingdom,* Cd 5422, 1910
Local Government Board, *Report on Venereal Diseases: by Dr R. W. Johnstone*
[Cd.7029], HMSO, 1913
Select Committee on Patent Medicines 1914 (414)
*Royal Commission on Venereal Diseases: First Report: Appendix; Minutes of Evidence
(1913–1914),* Cd 7475, 1914
Final Report, Cd 8189, 1916

Journals

The Adult
British Journal of Venereal Diseases
British Medical Journal
The Freewoman/The New Freewoman
Home Chat/Home Chat and Mother and Home
The Lancet
Lucky Star: The New Home Story Paper
Modern Home
Modern Woman (incorporating Leach's Newest Fashions)
Mother: The Home Magazine
The Nineteenth Century
The Pelican: A Journal of Today
The Practitioner
Shafts: A Journal for Women and the Working Classes
The Shield: The Journal of the Association for Moral and Social Hygiene

Silver Star: The Biggest and Best Home Story Paper
The Sporting Times: otherwise known as the Pink 'Un
Woman's Friend
Woman's Weekly
Woman's World: The Favourite Paper of a Million Homes

Other Published Sources

Mary Abbott, *Family Ties: English Families 1540–1920* (London and New York: Routledge, 1993).

William Acton, *The Functions and Disorders of the Reproductive Organs in Youth, Adult, Age, and Advanced Life, Considered in their Physiological, Social and Psychological Relations* (London: John Churchill, 1857; 3rd edn, 1862).

William Acton, *Prostitution Considered in its Moral, Social, and Sanitary Aspects in London and Other Large Cities: With Proposals for the Mitigation and Prevention of Its Attendant Evil* (London: J. Churchill, 1857; 2nd edn, ed. Peter Fryer, London: MacGibbon and Kee, 1968).

Paul Langford Adams, 'Health of the State: British and American. Public Health Policies in the Depression and World War II' (Unpublished dissertation for the Doctorate of Social Welfare, University of California Berkeley, 1979).

John Addy, *Sin and Society in the Seventeenth Century* (London and New York: Routledge, Chapman and Hall, 1989).

H. B. Adelmann, *Marcello Malpighi and the Evolution of Embryology*, 5 vols (Ithaca, NY: Cornell University Press, 1966).

Michael Adler, 'The Terrible Peril: A Historical Perspective on the Venereal Diseases', *British Medical Journal*, ii (1980), 202–211.

Peter Agate, *Sexual Economy as Taught by Charles Bradlaugh, M.P., with an Addendum by Saladin* (London: W. Stewart, n. d. ?1878).

'A Graduate', *A Lecture to Young Men on the Preservation of Health and Personal Purity of Life*, 7th edn (Pulvermacher's World Famed Galvanic Belt Co.) (London: H. Renshaw, 1892).

Johanna Alberti, *Beyond Suffrage: Feminists in War and Peace, 1914–1928* (London: Macmillan, 1989).

W. Alexander, *The History of Women from the Earliest Antiquity to the Present Times*, 2 vols in 1 (London: W. Strahan and T. Cadell, 1779).

H. A. Allbutt, *The Wife's Handbook: How a Woman Should Order Herself during Pregnancy, in the Lying-In Room, and After Delivery. With Hints on the Management of the Baby, and other Matters of Importance Necessary to be Known by Married Women* (London: W. J. Ramsay, 1886).

R. Alter, 'Tristram Shandy and the Game of Love', *American Scholar*, xxxvii (1968), 316–23.

Richard D. Altick, *The English Common Reader. A Social History of the Mass Reading Public 1800–1900* (Chicago: University of Chicago Press, 1957).

Richard D. Altick, *Victorian Studies in Scarlet* (London: J. M. Dent and Sons, 1972).

Richard D. Altick, *The Shows of London* (Cambridge, Mass. and London: Belknap Press of Harvard University Press, 1978).

Michael Anderson, *Approaches to the History of the Western Family, 1500–1914* (London: Macmillan, 1980).

[Anon.], *Descriptive Catalogue of the Liverpool Museum of Anatomy* (*c.* 1851?; Liverpool: John H. Matthews, 1877).

[Anon.], *Nature's Revelations for the Married Only*, printed for private circulation only, Electric Life Invigorator Co. (Gloucester: G. W. Ventnor, The Limes, Painswick Rd, ?1904).

[Anon.], *Onania, or the Heinous Sin of Self-Pollution and All its Frightful Conse quences in Both Sexes Consider'd with Spiritual and Physical Advice to those, Who Have Already Injur'd Themselves by This Abominable Practice. And Seasonable Admonition to the Youth of the Nation, (of both Sexes) and Those Whose Tuition They Are Under, Whether Parents, Guardians, Masters, or Mistresses*, 8th edn (London: ?1710; printed by E. Rumball for T. Crouch, 1723; facsimile reprint, New York and London: Ganand, 1986).

[Anon.], 'Piss Pot Science', *Journal of the History of Medicine*, x (1955), 121–3.

[Anon.], *Rare Verities: The Cabinet of Venus Unlocked, and Her Secrets Laid Open* (London: P. Briggs, 1657).

[Anon.], *A Supplement to the Onania* (London: n. d.).

Aristotle [pseud.], *The Works of Aristotle the Famous Philosopher, Containing his Complete Masterpiece, and Family Physician; His Experienced Midwife, His Book of Problems, and His Remarks on Physiognomy*, complete edn, with engravings (High Holborn, London: J. Smith, n. d., twentieth-century).

Aristotle [pseud.], *Aristotle's Master-piece* (London: F. L. for J. How, 1690).

Aristotle [pseud.], *Aristotle's Master-piece* (London: 12th edn, early eighteenth century).

Aristotle [pseud.], *Aristotle's Master-piece* (London: Printed for D. P., 1710).

Aristotle [pseud.], *Aristotle's Last Legacy or His Golden Cabinet of Secrets Opened for Youth's Delightful Pastime* (London: Thomas Norris, 1711).

Aristotle [pseud.], *Aristotle's Compleat Masterpiece. In Three Parts* (London: printed and sold by the booksellers, 1725).

Aristotle [pseud.], *The Works of Aristotle in Four Parts* (London: All the Booksellers, 1796).

Aristotle [pseud.], *The Works of Aristotle, the Famous Philosopher* (London: printed for Archibald Whisleton, Chiswell Street, n. d. but *c.* 1810).

John Armstrong, *The Oeconomy of Love* (London: T. Cooper, 1736; 3rd edn 1739).

Cynthia Asquith, Lady, *Diaries 1915–1918* (London: Hutchinson, 1968).

Jean Astruc, *A Treatise of the Venereal Disease*, trans. W. Barrowby (London: W. Innys and R. Manby, 1737).

Jean Astruc, *A Treatise on all the Diseases Incident to Women* (London: Cooper, 1743).

L. Babb, *Sanity in Bedlam: A Study of Robert Burton's 'Anatomy of Melancholy'* (East Lansing: Michigan State University Press, 1959).

Baden-Powell, Robert, Lord, *Scouting for Boys: A Handbook for Instruction in Good Citizenship* (London: C. Arthur Pearson, 1908; 10th edn 1922).

Baden-Powell, Robert, Lord, *Rovering to Success: A Book of Life-Sport for Young Men* (London: Herbert Jenkins, 1922).

Victor Bailey and Sheila Blackburn, 'The Punishment of Incest Act 1908: A

Case Study of Law Creation', *Criminal Law Review* (1979), 708–18.

Mikhail M. Bakhtin, *Rabelais and his World*, trans. H. Iswolsky (Cambridge, Mass.: MIT Press, 1968).

Kenneth Ballhatchet, *Race, Sex, and Class under the Raj: Imperial Attitudes and Policies and their Critics, 1793–1905* (London, Weidenfeld and Nicolson, 1980).

Honoré de Balzac, *La Physiologie du Mariage* (*The Physiology of Marriage*) (Paris: 1826; London: translation privately printed, 1904).

J. A. Banks, *Prosperity and Parenthood: A Study of Family Planning among the Victorian Middle Classes* (London: Routledge and Kegan Paul, 1954).

J. A. Banks, *Victorian Values: Secularism and the Size of Families* (London and Boston: Routledge and Kegan Paul, 1981).

G. J. Barker-Benfield, 'The Spermatic Economy: A Nineteenth-Century View of Sexuality', *Feminist Studies*, i (1972), 45–74.

G. J. Barker-Benfield, *The Horrors of the Half-Known Life: Male Attitudes toward Women and Sexuality in Nineteenth-Century America* (New York: Harper and Row, 1976).

G. J. Barker-Benfield, *The Culture of Sensibility: Sex and Society in Eighteenth-Century Britain* (Chicago: University of Chicago Press, 1992).

Barry Barnes, *Interests and the Growth of Knowledge* (London: Routledge and Kegan Paul, 1977).

Barry Barnes, 'Sociological Theories of Scientific Knowledge', in R. C. Olby, G. N. Cantor, J. R. R. Christie and M. J. S. Hodge (eds), *Companion to the History of Modern Science* (London: Routledge, 1990), 60–76.

Barry Barnes and Steven Shapin (eds), *Natural Order: Historical Studies of Scientific Culture* (Beverly Hills, Calif. and London: Sage Publications, 1979).

Arthur T. Barnett, 'The Testimony of Medical Men', in The White Cross League, *The Blanco Book* (London: White Cross League, 1913).

Françoise Barret-Ducrocq, *L'amour sous Victoria: sexualité et classes populaires à Londres au XIX siècle* (Paris: Plon, 1989); trans. John Howe, *Love in the Time of Victoria: Sexuality, Class, and Gender in Nineteenth-Century London* (London and New York: Verso, 1991).

Roland Barthes, *Mythologies*, trans. Annette Lavers (London: Jonathan Cape, 1972).

Roland Barthes, *The Fashion System*, trans. Matthew Ward and Richard Howard (New York: Hill and Wang, 1983).

'Dr' G. Courtenay Beale [pseud.], *Wise Wedlock: The Whole Truth: A Book of Counsel and Instruction for All Who Seek for Happiness in Marriage*, 2nd edn (London: Health Promotion, c. 1922).

Otho T. Beall Jr., *'Aristotle's Master-Piece* in America: A Landmark in the Folklore of Medicine', *William and Mary Quarterly*, 3rd ser. xx (1963), 207–22.

Thomas Beddoes, *Hygëia: or Essays Moral and Medical, on the Causes Affecting the Personal State of our Middling and Affluent Classes*, 3 vols (Bristol: J. Mills, 1802).

T. Beddoes, *Hygëia*, 3 vols (Bristol: Phillips, 1802–3).

Thomas Beddoes, *Manual of Health: or, the Invalid Conducted Safely through the Seasons* (London: Johnson, 1806).

W. Blair Bell, *The Sex Complex: A Study of the Relationships of the Internal Secretions to the Female Characteristics and Functions in Health and Disease* (London: Baillière, Tindall and Cox, 1916).

J. Miriam Benn, *The Predicaments of Love* (London: Pluto Press, 1992).

J. Benthall, *The Body Electric* (London: Thames and Hudson, 1976).

V. Berridge and P. Strong (eds), *AIDS and Contemporary History* (Cambridge: Cambridge University Press, 1993).

J. Bettley, 'Post *Voluptatem Misericordia:* The Rise and Fall of the London Lock Hospitals', *The London Journal*, x, 2 (1984), 167–75.

Cyril Bibby, *Sex Education: A Guide for Parents, Teachers and Youth Leaders* (London: Macmillan, 1946).

M. D. T. de Bienville, *Nymphomania, or, a Dissertation Concerning the Furor Uterinus* (London: J. Bew, 1775).

Lynda Birke, *Women, Feminism and Biology: The Feminist Challenge* (Brighton: Wheatsheaf Books, 1986).

Jeremy Black, *The English Press in the Eighteenth Century* (London: Croom Helm, 1986).

Janet Blackman, 'Popular Theories of Generation: The Evolution of *Aristotle's Works:* The Study of an Anachronism', in John Woodward and David Richards (eds), *Health Care and Popular Medicine in Nineteenth-Century England: Essays in the Social History of Medicine* (London: Croom Helm, 1977), 56–88.

Lucy Bland, 'Marriage Laid Bare: Middle-Class Women and Marital Sex c. 1880–1914', in Jane Lewis (ed.), *Labour and Love: Women's Experience of Home and Family, 1850–1940* (Oxford: Basil Blackwell, 1986), 122–46.

Iwan Bloch, *The Sexual Life of Our Time, in its Relations to Modern Civilisation*, trans. from the 6th German edn by M. Eden Paul (London: Rebman, 1909).

Iwan Bloch, *Sex Life in England Illustrated: As Revealed in its Obscene Literature and Art*, trans. Richard Deniston (New York: Falstaff, 1934).

Iwan Bloch, *A History of English Sexual Morals*, trans. William H. Forstern (London: Francis Aldor, 1936).

Iwan Bloch, *Sexual Life in England Past and Present*, trans. William H. Forstern (London: Arco, 1958).

R. Howard Bloch, *Medieval Misogyny and the Invention of Western Romantic Love* (Chicago: University of Chicago Press, 1991).

J. Blondel, *The Strength of Imagination in Pregnant Women Examin'd* (London: J. Peele, 1727).

D. Bloor, *Knowledge and Social Imagery* (London: Routledge and Kegan Paul, 1976).

Renate Blumenfeld-Kosinski, *Not of a Woman Born: Representations of Caesarean Birth in Medieval and Renaissance Culture* (Ithaca, NY: Cornell University Press, 1990).

James Blundell, *Observations on Some of the More Important Diseases of Women* (London: Cox, 1837).

John Boardman, *Eros in Greece* (London: John Murray, 1978).

Philip Boardman, *The Worlds of Patrick Geddes, Biologist, Town Planner, Re-educator, Peace-Warrior* (London and Boston: Routledge and Kegan Paul, 1978).

Alan Bold (ed.), *The Sexual Dimension in Literature* (London: Vision Press, 1982; Totowa, NJ: Barnes and Noble, 1983).

Meyrick Booth, *Youth and Sex: A Psychological Study* (London: Allen and Unwin, 1932).

Merriley Borrell, 'Organotherapy, British Physiology, and Discovery of the Internal Secretions', *Journal of the History of Biology*, ix (ii) (1976), 235–68.

Merriley Borell, 'Setting the Standards for a New Science: Edward Schäfer and Endocrinology', *Medical History*, xxii (1978), 282–90.

Merriley Borrell, 'Organotherapy and the Emergence of Reproductive Technology', *Journal of the History of Biology*, xviii (i) (1985), 1–30.

Merriley Borell, 'Biologists and the Promotion of Birth Control Research, 1918–1938', *Journal of the History of Biology*, xx (i) (1987), 51–88.

John Boswell, *Christianity, Social Tolerance, and Homosexuality: Gay People in Western Europe from the Beginning of the Christian Era to the Fourteenth Century* (Chicago: University of Chicago Press, 1980).

F. Bottomley, *Attitudes to the Body in Western Christendom* (London: Lepus Books, 1979).

P.-G. Boucé, 'Aspects of Sexual Tolerance and Intolerance in Eighteenth Century England', *British Journal for Eighteenth Century Studies*, iii (1980), 173–89.

P.-G. Boucé, 'Some Sexual Beliefs and Myths in Eighteenth Century Britain', in P.-G. Boucé (ed.), *Sexuality in Eighteenth Century Britain* (Manchester: Manchester University Press, 1982), 28–46.

P.-G. Boucé (ed.), *Sexuality in Eighteenth Century Britain* (Manchester: Manchester University Press, 1982).

P.-G. Boucé, '"The Secret Nexus": Sex and Literature in Eighteenth-Century Britain', in Alan Bold (ed.), *The Sexual Dimension in Literature* (Totowa, NJ: Barnes and Noble, 1983), 70–89.

P.-G. Boucé, 'Les Jeux interdits de l'imaginaire: onanisme et culpabilisations sexuelles en XVIIIe siècle', in J. Céard (ed.), *La Folie et le corps* (Paris: Presses de l'Ecole Normale Supérieure, 1985), 223–43.

Alain Boureau, *The Order of Books*, trans. Ludia M. Cochrane (Cambridge: Polity Press, 1993).

Alain Boureau and Roger Chartier (eds), *The Culture of Print: Power and the Uses of Print in Early Modern Europe* (Cambridge: Polity Press, 1989).

P. J. Bowler, 'Preformation and Pre-existence in the Seventeenth Century: A Brief Analysis', *Journal of the History of Biology*, iv (1971), 221–44.

Muriel Box (ed.), *The Trial of Dr Stopes* (London: Femina Books, 1967).

Muriel Box, *Rebel Advocate: A Biography of Gerald Gardiner* (London: Gollancz, 1983).

Thomas Boyle, *Black Swine in the Sewers of Hampstead: Beneath the Surface of Victorian Sensationalism* (New York: Viking, 1988; Harmondsworth: Penguin, 1989).

F. Brady, '*Tristram Shandy*, Sexuality, Morality, and Sensibility', *Eighteenth Century Studies*, iv (1970–1), 41–56.

P. Branca, *Women in Europe since 1750* (London: Croom Helm, 1978).

Ruth Brandon, *The New Women and the Old Men: Love, Sex and the Woman Question* (London: Secker and Warburg, 1990).

Leo Braudy, '*Fanny Hill* and Materialism', *Eighteenth Century Studies*, iv (1970–1), 21–40.

A. Bray, *Homosexuality in Renaissance England* (London: Gay Men's Press, 1982).

Edward M. Brecher, *The Sex Researchers* (London: André Deutsch, 1970).

John Brewer and Roy Porter (eds), *Consumption and the World of Goods* (London: Routledge, 1993).

Edward J. Bristow, *Vice and Vigilance: Purity Movements in Britain since 1700*

(Dublin: Gill and Macmillan, 1977).

William Brodum, *A Guide to Old Age or a Cure for the Indiscretions of Youth* (London: J. W. Myers, 1795).

Vincent Brome, *Havelock Ellis: Philosopher of Sex* (London and Boston: Routledge and Kegan Paul, 1979).

Barbara Brookes, *Abortion in England, 1900–1967* (London: Croom Helm, 1988).

Isaac Baker Brown, *On the Curability of Certain Forms of Insanity, Epilepsy, Catalepsy, and Hysteria in Females* (London: R. Hardwicke, 1866).

Peter Brown, *The Body and Society: Men, Women and Sexual Renunciation in Early Christianity* (New York: Columbia University Press, 1988).

F. W. Stella Browne, 'A New Psychological Society', *International Journal of Ethics*, xxviii (1917–18), 266–9.

F. W. Stella Browne, *The Sexual Variety and Variability among Women and their Bearing upon Social Reconstruction* (London: British Society for the Study of Sex Psychology, 1917).

Janet Browne, 'Botany for Gentlemen: Erasmus Darwin and *The Loves of the Plants*', *Isis*, lxxx (1989), 593–612.

Sir Thomas Browne, *Religio Medici*, in C. Sayle (ed.), *The Works of Sir Thomas Browne*, 3 vols (Edinburgh, 1912).

James A. Brundage, *Law, Sex and Christian Society in Medieval Europe* (Chicago: University of Chicago Press, 1988).

N. Bryson, *Word and Image* (Cambridge: Cambridge University Press, 1981).

W. Buchan, *Observations Concerning the Prevention and Cure of the Venereal Disease* (London: printed for T. Chapman, Fleet Street, and Mudie and Sons, Edinburgh, 1796).

V. Bullough, 'An Early American Sex Manual; or Aristotle Who?', *Early American Literature*, vii (1973), 236–46.

Vern L. Bullough and James Brundage, *Sexual Practices and the Medieval Church* (Buffalo, NY: Prometheus, 1982).

Martin Bulmer, 'The Development of Sociology and of Empirical Social Research in Britain', in Martin Bulmer (ed.), *Essays on the History of Sociological Research* (Cambridge: Cambridge University Press, 1985), 3–36.

Martin Bulmer, Kevin Bales and Kathryn Kish Sklar, 'The Social Survey in Historical Perspective 1880–1940', in Martin Bulmer, Kevin Bales and Kathryn Kish Sklar (eds), *The Social Survey in Historical Perspective 1880–1940* (Oxford: Oxford University Press, 1991), 1–48.

J. A. Burgess, 'Is a New Deal in the Control of Venereal Disease Necessary?' *British Journal of Venereal Diseases*, xx (1944), 19–30.

Peter Burke, 'Popular Culture in Seventeenth Century London', *London Journal*, iii (1977), 143–62.

Peter Burke, *Popular Culture in Early Modern Europe* (London: Temple Smith, 1978).

Peter Burke, 'Popular Culture between History and Ethnology', *Ethnologi Europaea*, xiv (1984), 5–13.

Peter Burke (ed.), *New Perspectives on Historical Writing* (Cambridge: Polity Press, 1991).

Peter Burke and Roy Porter (eds), *Language, Self and Society: The Social History of Language* (Cambridge: Polity Press, 1991).

Robert Burton, *The Anatomy of Melancholy*, Vol. I: *Text – 'Democritus Junior to the Reader' and 'The First Partition'*, ed. Thomas C. Faulkner *et al.* (Oxford: Oxford University Press, 1989).

Judith Butler, *Bodies that Matter: on the Discursive Limits of 'Sex'* (London: Routledge, 1993).

Caroline Walker Bynum, *Fragmentation and Redemption: Essays on Gender and the Human Body in Medieval Religion* (New York: Zone Books, 1991).

W. F. Bynum, 'Treating the Wages of Sin: Venereal Disease and Specialism in Eighteenth-Century Britain', in W. F. Bynum and R. Porter (eds), *Medical Fringe and Medical Orthodoxy, 1750–1850* (London: Croom Helm, 1987), 5–28.

Joan Cadden, *Meanings of Sex Difference in the Middle Ages: Medicine, Science and Culture* (Cambridge and New York: Cambridge University Press, 1993).

Angus Calder, 'Mass Observation 1937–1949', in Martin Bulmer (ed.), *Essays on the History of Sociological Research* (Cambridge: Cambridge University Press, 1985), 121–36.

Angus Calder and Dorothy Sheridan (eds), *Speak for Yourself: A Mass Observation Anthology 1937–1949* (Oxford: Oxford University Press, 1985).

D. J. Campbell, 'Venereal Diseases in the Armed Forces Overseas (2)', *British Journal of Venereal Diseases*, xxii (1946), 158–68.

Eva Cantarella, *Bisexuality in the Ancient World*, trans. Cormac Ó'Cuilleanáin (New Haven and London: Yale University Press, 1992).

G. N. Cantor and M. J. S. Hodge (eds), *Conceptions of Ether* (Cambridge: Cambridge University Press, 1982).

Edward Carpenter, *Love's Coming of Age. A Series of Papers on the Relation of the Sexes* (London: Allen and Unwin, 1896; 13th edn 1930).

Edward Carpenter, *Ioaus: An Anthology of Friendship* (London: Swann Sonnenschein, 1902).

Edward Carpenter, *The Intermediate Sex* (London: Swan Sonnenschein, 1908).

Edward Carpenter, *Intermediate Types among Primitive Folk* (London: G. Allen and Co., 1914).

W. Metcalfe Chambers, 'Prostitution and Venereal Diseases', *British Journal of Venereal Diseases*, ii (v) (1926), 68–75.

Francis Champneys, Sir, 'The Fight against Venereal Infection: A Reply to Sir Bryan Donkin', *The Nineteenth Century*, lxxxii (1917), 1044–54.

Francis Champneys, Sir, 'The Fight against Venereal Infection: A Further Reply to Sir Bryan Donkin', *The Nineteenth Century*, lxxxiii (1918), 611–18.

S. Chandrasekhar, *'A Dirty Filthy Book': The Writings of Charles Bradlaugh and Annie Besant on Reproductive Physiology and Birth Control, and an Account of the Bradlaugh–Besant Trial* (Berkeley, Calif.: University of California Press, 1981).

Enid Charles, *The Practice of Birth Control: An Analysis of the Birth-Control Experiences of Nine Hundred Women* (London: Williams and Norgate, 1932).

Roger Chartier, *Cultural History. Between Practices and Representations* (Ithaca, NY: Cornell University Press; Cambridge: Polity Press, 1988).

H. J. Chaytor, *From Script to Print* (Cambridge: Cambridge University Press, 1945).

Eustace Chesser, *Love without Fear: A Plain Guide to Sex Technique for Every Married Adult* (London: Rich and Cowan Medical Publications, 1941; revised 2nd edn July 1942).

Eustace Chesser, *Sexual Behaviour: Normal and Abnormal* (London: London Medical Publications, 1949).

Eustace Chesser, *Grow Up – and Live* (Harmondsworth: Penguin, 1949).

Eustace Chesser, Joan Maizels, Leonard Jones and Brian Emmett, *The Sexual, Marital and Family Relationships of the English Woman* (London: Hutchinson's Medical Publications, 1956).

Fenella Childs, 'Prescriptions for Manners in Eighteenth Century Courtesy Literature' (D.Phil. dissertation, Oxford University, 1984)

Johann L. Choulant, *History and Bibliography of Anatomic Illustration in its Relation to Anatomic Science and the Graphic Arts*, trans. Mortimer Frank (Chicago: University of Chicago Press, 1920; revised edn New York: Schuman's, 1945).

John Christie, 'Feminism in the History of Science', in R. Olby, G. Cantor, J. R. R. Christie and M. J. Hodge (eds), *Companion to the History of Modern Science* (London: Routledge, 1990), 100–9.

John Cleland, *Memoirs of a Woman of Pleasure* (London, 1749; edn quoted, Mayflower Books, London, 1977).

K. B. Clinton, 'Femme et Philosophe: Enlightenment Origins of Feminism', *Eighteenth Century Studies*, viii (1975), 283–300.

Claud Cockburn, *Bestseller: The Books that Everyone Read, 1900–1939* (London: Sidgwick and Jackson, 1972).

T. Coffin, *The Proper Book of Sexual Folklore* (New York: Seabury Press, 1978).

I. Bernard Cohen, *Revolution in Science* (Cambridge, Mass.: Belknap Press of Harvard University Press, 1985).

Patricia Cline Cohen, *A Calculating People: The Spread of Numeracy in Early America* (Chicago: University of Chicago Press, 1982).

Patricia Cline Cohen, 'Reckoning with Commerce: Numeracy in Eighteenth-Century America', in John Brewer and Roy Porter (eds), *Consumption and the World of Goods* (London and New York: Routledge, 1993), 320–34.

A. J. Cokkinis, *The Reproduction of Life: a Handbook of the Science of Reproduction in Nature and Man* (London: Baillière, 1926).

F. J. Cole, *Early Theories of Sexual Generation* (Oxford: Clarendon Press, 1930).

D. C. Coleman and R. S. Schofield, *The State of Population Theory: Forward from Malthus* (Oxford: Basil Blackwell, 1986).

W. Coleman, 'Health and Hygiene in the *Encyclopédie*: A Medical Doctrine for the Bourgeoisie', *Journal of the History of Medicine and Allied Sciences*, xxix (1974), 399–421.

R. Colie, *Paradoxia Epidemica* (Princeton, NJ: Princeton University Press, 1966).

Harry Collins, *Changing Order: Replication and Induction in Scientific Practice* (Beverly Hills and London: Sage Publications, 1985).

H. M. Collins and T. J. Pinch, *Frames of Meaning: The Social Construction of Extraordinary Science* (London: Routledge and Kegan Paul, 1982).

Alex Comfort, 'Sex Education in the Medical Curriculum', *International Journal of Sexology*, iii (1950), 175–7.

Alex Comfort, *The Anxiety Makers: Some Curious Preoccupations of the Medical Profession* (London: Nelson, 1967).

Alex Comfort, ed., *The Joy of Sex: A Gourmet Guide to Lovemaking* (London: Modsets Securities Ltd, 1972; Quartet Books, 1974).

Peter T. Cominos, 'Late Victorian Respectability and the Social System', *International Review of Social History*, viii (1963), 18–48 and 216–50.

H. F. B. Compston, *The Magdalen Hospital* (London: SPCK, 1917).

Edward le Comte, *Milton and Sex* (London: Macmillan, 1978).

Brian A. Connery, 'Self-Representation, Authority, and the Fear of Madness in the Works of Swift', *Studies in Eighteenth-Century Culture*, xx (1990), 165–82.

Harold J. Cook, 'Sir John Colbatch and Augustan Medicine: Experimentalism, Character and Entrepreneurialism', *Annals of Science*, xlvii (1991), 495–6.

Harold J. Cook, 'Good Advice and Little Medicine: The Professional Authority of Early Modern English Physicians', *Journal of British Studies*, xxxiii (1994), 1–31.

Arthur Cooper, *The Sexual Disabilities of Man and Their Treatment* (London: H. K. Lewis, 1908; 2nd edn 1910; 3rd edn 1916).

James Copland, *A Dictionary of Practical Medicine: Comprising General Pathology, the Nature and Treatment of Diseases, Morbid Structures and the Disorders Especially Incident to Climates, to the Sex, and to the Different Epochs of Life*, 4 vols (London: Longmans, 1844–58).

George W. Corner, 'The Early History of the Oestrogenic Hormones', *Journal of Endocrinology*, xxxi (1965), iii–xvii.

A. Costler, A. Willy and Norman Haire, *Encyclopaedia of Sexual Knowledge* (London: Encyclopaedic Press, 1934; 2nd edn 1952).

Nancy F. Cott, 'Passionlessness: An Interpretation of Victorian Sexual Ideology, 1790–1850', *Signs: Journal of Women in Culture and Society*, iv (1978), 219–36.

I. Couliano, *Eros and Magic in the Renaissance*, trans. Margaret Cook (Chicago and London: University of Chicago Press, 1987).

Sheila Cousins [pseud.], *To Beg I Am Ashamed: The Autobiography of a London Prostitute* (Paris: Obelisk Press, 1938).

P. Coveney, *Poor Monkey: The Child in Literature* (London: Rockliff, 1957).

D. A. Coward, 'Eighteenth-Century Attitudes to Prostitution', *Studies on Voltaire and the Eighteenth Century*, clxxxix (1980), 363–99.

Alec Craig, *Above All Liberties* (London: Allen and Unwin, 1942).

Alec Craig, 'Recent Developments in the Law of Obscene Libel', in A. Pillay and Albert Ellis (eds), *Sex, Society and the Individual: Selected Papers, Revised and Brought up to Date, from 'Marriage Hygiene' (1934–1937) and 'International Journal of Sexology' (1947–1952)* (Bombay: International Journal of Sexology, 1953), 302–27.

Patricia Crawford, 'Attitudes to Pregnancy from a Woman's Spiritual Diary, 1687–88', *Local Population Studies*, xxi (1978), 43–5.

Patricia Crawford, 'Attitudes to Menstruation in Seventeenth Century England', *Past and Present*, xci (1981), 47–73.

Patricia Crawford, 'Sexual Knowledge in England, 1500–1750', in Roy Porter and Mikuláš Teich (eds), *Sexual Knowledge, Sexual Science: The History of Attitudes to Sexuality* (Cambridge: Cambridge University Press, 1994), 82–106.

David Cressy, *Literacy and the Social Order: Reading and Writing in Tudor and Stuart England* (Cambridge: Cambridge University Press, 1980).

David Cressy, 'Literacy in Context: Meaning and Measurement in Early Modern England', in John Brewer and Roy Porter (eds), *Consumption and the World of Goods* (London and New York: Routledge, 1993), 305–19.

L. Crocker, *An Age of Crisis: Man and World in Eighteenth Century French Thought* (Baltimore, Md.: Johns Hopkins University Press, 1959).

Louis Crompton, *Byron and Greek Love: Homophobia in Nineteenth Century England*

(Berkeley: University of California Press, 1985).

Helkiah Crooke, *Microcosmographia* (London: W. Jaggard, 1615).

F. D. Crozier, *A Brass Hat in No-Man's Land: A Personal Record of the European War* (London: Jonathan Cape, 1930).

J. Culler, *On Deconstruction* (London: Routledge and Kegan Paul, 1983).

J. Culler, *Framing the Sign: Criticism and Its Institutions* (Norman: University of Oklahoma Press, 1988).

H. Cunningham, *Leisure in the Industrial Revolution* (London: Croom Helm, 1980).

L. A. Curtis, 'A Case Study of Defoe's Domestic Conduct Manuals Suggested by *The Family, Sex and Marriage in England 1500–1800*', *Studies in Eighteenth Century Culture*, x (1981), 409–28.

Ann Dally, *Women under the Knife: A History of Surgery* (London: Hutchinson Radius, 1991).

Sir Weldon Dalrymple-Champneys, 'The Epidemiological Control of Venereal Disease', *British Journal of Venereal Diseases*, xxiii (1947), 101–8.

Mary Daly, *Gyn/ecology* (Boston, Mass.: Beacon Press, 1978).

P. Darmon, *Le Mythe de la procréation à l'âge baroque* (Paris: J. J. Pauvert, 1977).

P. Darmon, *Le Tribunal de l'impuissance: virilité et défaillances conjugales dans l'ancienne France* (Paris: Editions du Seuil, 1979).

R. Darnton, 'The High Enlightenment and the Low-Life of Literature in Pre-revolutionary France', *Past and Present*, li (1971), 81–115; reprinted in his *The Literary Underground of the Old Regime* (Cambridge, Mass.: Harvard University Press, 1982), 1–40.

R. Darnton, *The Literary Underground of the Old Regime* (Cambridge, Mass.: Harvard University Press, 1982).

R. Darnton, *The Great Cat Massacre and other Episodes in French Cultural History* (New York: Basic Books, 1984; Harmondsworth: Penguin, 1985).

R. Darnton and Daniel Roche (eds), *Revolution in Print: The Press in France 1775–1800* (Berkeley: University of California Press, 1989).

Robert Darnton, *The Business of Enlightenment* (Cambridge, Mass., 1979).

Erasmus Darwin, *The Botanic Garden* (London: J. Johnson, 1791).

Erasmus Darwin, *Zoonomia*, 2 vols (London: J. Johnson, 1794–6).

Erasmus Darwin, *Phytologia* (London: J. Johnson, 1800).

Erasmus Darwin, *The Temple of Nature* (London: J. Johnson, 1803).

Richard Davenport-Hines, *Sex, Death, and Punishment: Attitudes to Sex and Sexuality in Britain since the Renaissance* (London: Collins, 1990).

Claire Davey, 'Birth Control in Britain during the Inter-War Years: Evidence from the Stopes Correspondence', *Journal of Family History*, xiii (iii) (1988), 329–45.

Leonore Davidoff, 'The Family in Britain', in F. M. L. Thompson (ed.), *The Cambridge Social History of England 1750–1950*, Vol. II (Cambridge: Cambridge University Press, 1990), 76–109.

Leonore Davidoff and Catherine Hall, *Family Fortunes: Men and Women of the English Middle Class, 1780–1850* (London: Hutchinson, 1987; London: Routledge, 1987).

Arnold Davidson, 'Sex and the Emergence of Sexuality', *Critical Inquiry*, xiv (1987), 16–48.

Margaret Llewelyn Davies (ed.), *Maternity: Letters from Working Women Collected by the Women's Co-operative Guild* (London: G. Bell and Sons, 1915; London: Virago, 1978).

Margaret Llewelyn Davies (ed.), *Life as We Have Known It, by Co-operative Working Women* (London: Hogarth Press, 1931; London: Virago, 1977).

Katherine B. Davis, *Factors in the Sex Life of Twenty-two Hundred Women* (New York: Harper and Bros, 1929).

N. Davis, *Society and Culture in Early Modern France* (London: Duckworth, 1975).

Lee Davison, Tim Hitchcock, Tim Keirn and Robert B. Shoemaker (eds), *Stilling the Grumbling Hive: The Response to Social and Economic Problems in England, 1689–1750* (Stroud: Alan Sutton; New York: St Martin's Press, 1992).

R. Dawson, *An Essay on Marriage, Being a Microscopic Investigation into its Physiological and Physical Relations, with Observations on the Nature, Causes and Treatment of Spermatorrhoea* (London: Hughes, 1845).

Allen G. Debus, 'Scientific Truth and Occult Tradition: The Medical World of Ebenezer Sibly (1751–1799)', *Medical History*, xxvi (1982), 259–78.

S. Delamont and L. Duffin (eds), *The Nineteenth Century Woman. Her Cultural and Physical World* (London: Croom Helm, 1978).

Paul Delany, *The Neo-Pagans: Friendship and Love in the Rupert Brooke Circle* (London: Macmillan, 1987).

M. Delon, 'Le Prétexte anatomique', *Dix-Huitième Siècle*, xii (1980), 35–48.

Jean Delumeau, *Sin and Fear. The Emergence of a Western Guilt Culture, 13th–18th Centuries* (New York: St Martin's Press, 1990).

L. DeMause, 'The Evolution of Childhood', in L. DeMause (ed.), *The History of Childhood* (New York: Psychohistory Press, 1974), 1–73.

I. Diamond and L. Quinby (eds), *Feminism and Foucault: Reflections on Resistance* (Boston, Mass.: Northeastern University Press, 1988).

Robert L. Dickinson and Lura Beam, *A Thousand Marriages* (Baltimore, Md.: Williams and Wilkins, 1932).

B. Dijkstra, *Idols of Perversity: Fantasies of Feminine Evil in Fin-de-Siècle Culture* (Oxford and New York: Oxford University Press, 1986).

Francis Doherty, *A Study in Eighteenth-Century Advertising Methods: The Anodyne Necklace* (Lewiston/Queenston/Lampeter: Edwin Mellen Press, 1992).

Jonathan Dollimore, *Sexual Dissidence: Augustine to Wilde, Freud to Foucault* (Oxford: Clarendon Press, 1991).

Bryan Donkin, 'The Fight against Venereal Infection', *The Nineteenth Century*, lxxxii (1917), 580–95.

Bryan Donkin, 'The Fight against Venereal Infection: A Rejoinder', *The Nineteenth Century*, lxxxiii (1918), 184–90.

Jean Donnison, *Midwives and Medical Men: A History of Inter-Professional Rivalries and Women's Rights* (London: Heinemann Educational, 1977).

Emma Donoghue, *Passions between Women: British Lesbian Culture 1668–1801* (London: Scarlet Press, 1993).

Mary Douglas, *Purity and Danger* (London: Routledge and Kegan Paul, 1966).

Mary Douglas, *Implicit Meanings* (London: Routledge and Kegan Paul, 1975).

Kenneth J. Dover, *Greek Homosexuality* (Cambridge, Mass.: Harvard University Press, 1978; updated with a new postcript 1989).

George Drysdale, *Elements of Social Science: or Physical, Sexual, and Natural Religion, an Exposition of the True Cause and Only Cure of the Three Primary Social*

Evils: Poverty, Prostitution, and Celibacy, by a Doctor of Medicine (London: [anonymously], E. Truelove, 1854; London: G. Standring, 1905).

F. Duchesneau, *La Physiologie des lumières* (The Hague: M. M. Nijhoff, 1982).

Barbara Duden, *The Woman beneath the Skin: A Doctor's Patients in Eighteenth-Century Germany*, trans. Thomas Dunlap (Cambridge, Mass. and London: Harvard University Press, 1991).

Andrea Dworkin, *Intercourse* (London: Secker and Warburg, 1987).

Carol Dyhouse, *Feminism and the Family in England 1880–1939* (Oxford: Basil Blackwell, 1989).

William Eamon, *Science and the Secrets of Nature. Books of Secrets in Medieval and Early Modern Culture* (Princeton: Princeton University Press, 1994).

Peter Earle, *The Making of the English Middle Class: Business, Society and Family Life in London, 1660–1730* (London: Methuen, 1989).

Brian Easlea, *Science and Sexual Oppression: Patriarchy's Confrontation with Women and Nature* (London: Weidenfeld and Nicolson, 1981).

Peter Eaton and Marilyn Warnick, *Marie Stopes: A Checklist of Her Writings* (London: Croom Helm, 1977).

Audrey Eccles, *Obstetrics and Gynaecology in Tudor and Stuart England* (London: Croom Helm, 1982).

Barbara Ehrenreich and Deirdre English, *Complaints and Disorders* (Old Westbury, NY: Feminist Press, 1973; London: Compendium, 1974).

Barbara Ehrenreich and Deirdre English, *Witches, Midwives and Nurses: A History of Women Healers*, 2nd edn (Old Westbury, NY: Feminist Press, 1973).

Barbara Ehrenreich, Elizabeth Hess and Gloria Jacobs, *Remaking Love: The Feminization of Sex* (Garden City, NY: Anchor Press/Doubleday, 1986; London: Fontana, 1987).

Elizabeth Eisenstein, 'On Revolution and the Printed Word', in Roy Porter and Mikuláš Teich (eds), *Revolution in History* (Cambridge: Cambridge University Press, 1986), 186–205.

R. Elbourne, *Music and Tradition in Early Industrial Lancashire* (Woodbridge: Brewer for the Folklore Society, 1980).

Ethel M. Elderton, *Report on the English Birthrate. Part I. England, North of Humber*, Eugenics Laboratory Memoirs, nos 19 and 20 (London: University of London, 1914).

Havelock Ellis, *Man and Woman: A Study of Human Secondary Sexual Characters*, Contemporary Science Series (London: Walter Scott, 1894).

Havelock Ellis, *The Evolution of Modesty: The Phenomena of Sexual Periodicity: Auto-Erotism, Studies in the Psychology of Sex Volume I* (Leipzig and Watford, 1899; Philadelphia: F. A. Davis, 1901; 3rd edn 1910; New York: omnibus edn, Vol. I, Random House, 1937).

Havelock Ellis [and J. Addington Symonds], *Sexual Inversion, Studies in the Psychology of Sex Volume II* (Leipzig and Watford, 1897; Philadelphia: F. A. Davis, 1901; 3rd edn 1915; New York: omnibus edn, Vol. I, Random House, 1937).

Havelock Ellis, *The Analysis of the Sexual Impulse: Love and Pain: The Sexual Impulse in Women. Studies in the Psychology of Sex Volume III* (Philadelphia: F. A. Davis, 1903: omnibus edn, New York: Random House, 1937).

Havelock Ellis, *Sexual Selection in Man, Studies in the Psychology of Sex Volume IV* (Philadelphia: F. A. Davis, 1905; omnibus edn, vol. I, New York: Random House, 1937).

Havelock Ellis, *Erotic Symbolism: The Mechanism of Detumescence: The Psychic State in Pregnancy, Studies in the Psychology of Sex Volume V* (Philadelphia: F. A. Davis, 1906).

Havelock Ellis, *Sex in Relation to Society, Studies in the Psychology of Sex Volume VI* (Philadelphia: F. A. Davis, 1910; London: Heinemann Medical Books, 1937; War Economy edn, 1946).

Havelock Ellis, *Eonism and Other Supplementary Studies, Studies in the Psychology of Sex Volume VII* (Philadelphia: F. A. Davis, 1928).

Havelock Ellis, *Essays in War-Time: First Series* (London: Constable, 1916).

Havelock Ellis, *The Erotic Rights of Women and The Objects of Marriage* (London: British Society for the Study of Sex Psychology, 1918).

Havelock Ellis, *The Philosophy of Conflict, and Other Essays in War-Time: Second Series* (London: Constable, 1919).

Havelock Ellis, *The Play-Function of Sex* (London: British Society for the Study of Sex Psychology, 1921).

Havelock Ellis, *Little Essays of Love and Virtue* (London: A. and C. Black, 1922).

Havelock Ellis, *More Essays of Love and Virtue* (London: Constable, 1931).

Havelock Ellis, *Psychology of Sex. The Biology of Sex – The Sexual Impulse in Youth – Sexual Deviation – The Erotic Symbolisms – Homosexuality – Marriage – The Art of Love* (London: Heinemann, 1933; 12th impression 1948).

Antoinette Emch-Dériaz, *Tissot: Physician of the Enlightenment* (New York: Peter Lang, 1992).

H. Tristram Engelhardt Jr, 'The Disease of Masturbation: Values and the Concept of Disease', *Bulletin of the History of Medicine*, xlviii (1974), 234–48.

Leonard England, 'A British Sex Survey', in A. Pillay and Albert Ellis (eds), *Sex Society and the Individual: Selected Papers, Revised and Brought up to Date, from 'Marriage Hygiene' (1934–1937) and 'International Journal of Sexology' (1947–1952)* (Bombay: International Journal of Sexology, 1953), 360–7.

Laura Engelstein, *The Key to Happiness: Sex and the Search for Modernity in Fin de Siècle Russia* (Ithaca, NY: Cornell University Press, 1992).

W. H. Epstein, *John Cleland, Images of a Life* (New York: Columbia University Press, 1974).

Nina C. Epton, *Love and the English* (Cleveland, NY: World Publishing; London: Cassell, 1960).

Robert A. Erickson, 'The Books of Generation: Some Observations on the Style of the English Midwife Books, 1671–1764', in P.-G. Boucé (ed.), *Sexuality in Eighteenth Century Britain* (Manchester and Totowa, NJ: Manchester University Press, 1982), 74–95.

'Ellis Ethelmer' [Mrs Wolstenholme Elmy], *Woman Free* (Congleton: Woman's Emancipation Union, 1893).

'Ellis Ethelmer' [Mrs Wolstenholme Elmy], *The Human Flower* (Congleton: Mrs Wolstenholme Elmy, 1894).

'Ellis Ethelmer' [Mrs Wolstenholme Elmy], *Baby Buds* (Congleton: Mrs Wolstenholme Elmy, 1895).

Barbara Evans, *Freedom to Choose: The Life and Work of Dr Helena Wright, Pioneer of Contraception* (London: Bodley Head, 1984).

M[argaret] Leonora Eyles, *The Woman in the Little House* (London: Grant Richards, 1922).

M[argaret] Leonora Eyles, *Commonsense about Sex* (London: Gollancz, 1933).

Lillian Fadermann, *Surpassing the Love of Men: Romantic Friendship and Love between Women form the Renaissance to the Present* (New York: Morrow, 1981; London: Junction Books, 1982).

Lillian Fadermann, *Scotch Verdict: Dame Gordon vs. Pirie and Woods* (New York: Morrow, 1983).

C. Fairchilds, 'Female Sexual Attitudes and the Rise of Illegitimacy: a Case Study', *Journal of Interdisciplinary History*, viii (1978), 627–67.

J. Feather, 'The Commerce of Letters: The Study of the Eighteenth Century Book Trade', *Eighteenth Century Studies*, xvii (1984), 405–24.

Feminist Review, *Sexuality: A Reader* (London: Virago, 1987).

Marjorie Ferguson, *Forever Feminine: Women's Magazines and the Cult of Femininity* (London: Heinemann, 1983).

Jacques Ferrand, *A Treatise on Lovesickness*, trans. and ed. Donald A. Beecher and Massimo Ciavolella (Syracuse, NY: Syracuse University Press, 1990).

Paul Ferris, *Sex and the British: A Twentieth Century History* (London: Michael Joseph, 1993).

A. Fessler, 'Advertisements on the Treatment of Venereal Disease and the Social History of Venereal Disease', *British Journal of Venereal Diseases*, xxv (1949), 84–7.

A. Fessler, 'Venereal Disease and Prostitution in the Reports of the Poor Law Commissioners, 1834–1850', *British Journal of Venereal Diseases*, xxvii (1951), 154–7.

A. Fessler and R. S. France, 'Syphilis in Seventeenth-Century Lancashire', *British Journal of Venereal Disease*, ii (1945), 177–8.

L. Fiedler, *Freaks* (New York: Simon and Schuster, 1978).

Henry Fielding, *An Enquiry into the Causes of the Late Increase in Robberies* (London: A. Miller, 1751).

Karl M. Figlio, 'Chlorosis and Chronic Disease in Nineteenth-Century Britain: The Social Constitution of Somatic Illness in a Capitalist Society', *Social History*, iii (1978), 167–97.

Frances Finnegan, *Poverty and Prostitution: A Study of Victorian Prostitutes in York* (Cambridge and New York: Cambridge University Press, 1979).

Ruth First and Anne Scott, *Olive Schreiner* (London: André Deutsch, 1980).

Mary E. Fissell, 'Readers, Texts and Contexts: Vernacular Medical Works in Early Modern England', in Roy Porter (ed.), *The Popularization of Medicine, 1650–1850* (London and New York: Routledge, 1992), 72–96.

Jean-Louis Flandrin, *Le Sexe et l'Occident* (Paris: Seuil, 1981).

Jean Flouret, *Nicolas Venette: Médecin Rochelais 1633–1698* (La Rochelle: Éditions Rupella, 1992).

Brown K. Ford, *Fathers of the Victorians: The Age of Wilberforce* (Cambridge: Cambridge University Press, 1961).

Michel Foucault, *Histoire de la sexualité*, Vol. I: *La Volonté de savoir* (Paris: Gallimard, 1976); trans. Robert Hurley, *The History of Sexuality: An Introduction* (London: Allen Lane, 1978; New York: Vintage Books, 1985).

Michel Foucault, *Histoire de la sexualité*, Vol. II: *L'usage des plaisirs* (Paris: Gallimard, 1984); trans. Robert Hurley, *The Use of Pleasure* (New York: Random House, 1985; London: Viking, 1986; Harmondsworth: Penguin, 1987).

Michel Foucault, *Histoire de la sexualité*, Vol. III: *Le Souci de soi* (Paris: Gallimard, 1984); trans. Robert Hurley, *The Care of the Self* (New York: Pantheon Books,

1986; Random House, 1987).

John C. Fout (ed.), *Forbidden History: The State, Society, and the Regulation of Sexuality in Modern Europe* (Chicago: University of Chicago Press, 1992).

John C. Fout, 'Sexual Politics in Wilhelmine Germany: The Male Gender Crisis, Moral Purity, and Homophobia', in John C. Fout (ed.), *Forbidden History: The State, Society, and the Regulation of Sexuality in Modern Europe* (Chicago: University of Chicago Press, 1992).

Bridget Fowler, 'True to Me Always: An Analysis of Women's Magazine Fiction', in Christopher Pawling (ed.), *Popular Fiction and Social Change* (London: Macmillan, 1984), 99–126.

O. S. Fowler, *Creative and Sexual Science; or, Manhood, Womanhood and Their Mutual Interrelations; Love, its Laws, Power, etc.; Selection, or Mutual Adaptation; Courtship, Married Life and Perfect Children; Their Generation, Endowment, Paternity, Maternity, Bearing, Nursing and Rearing; together with Puberty, Boyhood, Girlhood, etc., Sexual Impairments Restored, Male Vigour and Female Health and Beauty Perpetuated and Augmented, etc., as Taught by Phrenology and Physiology* (New York: O. S. Fowler, 1870; 2nd edn *c.* 1900).

David Foxon, *Libertine Literature in England 1660–1745: With an Appendix on the Publication of John Cleland's 'Memoirs of a Woman of Pleasure', Commonly Known as 'Fanny Hill'* (New York: University Books, 1965).

A. D. Frazer, 'The Problem of the Defaulter', *British Journal of Venereal Diseases*, viii (1932), 56–8.

Sigmund Freud, 'Fragment of the Analysis of a Case of Hysteria', in *The Standard Edition of the Complete Psychological Works of Sigmund Freud*, trans. and ed. James Strachey *et al.* (London: Hogarth Press and the Institute of Psycho-Analysis, 1953–74), Vol. VII, 1–122.

T. R. Frosch, *The Awakening of Albion: The Renovation of the Body in the Poetry of William Blake* (Ithaca, NY: Cornell University Press, 1974).

Peter Fryer, *The Birth Controllers* (London: Secker and Warburg, 1965).

Peter Fryer, *Forbidden Books of the Victorians: Henry Spencer Ashbee's Bibliographies of Erotica Abridged and Edited, with an Introduction and Notes* (London: Odyssey Press, 1970).

Catherine Gallagher, 'The Body versus the Social Body in the Works of Thomas Malthus and Henry Mayhew', in Catherine Gallagher and Thomas Laqueur (eds), *The Making of the Modern Body: Sexuality and Society in the Nineteenth Century* (Berkeley and Los Angeles: University of California Press, 1987), 83–106.

Walter Gallichan, *The Poison of Prudery: An Historical Survey* (London: T. Werner Laurie, 1929).

A. K. Gardner, *The Conjugal Relationship as Regards Personal Health and Hereditary Well-Being Practically Treated* (New York: G. J. Moulton, 1892; Glasgow: T. D. Morison, 1892; London: Simpkin, Marshall, Hamilton and Kent, 1894).

Elizabeth Gasking, *Investigations into Generation, 1651–1828* (London: Hutchinson, 1967).

Peter Gay, *The Enlightenment: An Interpretation*, Vol. I: *Rise of Modern Paganism* (London: Weidenfeld & Nicolson, 1967); Vol. II: *The Science of Freedom* (London: Weidenfeld & Nicolson, 1969).

Peter Gay, *The Party of Humanity: Essays in the French Enlightenment* (New York: Norton, 1971).

Peter Gay, 'Victorian Sexuality: Old Texts and New Insights', *American Scholar*, xlix (1980), 372–7.

Peter Gay, *The Bourgeois Experience – Victoria to Freud*, Vol. I: *Education of the Senses* (London and New York: Oxford University Press, 1983).

Peter Gay, *The Bourgeois Experience – Victoria to Freud*, Vol. II: *The Tender Passion* (London and New York: Oxford University Press, 1986).

Patrick Geddes and J. Arthur Thomson, *The Evolution of Sex*, Contemporary Science Series, ed. Havelock Ellis (London: Walter Scott, 1889; 2nd edn 1901).

Patrick Geddes and J. Arthur Thomson, *Sex*, Home University Library (London: Williams and Norgate, 1914).

T. Gelfand, *Professionalizing Modern Medicine* (Westport, Conn.: Greenwood Press, 1980).

Kent Gerard and Gert Hekma (eds), *The Pursuit of Sodomy: Male Homosexuality in Renaissance and Enlightenment Europe* (New York: Harrington Park, 1989).

T. Gibson, *The English Vice: Beating, Sex and Shame in Victorian England and After* (London: Duckworth, 1978).

Anthony Giddens, *The Transformation of Intimacy: Sexuality, Love and Eroticism in Modern Societies* (Cambridge: Polity Press, 1992).

A. N. Gilbert, 'Sexual Deviance and Disaster during the Napoleonic Wars', *Albion*, ix (1977), 98–113.

S. Gilbert and S. Gubar, *The Madwoman in the Attic: The Woman Writer and the Nineteenth-Century Imagination* (New Haven and London: Yale University Press, 1979).

John R. Gillis, *For Better, For Worse: British Marriages, 1600 to the Present* (New York and Oxford: Oxford University Press, 1985).

John R. Gillis, 'Married but Not Churched: Plebeian Sexual Relations and Marital Nonconformity in Eighteenth-Century Britain', in R. P. Maccubbin (ed.), *Unauthorized Sexual Behaviour during the Enlightenment* (Williamsburg, Va.: College of William and Mary, 1985), 31–42.

Sander Gilman, *Sexuality: An Illustrated History* (New York: Wiley, 1989).

Diana Gittins, *Fair Sex: Family Size and Structure 1900–1939* (London: Hutchinson, 1982).

Victoria Glendinning, *Vita* (Harmondsworth: Penguin, 1985).

Victoria Glendinning, *Rebecca West: A Life* (London: Weidenfeld and Nicolson, 1987).

W. Godwin, *Enquiry concerning Political Justice*, ed. I. Kramnick (Harmondsworth: Penguin, 1978).

John M. Golby and A. W. Purdue, *The Civilization of the Crowd: Popular Culture in England, 1750–1900* (London: Batsford Academic and Educational, 1984).

Jonathan Goldberg, *Sodometries: Renaissance Texts, Modern Sexualities* (Stanford, Calif.: Stanford University Press, 1992).

Rita Goldberg, *Sex and Enlightenment. Women in Richardson and Diderot* (Cambridge: Cambridge University Press, 1984).

J. E. Gordon, 'The Control of Venereal Disease: An Epidemiological Approach', *The Lancet*, ii (1944), 711–15.

Michael Gordon, 'From an Unfortunate Necessity to a Cult of Mutual Orgasm: Sex in American Marital Education Literature 1830–1940', in J. Henslin (ed.), *Studies in the Sociology of Sex* (New York: Appleton-Century Crofts,

1975), 53–77.

D. Gorham, *The Victorian Girl and the Feminine Ideal* (London: Croom Helm, 1982).

S. Gould, *A Brief Treatise on Venereal Disease and Spermatorrhoea, its Cause and Cure (For Private Circulation Only. Entered at Stationers' Hall.) Manhood, How Lost, by Acquired Diseases; How Regained, by Vegetable Compounds* (Bradford? *c.* 1910).

Jean-Marie Goulemot, *Reading the Erotic: The Uses of Pornographic Literature in Eighteenth-Century France* (Cambridge: Polity Press, 1994).

James Graham, *Lecture on the Generation, Increase and Improvement of the Human Species* (London: M. Smith, 1780).

James Graham, *A New and Curious Treatise of the Nature and Effects of Simple Earth, Water and Air* (London and Bath: Cruttwell, 1780).

James Graham, *A Sketch, or Short Description of Dr Graham's Medical Apparatus* (London: Almon, 1780).

James Graham, *A Discourse Delivered August 17, 1783 in Edinburgh* (Hull: Briggs, 1787).

James Graham, *Proposals for the Establishment of a New and True Christian Church* (Bath: Cruttwell, 1788).

James Graham, *The General State of Medical and Chirurgical Practice Exhibited* (London, Almon, 1779).

James Graham, *A Short Treatise on the All-Cleansing Earth* (Newcastle: Hall, 1790).

Thomas J. Graham, *The Diseases Peculiar to Females* (London: Simkin and Marshall, 1834).

Linda Grant, *Sexing the Millennium: A Political History of the Sexual Revolution* (London: Harper Collins, 1993).

Robert Graves and Alan Hodge, *The Long Weekend: A Social History of Great Britain 1918–1939* (London: Faber and Faber, 1940).

Rev. A. Herbert Gray, *Men, Women, and God. A Discussion of Sex Questions from the Christian Point of View* (London: Student Christian Movement, 1923; Worthing: Churchman, 1987).

Rev. A. Herbert Gray, *Sex Teaching* (London: National Sunday School Union, [n. d. 1929]).

Jonathan Green, *It: Sex since the Sixties* (London: Secker and Warburg, 1993).

David F. Greenberg, *The Construction of Homosexuality* (Chicago: University of Chicago Press, 1988).

Germaine Greer, *The Female Eunuch* (London: MacGibbon and Kee, 1970).

Germaine Greer, *Sex and Destiny* (London: Secker and Warburg, 1984).

Germaine Greer, *The Change* (London: Hamish Hamilton, 1991).

J. Greig (ed.), *The Letters of David Hume,* 2 vols (Oxford: Clarendon Press, 1932).

Edward F. Griffith, *Modern Marriage and Birth Control* (London: Gollancz, 1935).

Edward F. Griffith, *The Pioneer Spirit* (Upton Grey, Hants: Green Leaves Press, 1981).

F. Grose, *A Guide to Health, Beauty, Riches and Honour* (London: Hooper and Wigstead, 1796).

Phyllis Grosskurth, *Havelock Ellis: A Biography* (London: Allen Lane, 1980).

Jean H. Hagstrum, *Sex and Sensibility. Ideal and Erotic Love from Milton to Mozart* (Chicago and London: University of Chicago Press, 1980).

Paul Hair (ed.), *Before the Bawdy Court: Selections from the Church Court and Other Records Relating to the Correction of Moral Offences in England, Scotland and New*

England, 1300–1800 (London: Paul Elek, 1972).

Paul Hair, 'Bridal Pregnancy in Britain: The Limits of "Establishment" Social Control?', in Ad van der Woude (ed.), *The Role of the State and Public Opinion in Sexual Attitudes and Demographic Behaviour* (Paris: International Commission of Historical Demography, 1990), 35–48.

Norman Haire, *Hymen, or the Future of Marriage* (New York: E. P. Dutton, 1928).

E. Halévy, *The Growth of Philosophic Radicalism*, trans. M. Morris (London: Faber and Faber, 1928).

Diana Long Hall, 'Biology, Sex Hormones and Sexism in the 1920s', *Philosophical Quarterly*, v (1973–4), 81–96.

Gladys M. Hall, *Prostitution: a Survey and a Challenge* (London: Williams and Norgate, 1933).

Lesley A. Hall, 'The Stopes Collection in the Contemporary Medical Archives Centre of the Wellcome Institute for the History of Medicine', *Bulletin of the Society for the Social History of Medicine*, xxxii (1983), 50–1.

Lesley A. Hall, ' "Somehow very distasteful": Doctors, Men and Sexual Problems between the Wars', *Journal of Contemporary History*, xx (iv) (1985), 553–74.

Lesley A. Hall, 'From *Self-Preservation* to *Love Without Fear*: Medical and Lay Writers of Sex Advice from William Acton to Eustace Chesser', *Bulletin of the Society for the Social History of Medicine*, xxxix (1986), 20–3.

Lesley A. Hall, 'Illustrations from the Wellcome Institute Library: The Eugenics Society Archive in the Contemporary Medical Archives Centre', *Medical History*, xxxiv (1990), 327–33.

Lesley A. Hall, 'Medical Attitudes to the Sexual Disorders of the "Normal" Male in Britain 1900–1950' (PhD thesis, University of London, 1990).

Lesley A. Hall, *Hidden Anxieties: Male Sexuality, 1900–1950* (Cambridge: Polity Press, 1991).

Lesley A. Hall, 'Forbidden by God, Despised by Men: Masturbation, Medical Warnings, Moral Panic and Manhood in Great Britain, 1850–1950', *Journal of the History of Sexuality*, ii (iii) (1992), 365–87.

Lesley A. Hall, ' "The Cinderella of Medicine": Sexually-Transmitted Diseases in Britain in the Nineteenth and Twentieth Centuries', *Genitourinary Medicine*, lxix (1993), 314–19.

Lesley A. Hall, 'Uniting Science and Sensibility: Marie Stopes and the Narratives of Marriage in the 1920s', in A. Ingram and D. Patai (eds), *Rediscovering Forgotten Radicals: British Women Writers, 1880–1939* (Chapel Hill: University of North Carolina Press, 1993), 118–36.

Lesley A. Hall, ' "The English Have Hot-Water Bottles": The Morganatic Marriage of Medicine and Sexology in Britain since William Acton', in Roy Porter and Mikuláš Teich (eds), *Sexual Knowledge, Sexual Science: The History of Attitudes to Sexuality* (Cambridge University Press, 1994), 350–66.

Lesley A. Hall, ' "Disinterested Enthusiasm for Sexual Misconduct": The British Society for the Study of Sex Psychology 1913–1947', article forthcoming in *Journal of Contemporary History*.

Lesley A. Hall, 'A New Man in the 1920s? Questions of Social/Sexual Change' (unpublished paper circulated at conference 'Sexual Cultures in Europe', Amsterdam, 24–26 June 1992, Papers Group C: Sexual Codes and Practices, 51–61).

Marie Boas Hall, *Nature and Nature's Laws* (New York: Harper and Row, 1970).

Ruth Hall, *Marie Stopes: A Biography* [*Passionate Crusader: The Life of Marie Stopes in the USA*], (London: André Deutsch, 1977; New York: Harcourt Bracc Jovanovich, 1977).

Ruth Hall (ed.), *Dear Dr Stopes: Sex in the 1920s* (London: André Deutsch, 1978).

John S. Haller, Sr, 'From Maidenhead to Menopause: Sex Education for Women in Victorian America', *Journal of Popular Culture*, vi (1972), 49–69.

G. V. T. Hamilton, *A Research in Marriage* (New York: A. & C. Boni, 1929).

A. James Hammerton, *Cruelty and Companionship: Conflict in Nineteenth Century Married Life* (London and New York: Routledge, 1992).

E. H. Hare, 'Masturbatory Insanity: The History of an Idea', *Journal of Mental Science*, cviii (1962), 1–25.

Brian Harrison, 'Underneath the Victorians', *Victorian Studies*, x (1967), 239–62.

Fraser Harrison, *The Dark Angel: Aspects of Victorian Sexuality* (London: Sheldon Press, 1977).

L. W. Harrison, 'The Public Health Services and Venereal Diseases', *British Journal of Venereal Diseases*, i (1925), 12–22.

L. W. Harrison, 'Those Were the Days! or Random Notes on Then and Now in VD', *Bulletin of the Institute of Technicians in Venereology*, Wellcome Institute Library Reprint Collection (n. d. ?1950s), 1–7.

L. W. Harrison, 'Some Lessons Learnt in Fifty Years' Practice in Venereology', *British Journal of Venereal Diseases*, xxx (1954), 184–90.

Mark Harrison, 'The Politics of Venereal Disease Control and the British Army, 1914–1918,' *Medical History* (forthcoming).

Tom Harrisson, *Britain Revisited* (London: Gollancz, 1961).

Mary S. Hartmann, *Victorian Murderesses: A True History of Thirteen Respectable French and English Women Accused of Unspeakable Crimes* (London: Robson Books; New York: Schocken Books, 1977).

A. D. Harvey, 'Prosecution for Sodomy in England at the Beginning of the Nineteenth Century', *Historical Journal*, xxi (1978), 939–48.

Cate Haste, *Rules of Desire: Sex in Britain, World War I to the Present* (London: Chatto and Windus, 1992).

Walter Heape, *Sex Antagonism* (London: Constable, 1913).

Stephen Heath, *The Sexual Fix* (New York: Schocken; London: Macmillan, 1982).

A. R. Henderson, 'Female Prostitution in London, 1730–1830' (PhD dissertation, University of London, 1992).

Mrs S. Herbert, *Sex-Lore: A Primer on Courtship, Marriage and Parenthood* (London: A. & C. Black, 1918).

J. B. Hess and L. Nochlin, *Women as Sex Objects* (London: Allen Lane, 1973).

Boyd Hilton, *The Age of Atonement: the Influence of Evangelicalism on Social and Economic Thought, 1750–1865* (Oxford: Clarendon Press; New York: Oxford University Press, 1988).

Norman E. Himes, *The Medical History of Contraception* (Baltimore, Md.: Williams and Wilkins, 1936).

Gertrude Himmelfarb, *The Idea of Poverty: England in the Early Industrial Age* (London: Faber and Faber; New York: Knopf, 1984).

Magnus Hirschfeld, *Sexual Anomalies and Perversions: Physical and Psychological Development and Treatment, A Summary of the Works of the Late Professor Dr Magnus Hirschfeld, Compiled as a Humble Memorial by His Pupils* (London:

Torch Publishing, 1936).

D. Hirst, *Hidden Riches* (London: Eyre and Spottiswoode, 1964).

History of the Great War Based on Official Documents: Medical Services: Diseases of the War Volume II (London: HMSO, 1923).

History of the Second World War: United Kingdom Medical Series; The Army Medical Services: Administration II, ed. F. A. E. Crew (London: HMSO, 1955).

Paul Hoffman, *La Femme dans la pensée des lumières* (Paris: Ophrys, 1977).

Ellen Holtzmann, 'The Pursuit of Married Love: Women's Attitudes towards Sexuality and Marriage in Great Britain, 1918–1939', *Journal of Social History*, xvi (1982), 39–52.

M. A. Hopkins, *Hannah More and her Circle* (New York: Longmans, Green, 1947).

W. E. Houghton, *The Victorian Frame of Mind 1830–1870* (New Haven: Yale University Press, 1957).

Ralph Houlbrooke, *The English Family, 1450–1700* (London: Longman, 1984).

[Laurence Housman], *Policy and Principles: General Aims* (London: British Society for the Study of Sexual Psychology [Publication no. 1], 1914; 2nd edn 1929).

R. A. Houston, *Literacy in Early Modern Europe: Culture and Education, 1500–1800* (London: Longman, 1988).

Marie-Hélène Huet, *Monstrous Imagination* (Cambridge, Mass.: Harvard University Press, 1993).

Geoffrey Hughes, *Swearing. A Social History of Foul Language, Oaths and Profanity in English* (Oxford: Basil Blackwell, 1991).

M. Huhner, *A Practical Treatise on Disorders of the Sexual Function in the Male and Female* (Philadelphia: F. A. Davis, 1916; 3rd edn 1929).

David Hume: *A Treatise of Human Nature*, ed. L. A. Selby-Bigge (Oxford: Clarendon Press, 1978).

Steve Humphries, *A Secret World of Sex: Forbidden Fruit, the British Experience 1900–1950* (London: Sidgwick and Jackson, 1988).

Lynn Hunt (ed.), *The Invention of Pornography, 1500–1800* (New York: Zone Books, 1993).

Morton M. Hunt, *The Natural History of Love* (New York: Knopf, 1959; London: Hutchinson, 1960).

Francis Hutcheson, *A System of Moral Philosophy*, 2 vols (Glasgow: published by his son F. Hutcheson, 1755).

K. Hutchinson, 'What Happened to Occult Qualities in the Scientific Revolution?', *Isis*, lxxiii (1982), 233–53.

Isabel Elmslie Hutton, *The Hygiene of Marriage* (London: Heinemann Medical Books, 1923; 4th edn 1933).

Isabel Elmslie Hutton, *Memories of a Doctor in War and Peace* (London: Heinemann, 1960).

H. Montgomery Hyde, *The Other Love* (London: Heinemann, 1970).

H. Montgomery Hyde, *A Tangled Web: Sex Scandals in British Politics and Society* (London: Constable, 1986).

Samuel Hynes, *The Edwardian Turn of Mind* (Princeton, NJ: Princeton University Press, 1968; London: Pimlico Press, 1991).

Samuel Hynes, *The Auden Generation: Literature and Politics in England in the 1930s* (London: Bodley Head, 1976; Pimlico Press, 1992).

Samuel Hynes, *A War Imagined: The First World War and English Culture* (London: Bodley Head, 1990).

M. Ignatieff, 'Homo Sexualis', *London Review of Books*, 4–17 March 1982.

Martin Ingram, *Church Courts, Sex and Marriage in England 1570–1640* (Cambridge: Cambridge University Press, 1987).

Janice M. Irvine, *Disorders of Desire: Sex and Gender in Modern American Sexology* (Philadelphia: Temple University Press, 1990).

M. Jackson, *The Real Facts of Life: Feminism and the Politics of Sexuality c. 1850–1940* (London: Taylor and Francis, 1994).

M. C. Jacob, *The Radical Enlightenment* (London: Allen and Unwin, 1981).

E. Jacobs, W. H. Barber, J. H. Bloch, F. W. Leakey and E. Le Breton (eds), *Woman and Society in Eighteenth Century France* (London: Athlone Press, 1980).

Mary Jacobus, Evelyn Fox Keller and Sally Shuttleworth (eds), *Body/Politics: Women and the Discourses of Science* (New York: Routledge, 1990).

Danielle Jacquart and Claude Thomasset, *Sexualité et savoir medical au Moyen Age* (Paris: Presses Universitaires de France, 1985), trans. Matthew Adamson as *Sexuality and Medicine in the Middle Ages* (Cambridge: Polity Press, 1989).

M. Jaeger, *Before Victoria* (London: Chatto and Windus, 1956).

Pat Jalland, *Women, Marriage, and Politics, 1860–1914* (Oxford: Oxford University Press, 1986).

Patricia James, *Population Malthus: His Life and Times* (London: Routledge and Kegan Paul, 1979).

Stephen Jeffrey-Poulter, *Peers, Queers and Commons: The Struggle for Gay Law Reform from 1950 to the Present* (London: Routledge, 1991).

Sheila Jeffreys, 'Sex Reform and Anti-Feminism in the 1920s', in London Feminist History Group, *The Sexual Dynamics of History: Men's Power, Women's Resistance* (London: Pluto Press, 1983), 177–202.

Sheila Jeffreys, *The Spinster and Her Enemies: Feminism and Sexuality 1880–1930* (London: Pandora Press, 1985).

Sheila Jeffreys, *Anti-climax: A Feminist Perspective on the Sexual Revolution* (London: Women's Press, 1990).

Maroula Joannou, ' "The Woman in the Little House": Leonora Eyles and Socialist Feminism', in A. Ingram and D. Patai (eds), *Rediscovering Forgotten Radicals: British Women Writers 1880–1939* (Chapel Hill: University of North Carolina Press, 1993), 75–89.

Hilda M. Johns, 'The Social Aspect of the Venereal Diseases: Contact Tracing', *British Journal of Venereal Diseases*, xxi (1945), 15–17.

A. M. Johnson *et al.*, *Sexual Attitudes and Lifestyles* (Oxford: Blackwell Scientific Publications, 1994).

Thomas H. Johnson, 'Jonathan Edwards and the "Young Folks' Bible" ', *The New England Quarterly*, v (1932), 37–54.

R. F. Jones, *Ancients and Moderns* (St Louis: Washington University Press, 1961).

Vivien Jones (ed.), *Women in the Eighteenth Century: Constructions of Femininity* (London: Routledge, 1990).

Ludmilla Jordanova, 'Natural Facts: a Historical Perspective on Science and Sexuality', in C. MacCormack and M. Strathern (eds), *Nature, Culture and Gender* (Cambridge: Cambridge University Press, 1980), 42–69.

Ludmilla Jordanova (ed.), *Languages of Nature: Critical Essays on Science and Literature* (London: Free Association Books, 1986).

Ludmilla Jordanova, 'The Popularisation of Medicine: Tissot on Onanism', *Textual Practice*, i (1987), 68–80.

Ludmilla Jordanova, *Sexual Visions* (Hemel Hempstead: Harvester, 1989).

Raymond Kent, 'The Emergence of the Sociological Survey, 1887–1939', in Martin Bulmer (ed.), *Essays on the History of Sociological Research* (Cambridge: Cambridge University Press, 1985), 52–69.

Eva Keuls, *The Reign of the Phallus: Sexual Politics in Ancient Athens* (New York: Harper and Row, 1985).

Ambrose King, 'These Dying Diseases: Venereology in Decline?', *The Lancet*, i (1958), 651–7.

Ambrose King, 'The First Harrison Lecture, 1974: The Life and Times of Colonel Harrison', *British Journal of Venereal Diseases*, 1 (1974), 391–403.

L. S. King, *The Road to Medical Enlightenment 1650–1695* (London: Macdonald, 1970).

L. S. King, *The Medical World of the Eighteenth Century* (New York: Kreiger, 1971).

D. King-Hele, *The Essential Writings of Erasmus Darwin* (London: MacGibbon and Kee, 1968).

D. King-Hele, *Doctor of Revolution* (London: Faber and Faber, 1977).

Alfred C. Kinsey, *et al.*, *Sexual Behaviour in the Human Male* (Philadelphia and London: W. B. Saunders Co. Ltd, 1948).

Paddy Kitchen, *A Most Unsettling Person: An Introduction to the Ideas and Life of Patrick Geddes* (London: Gollancz, 1975).

Henry Thomas Kitchener, *Letters on Marriage, on the Causes of Matrimonial Infidelity, and on the Reciprocal Relations of the Sexes*, 2 vols (London: Chapple, 1812).

C. Knowlton, *Fruits of Philosophy: An Essay on the Population Question*, new edn, with notes, ed. G. Drysdale printed by Charles Bradlaugh and Annie Besant (London: Freethought Publishing [1877]; first published USA, 1847).

Elizabeth Kowaleski-Wallace, *Their Fathers' Daughters: Hannah More, Maria Edgeworth, and Patriarchal Complicity* (Oxford and New York: Oxford University Press, 1991).

Richard von Krafft-Ebing, *Psychopathia Sexualis: With Especial Reference to the Antipathetic Sexual Instinct. A Medico-Forensic Study* (Stuttgart: Erke, 1886; Philadelphia and London: F. A. Davis, 1892; Philadelphia: F. A. Davis, 1893).

W. E. Kruck, *Looking for Dr Condom* (Alabama: University of Alabama Press, 1981).

Samuel La'mert, *Self-Preservation: A Medical Treatise on Nervous and Physical Debility, Spermatorrhoea, Impotence and Sterility, with Practical Observations on the Use of the Microscope in the Treatment of Diseases of the Generative System*, '64th edn' (London: 'Published by the Author and sold at all Booksellers', *c.* 1850s–60s).

Elsa Lanchester, *Elsa Lanchester Herself* (London: Michael Joseph, 1983).

Coral Lansbury, *The Old Brown Dog: Women, Workers and Vivisection in Edwardian England* (Madison: University of Wisconsin Press, 1985).

Thomas W. Laqueur, 'Orgasm, Generation, and the Politics of Reproductive Biology', in C. Gallagher and T. Laqueur (eds), *The Making of the Modern Body* (Berkeley: California University Press, 1987), 1–41.

Thomas W. Laqueur, *Making Sex. Gender and the Body from Aristotle to Freud* (Cambridge, Mass.: Harvard University Press, 1990).

Thomas W. Laqueur, 'The Social Evil, the Solitary Vice and Pouring Tea', in Paula Bennett and Vernon A. Rosario II (eds), *Eros and Masturbation: The*

Historical, Theoretical and Literary Discourses of Autoeroticism (London: Routledge, forthcoming).

Peter Laslett, *The World We have Lost* (London: Methuen, 1965).

Peter Laslett, Karla Oosterveen and Richard M. Smith (eds), *Bastardy and its Comparative History* (London: Edward Arnold, 1980).

R. Latham and W. Matthews (eds), *The Diary of Samuel Pepys*, 11 vols (London: Bell and Hyman, 1970–83).

Brian Lawn (ed.), *The Prose Salernitan Questions* (London: Oxford University Press, 1979).

Nicky Leap and Billie Hunter, *The Midwife's Tale: An Oral History from Handywoman to Professional Midwife* (London: Scarlet Press, 1993).

Audrey Leathard, *The Fight for Family Planning* (London: Macmillan, 1980).

Rosina Ledbetter, *A History of the Malthusian League, 1877–1927* (Columbus: Ohio State University Press, 1976).

Robert Lees, 'Venereal Diseases in the Armed Forces Overseas (1)', *British Journal of Venereal Diseases*, xxii (1946), 149–58.

M. LeGates, 'The Cult of Womanhood in Eighteenth Century Thought', *Eighteenth Century Studies*, x (1976), 21–40.

Helen Rodnite Lemay, 'Human Sexuality in Twelfth through Fifteenth Century Scientific Writings', in Vern L. Bullough (ed.), *Sexual Practices and the Medieval Church*, 187–205 (Buffalo, NY: Prometheus, 1982).

Helen Rodnite Lemay, *Women's Secrets: A Translation of Pseudo-Albertus Magnus's 'De Secretis Mulierum' with Commentaries* (Albany, NY: State University of New York Press, 1992).

Alexandre Leupin, *Barbarolexis: Medieval Writing and Sexuality*, trans. Kate Cooper (Cambridge, Mass.: Harvard University Press, 1989).

David Levine, *Family Formation in an Age of Nascent Capitalism* (New York: Academic Press, 1977).

C. S. Lewis, *The Allegory of Love: A Study in Medieval Tradition* (Oxford: Clarendon Press, 1936).

Jane Lewis, *Women in England 1870–1950: Sexual Divisions and Social Change* (Brighton: Wheatsheaf, 1984).

Jane Lewis, David Clark and David Morgan, *Whom God Hath Joined Together: The Work of Marriage Guidance* (London: Routledge, 1992).

E. Lewis-Faning, *Papers from the Royal Commission on Population, Vol. 1: Report on an Enquiry into Family Limitation and its Influence on Human Fertility during the Past Fifty Years Conducted at the Request of the Royal Commission on Population* (London: HMSO, 1949).

Jane Lidderdale and Mary Nicholson, *Dear Miss Weaver: Harriet Shaw Weaver 1876–1961* (London: Faber and Faber, 1970).

A. Lloyd, *The Wickedest Age* (Newton Abbot: David and Charles, 1971).

I. Loudon, 'Chlorosis, Anaemia and Anorexia Nervosa', *British Medical Journal*, cclxxxi (1980), 1–19.

I. Loudon, 'The Diseases called Chlorosis', *Psychological Medicine*, xiv (1984), 27–36.

C. Lougée, *Le Paradis des Femmes: Women, Salons and Social Stratification in Seventeenth Century France* (Princeton, NJ: Princeton University Press, 1976).

A. O. Lovejoy, *The Great Chain of Being* (Cambridge, Mass.: Harvard University Press, 1936).

Thomas Power Lowry (ed.), *The Classic Clitoris: Historic Contributions to Scientific Sexuality* (Chicago: Nelson-Hall, 1978).

Arthur P. Luff, *Textbook of Forensic Medicine and Toxicology* (London: Longmans, Green, 1895).

E. Lyttelton (Hon.), *The Causes and Prevention of Immorality in Schools* (London: Social Purity Alliance, printed for private circulation, 1887).

Joseph McAleer, *Popular Reading and Publishing in Britain 1914–1950* (Oxford: Clarendon Press, 1992).

Ida Macalpine and Richard Hunter, *George III and the Mad Business* (London: Allen Lane, 1969).

I. D. McCalman, *Radical Underworld: Prophets, Revolutionaries and Pornographers in London, 1795–1840* (Cambridge: Cambridge University Press, 1988).

R. A. McCance, M. C. Luff and E. E. Widdowson, 'Physical and Emotional Periodicity in Women', *Journal of Hygiene,* xxxvii (1937), 571–611.

Robert Purks Maccubbin, *'Tis Nature's Fault: Unauthorized Sexuality during the Enlightenment* (New York and Cambridge: Cambridge University Press, 1987).

Robert H. MacDonald, 'The Frightful Consequences of Onanism: Notes on the History of a Delusion', *Journal of the History of Ideas,* xxviii (1967), 423–31.

Gilbert D. McEwen, *The Oracle of the Coffee-House: John Dunton's 'Athenian Mercury'* (The Huntington Library, San Marino, Ca.: 1972).

Bernarr A. MacFadden, *The Virile Powers of Superb Manhood: How Developed, How Lost, How Regained,* originally issued during the 1890s (New York: Physical Culture Publishing, 1900).

Alan Macfarlane, *Marriage and Love in England: Modes of Reproduction, 1300–1840* (Oxford: Basil Blackwell, 1986).

H. MacGregor, 'Eighteenth-Century V.D. Publicity', *British Journal of Venereal Diseases,* xxxi (1955), 117–18.

O. M. McGregor, *Divorce in England: A Centenary History* (London: Heinemann, 1957).

Paul McHugh, *Prostitution and Victorian Social Reform* (London: Croom Helm, 1980).

Neil McKendrick, John Brewer and J. H. Plumb, *The Birth of a Consumer Society: The Commercialization of Eighteenth-Century England* (London: Europa, 1982).

Angus McLaren, *Birth Control in Nineteenth Century England* (London: Croom Helm, 1978).

Angus McLaren, *Reproductive Rituals: The Perception of Fertility in England from the Sixteenth to the Nineteenth Century* (London and New York: Methuen, 1984).

Angus McLaren, 'The Pleasures of Procreation', in W. F. Bynum and Roy Porter (eds), *William Hunter and the Eighteenth Century Medical World* (Cambridge: Cambridge University Press, 1985), 323–420.

Angus McLaren, 'Clever Practices: Fertility Control Methods from the 18th to 20th Centuries', in Ad van der Woude (ed.), *The Role of the State and Public Opinion in Sexual Attitudes and Demographic Behaviour* (Paris: International Commission of Historical Demography, 1990), 425–40.

Angus McLaren, *A History of Contraception from Antiquity to the Present Day* (Oxford: Basil Blackwell, 1991).

Angus McLaren, 'Sex Radicalism in the Canadian Pacific Northwest, 1890–1920', *Journal of the History of Sexuality,* ii (iv) (1992), 527–46.

Angus McLaren and Arlene Tiger McLaren, *The Bedroom and the State: The*

Changing Practices and Politics of Contraception and Abortion in Canada, 1880–1980 (Toronto: McLelland and Stewart, 1986).

Ian MacLean, *Woman Triumphant* (Oxford: Clarendon Press, 1977).

Ian MacLean, *The Renaissance Notion of Women: A Study in the Fortunes of Scholasticism and Medical Science in European Intellectual Life* (Cambridge and New York: Cambridge University Press, 1980).

Lois McNay, *Foucault and Feminism: Power, Gender and the Self* (Cambridge: Polity Press, 1992).

John Macnicol, 'Eugenics and the Campaign for Voluntary Sterilization in Britain between the Wars', *Social History of Medicine*, ii (1989), 147–69.

John Macnicol, 'The Voluntary Sterilization Campaign in Britain, 1918–1939', in John C. Fout (ed.), *Forbidden History: The State, Society and the Regulation of Sexuality in Modern Europe: Essays from 'The Journal of the History of Sexuality'* (Chicago: University of Chicago Press, 1992), 317–33.

A. C. A. Magian, *Handbook of Venereal Diseases, Being an Outline of These Affections and of Their History and Treatment* (Manchester and London: John Heywood, 1909).

Linda Mahood, *The Magdalenes: Prostitution in the Nineteenth Century* (London and New York: Routledge, 1990).

T. R. Malthus, *An Essay on the Principle of Population*, 1st edn (London: Johnson, 1798).

F. E. and F. P. Manuel, *Utopian Thought in the Western World* (Cambridge, Mass.: Belknap Press of Harvard University Press, 1979).

Norah March, *Toward Racial Health, A Handbook for Parents, Teachers and Social Workers on the Training of Boys and Girls*, with a foreword by J. Arthur Thomson (London: George Routledge and Sons, 1915; 4th revised edn 1920).

Steven Marcus, *The Other Victorians: A Study of Sexuality and Pornography in Mid-Nineteenth Century England* (New York: Basic Books, 1964; London: Weidenfeld and Nicolson, 1966).

Catherine Marsh, *The Survey Method: The Contribution of Surveys to Sociological Explanation* (London: Allen and Unwin, 1982).

Catherine Marsh, 'Informants, Respondents and Citizens', in Martin Bulmer (ed.), *Essays on the History of Sociological Research* (Cambridge: Cambridge University Press, 1985), 206–27.

Francis H. A. Marshall, *The Physiology of Reproduction* (London, New York, Bombay and Calcutta: Longmans, Green, 1910).

John Marten, *A Treatise Of all the Degrees and Symptoms of the Venereal Disease In both Sexes*, 6th edn (London: S. Crouch, 1708).

John Marten, *Gonosologium Novum; or, A New System of all the Secret Infirmities and Diseases, Natural, Accidental, and Venereal in Men and Women*, 6th edn (London: Crouch, 1709).

Robert Martensen, 'The Transformation of Eve: Women's Bodies, Medicine, and Culture in Early Modern England', in Roy Porter and Mikuláš Teich (eds), *Sexual Knowledge, Sexual Science: The History of Attitudes to Sexuality* (Cambridge: Cambridge University Press, 1994), 107–33.

Arthur Marwick, *The Deluge: British Society and the First World War* (London, Bodley Head, 1965).

M. H. Mason, 'Public Morality: Some Constructive Suggestions', *The Nineteenth Century*, lxxxii (1917), 185–94.

Michael Mason, *The Making of Victorian Sexuality* (Oxford: Oxford University Press, 1994).

John Maubray, *The Female Physician* (London: J. Holland, 1724).

R. Mauzi, *L'idée du bonheur dans la littérature et la pensée françaises au XVIIIe siècle* (Paris: Colin, 1960).

Henry Mayhew, *London Labour and the London Poor*, Vol. IV: *Those That Will Not Work, comprising Prostitutes, Thieves, Swindlers, and Beggars, by Several Contributors* (London: Griffin, Bohn, 1861–2; New York: Dover Publications, 1968).

John Maynard, *Victorian Discourses on Sexuality and Religion* (Cambridge: Cambridge University Press, 1993).

R. L. Meade-King, 'Notes from a Seventeenth Century Textbook of Medicine', *British Medical Journal*, ii (1906), 433–5.

Jay Mechling, 'Advice to Historians on Advice to Mothers', *Journal of Social History*, ix (1975–6), 44–57.

'Medica' [Joan Malleson], *Any Wife or Any Husband: A Book for Couples who have met Sexual Difficulties and for Doctors* (London: Heinemann Medical Books, 1950).

Victor Cornelius Medvei, *A History of Endocrinology* (Lancaster, Boston and The Hague: MTP Press, 1982).

Billie Melman, *Woman and the Popular Imagination in the 1920s: Flappers and Nymphs* (London: Macmillan, 1988).

Susan Mendus and Jane Rendall (eds), *Sexuality and Subordination: Interdisciplinary Studies of Gender in the Nineteenth Century* (London: Routledge, 1989).

Carolyn Merchant, *The Death of Nature: Women, Ecology and the Scientific Revolution* (New York: Harper and Row, 1980; London: Wildwood House, 1982).

Mandy Merck, *Perversions: Deviant Readings* (London: Virago, 1993).

C. Mills, 'Collaboration between the Venereal Disease and Other Departments', *British Journal of Venereal Diseases*, x (1934), 233–48.

John Laws Milton, 'On the Nature and Treatment of Spermatorrhœa', *The Lancet*, i (1854).

John Laws Milton, *On Spermatorrhoea: Its Results and Complications*, 9th edn (London: Robert Hardwicke, 1872; from original papers in *The Lancet*, 1852 and *The Medical Circular*, 1858).

Naomi Mitchison, *All Change Here: Girlhood and Marriage* (London: Bodley Head, 1975).

Naomi Mitchison, *You May Well Ask: A Memoir 1920–1940* (London: Gollancz, 1979; Flamingo edn 1986).

Rosalind Mitchison and Leah Leneman, *Sexuality and Social Control: Scotland 1660–1780* (Oxford: Basil Blackwell, 1989).

Tania Modleski, *Loving with a Vengeance. Mass-Produced Fantasies for Women* (London: Methuen, 1984).

John Money, 'Teaching in the Market-Place, or "Caesar adsum jam forte aderat": The Retailing of Knowledge on Provincial England during the Eighteenth Century', in John Brewer and Roy Porter (eds), *Consumption and the World of Goods* (London and New York: Routledge, 1993), 335–79.

S. Moravia, *Il Pensiero degli Idéologues: Scienza e filosofia in Francia 1780–1815* (Firenze: La Nuova Italia, 1974).

S. Moravia, 'From *Homme Machine* to *Homme Sensible*: Changing Eighteenth Century Models of Man's Image', *Journal of the History of Ideas*, xxxix (1978),

45–60.

S. Moravia, 'The Enlightenment and the Sciences of Man', *History of Science*, xviii (1980), 247–68.

Johannes Morsink, *Aristotle on the Generation of Animals: a Philosophical Study* (Washington, DC: University Press of America, 1982).

Frank Mort, 'Purity, Feminism and the State: Sexuality and Moral Politics, 1880–1914', in M. Langon and B. Schwarz (eds), *Crises in the British State 1880–1930* (London: Hutchinson, 1985), 209–25.

Frank Mort, *Dangerous Sexualities: Medico-Moral Politics in England since 1830* (London and New York: Routledge and Kegan Paul, 1987).

Ornella Moscucci, *The Science of Woman: Gynaecology and Gender in England 1800–1929* (Cambridge: Cambridge University Press, 1990).

Guillaume de la Motte, *A General Treatise of Midwifery* (London: J. Waugh, 1746).

Stanley D. Nash, 'Prostitution and Charity: The Magdalen Hospital, a Case Study', *Journal of Social History*, xvii (1984), 617–28.

National Birth-Rate Commission, *The Declining Birth-Rate: its Causes and Effects, Being the Report of and the Chief Evidence Taken by the National Birth-rate Commission, Instituted, with Official Recognition, by the National Council of Public Morals – for the Promotion of Race Regeneration – Spiritual, Moral and Physical*, ed. Sir James Marchant (London: Chapman and Hall for the National Birth-Rate Commission, 1916).

National Birth-Rate Commission, *Problems of Population and Parenthood, Being the Second Report of and the Chief Evidence Taken by the National Birth-Rate Commission, 1918–1920* (London: Chapman and Hall, 1920).

National Birth-Rate Commission, *Youth and the Race: The Development and Education of Young Citizens for Worthy Parenthood, Being the Fourth Report of and the Chief Evidence Taken*, ed. Sir James Marchant (London: Kegan Paul, Trench Trubner, for the National Birth-Rate Commission, 1923).

Lynda Nead, *Myths of Sexuality: Representations of Women in Victorian Britain* (Oxford: Basil Blackwell, 1988).

Lynda Nead, *The Female Nude: Art, Obscenity, and Sexuality* (New York: Routledge, 1992).

J. Needham, *A History of Embryology* (Cambridge: Cambridge University Press, 1934; 2nd edn 1959).

A. Neilans, 'The Protection of Soldiers', *The Shield*, 3rd series, i (1916–17).

E. Neuburg, *Popular Literature: A History and Guide* (Harmondsworth: Penguin, 1977).

M. New, 'At the Backside of the Door of Purgatory', in V. Grosvenor-Myer (ed.), *Lawrence Sterne: Riddles and Mysteries* (London: Vision, 1984), 15–23.

Sir Arthur Newsholme, 'The Decline in Registered Mortality from Syphilis in England. To What is it Due?', *Journal of Social Hygiene*, xii (1926), 514–23.

T. L. Nichols, *Esoteric Anthropology (The Mysteries of Man) A Comprehensive and Confidential Treatise on the Structure, Functions, Passional Attractions, and Perversions, True and False Physical and Social Conditions and the Most Intimate Relations of Men and Women. Anatomical, Physiological, Pathological, Therapeutical and Obstetrical. Hygienic and Hydropathic. From the American Stereotype Edition, Revised and Rewritten* (Hygienic Institute, Museum St, London WC: the author, n. d. c. 1873).

S. Nissenbaum, *Sex, Diet, and Debility in Jacksonian America: Sylvester Graham and*

Health Reform (Westport, Conn. and London: Greenwood Press, 1980).

H. J. Norman, 'John Bulwer and his *Anthropometamorphosis*', in E. Ashworth Underwood (ed.), *Science, Medicine and History. Essays on the Evolution of Scientific Thought and Medical Practice*, Vol. II (Oxford: Oxford University Press, 1953), 80–99.

Rictor Norton, *Mother Clap's Molly House: The Gay Subculture in England 1700–1830* (London: Gay Men's Press, 1992).

Robert A. Nye, *Masculinity and Male Codes of Honor in Modern France* (Oxford: Oxford University Press, 1993).

D. O'Keefe, *Stolen Lightning* (Oxford: Martin Robertson, 1982).

Hugh Ormsby-Lennon, 'Swift's Spirit Reconjured: Das Dong-An-Sich', *Swift Studies*, iii (1988), 9–78.

Rebecca O'Rourke, *Reflecting on 'The Well of Loneliness'*, 'Heroines' series (London: Routledge, 1989).

Lawrence Osborne, *The Poisoned Embrace: A Brief History of Sexual Pessimism* (London: Bloomsbury, 1993).

Jean Frédéric Osterwald, *Traité contre l'impureté*, Amsterdam: T. Lombrail, 1707; trans. as *The Nature of Uncleanness Consider'd . . . to which is added A Discourse Concerning the Nature of Chastity and the Means of Obtaining it* (London: R. Bonwicke, 1708).

Nelly Oudshoorn, 'Endocrinologists and the Conceptualization of Sex, 1920–1940', *Journal of the History of Biology*, xxiii (ii) (1990), 163–86.

Nelly Oudshoorn, 'On the Making of Sex Hormones: Research Material and the Production of Knowledge', *Social Studies of Science*, xx (i) (1990), 5–33.

Nelly Oudshoorn, 'On Measuring Sex Hormones: The Role of Biological Assays in Sexualizing Chemical Substances', *Bulletin of the History of Medicine*, lxiv (1990), 243–61.

Dorinda Outram, *The Body and the French Revolution: Sex, Class and Political Culture* (New Haven: Yale University Press, 1989).

Alex Owen, *The Darkened Room: Women, Power and Spiritualism in Late Victorian England* (London: Virago, 1989).

E. L. Packer, 'Aspects of Working Class Marriage', *Pilot Papers: Social Essays and Documents*, ii (i) (1947), 92–104.

Sir James Paget, 'Sexual Hypochondriasis', in his *Clinical Lectures and Essays* (London: Longmans Green, 1875; 2nd edn 1879), 275–98.

Camille Paglia, *Sexual Personae* (New Haven: Yale University Press, 1990).

Christabel Pankhurst, *The Great Scourge and How to End It* (London: E. Pankhurst, 1913).

Jeannette Parisot, *Johnny Come Lately: A Short History of the Condom*, trans. and enlarged by Bill McCann (London: Journeyman Press, 1987).

Katherine Park and Lorraine J. Daston, 'Unnatural Conceptions: The Study of Monsters in Sixteenth Century France and England', *Past and Present*, xcii (1981), 20–54.

Sir Alan Parkes, *Sex, Science and Society: Addresses, Lectures and Articles* (Newcastle-upon-Tyne: Oriel Press, 1966).

S. Parks, *John Dunton and the English Book Trade: a Study of his Career with a Checklist of his Publications* (New York: Garland, 1976).

A. Parreaux, *Daily Life in England in the Reign of George III*, trans. C. Congreve (London: Allen and Unwin, 1969).

J. Passmore, *The Perfectibility of Man* (London: Duckworth, 1970).

Gail Kern Paster, *The Body Embarrassed: Drama and the Disciplines of Shame in Early Modern England* (Ithaca, NY: Cornell University Press, 1993).

Ronald Paulson, *Representations of Revolution 1789–1820* (New Haven: Yale University Press, 1983).

Pierre J. Payer, *The Bridling of Desire: Views of Sex in the Later Middle Ages* (Toronto: Toronto University Press, 1993).

Ronald Pearsall, *The Worm in the Bud: The World of Victorian Sexuality* (London: Weidenfeld and Nicolson, 1969; Harmondsworth: Penguin, 1971).

N. Perrin, *Dr Bowdler's Legacy – A History of Expurgated Books in England and America* (New York: Atheneum, 1969; London: Macmillan, 1970).

M. Jeanne Peterson, *The Medical Profession in Mid-Victorian London* (Berkeley, Calif.: University of California Press, 1978).

M. Jeanne Peterson, 'No Angels in the House: The Victorian Myth and the Paget Women', *American Historical Review*, lxxxix (iii) (1984), 677–708.

M. Jeanne Peterson, 'Dr Acton's Enemy: Medicine, Sex, and Society in Victorian England', *Victorian Studies*, xxix (iv) (1986), 569–90.

M. Jeanne Peterson, *Family, Love and Work in the Lives of Victorian Gentlewomen* (Bloomington and Indianapolis: Indiana University Press, 1989).

S. Pickering, Jr, *John Locke and Children's Books in Eighteenth Century England* (Knoxville: University of Tennesee, 1981).

Philip Pinkus, *Grub Street Stripped Bare* (London: Constable, 1980).

J. H. Plumb, *The Commercialization of Leisure in Eighteenth Century England* (Reading: University of Reading Press, 1973).

J. H. Plumb, *Georgian Delights* (London: Weidenfeld and Nicolson, 1980).

Frank Poller, *Holmes of Hanney*, Hanney History Group, Occasional Paper no. 1 (E. Hanney, Oxon.: Hanney History Group, 1993).

George Vivian Poore, *A Treatise in Medical Jurisprudence* (London: John Murray, 1901).

Mary Poovey, ' "Scenes of an Indelicate Character": The Medical "Treatment" of Victorian Women', *Representations*, xiv (1986), 152.

Mary Poovey, *Uneven Developments: The Ideological Work of Gender in Mid-Victorian England* (London: Virago, 1989).

Mary Poovey, 'Speaking of the Body: Mid-Victorian Constructions of Female Desire', in Mary Jacobus, Evelyn Fox Keller and Sally Shuttleworth (eds), *Body/Politics: Women and the Discourses of Science* (New York and London: Routledge, 1990), 29–46.

A. Portal, *Histoire de l'anatomie et de la chirurgie* (Paris: Didot le Jeuen, 1770–3).

Kevin Porter and Jeffrey Weeks, *Between the Acts: Lives of Homosexual Men 1885–1967* (London: Routledge, 1991).

Roy Porter, 'The Sexual Politics of James Graham', *British Journal for Eighteenth Century Studies*, v (1982), 119–6.

Roy Porter, 'Mixed Feelings: the Enlightenment and Sexuality in Eighteenth Century Britain', in P.-G. Boucé (ed.), *Sexuality in Eighteenth Century Britain* (Manchester: Manchester University Press, 1982), 1–27.

Roy Porter, 'Against the Spleen', in Valerie Grosvenor Myer (ed.), *Laurence Sterne: Riddles and Mysteries* (London and New York: Vision, 1984), 84–99.

Roy Porter, 'Spreading Carnal Knowledge or Selling Dirt Cheap? Nicolas Venette's *Tableau de l'amour conjugal* in Eighteenth Century England', *Journal of European Studies*, xiv (1984), 233–55.

Roy Porter, 'Lay Medical Knowledge in the Eighteenth Century: the Case of the *Gentleman's Magazine*', *Medical History*, xxix (1985), 138–68.

Roy Porter, 'Laymen, Doctors and Medical Knowledge in the Eighteenth Century: The Evidence of the *Gentleman's Magazine*', in Roy Porter (ed.), *Patients and Practitioners: Lay Perceptions of Medicine in Pre-Industrial Society* (Cambridge: Cambridge University Press, 1985), 283–314.

Roy Porter, 'Making Faces: Physiognomy and Fashion in Eighteenth Century England', *Etudes Anglaises*, xxxviii (Oct.–Dec. 1985), 385–96.

Roy Porter, '"The Secrets of Generation Display'd": *Aristotle's Master-piece* in Eighteenth-Century England', in R. P. Maccubbin (ed.), *Unauthorized Sexual Behaviour during the Enlightenment* (special issue of *Eighteenth Century Life*), Vol. IX, ns, (iii) (May 1985), 1–21.

Roy Porter, 'The Scientific Revolution: a Spoke in the Wheel?', in R. Porter and M. Teich (eds), *Revolution in History* (Cambridge: Cambridge University Press, 1986), 290–316.

Roy Porter, 'A Touch of Danger: The Man-Midwife as Sexual Predator', in G. S. Rousseau and R. Porter (eds), *Sexual Underworlds of the Enlightenment* (Manchester: Manchester University Press, 1988), 206–32.

Roy Porter, 'The Exotic as Erotic: Captain Cook at Tahiti', in G. S. Rousseau and Roy Porter (eds), *Exoticism in the Enlightenment* (Manchester: Manchester University Press, 1989), 117–44.

Roy Porter, *Health for Sale: Quackery in England 1650–1850* (Manchester: Manchester University Press, 1989).

Roy Porter, '"The Whole Secret of Health": Mind, Body and Medicine in *Tristram Shandy*', in John Christie and Sally Shuttleworth (eds), *Nature Transfigured* (Manchester: Manchester University Press, 1989), 61–84.

Roy Porter, 'Libertinism and Promiscuity', in J. Miller (ed.), *The Don Giovanni Book: Myths of Seduction and Betrayal* (London: Faber and Faber, 1990), 1–19.

Roy Porter, 'Love, Sex and Medicine: Nicolas Venette and his *Tableau de l'amour conjugal*', in Peter Wagner (ed.), *Erotica and the Enlightenment* (Frankfurt: Lang, 1990), 90–122.

Roy Porter, 'Civilization and Disease: Medical Ideology in the Enlightenment', in J. Black and J. Gregory (eds), *Culture, Politics and Society in Britain 1660–1800* (Manchester: Manchester University Press, 1991), 154–83.

Roy Porter, *Doctor of Society: Thomas Beddoes and the Sick Trade in Late Enlightenment England* (London: Routledge, 1991).

Roy Porter, 'Is Foucault Useful for Understanding Eighteenth and Nineteenth Century Sexuality?', *Contention*, i (1991), 61–82.

Roy Porter (ed.), *The Popularization of Medicine, 1650–1850* (London: Routledge, 1992).

Roy Porter, 'The Rise of Physical Examination', in W. F. Bynum and Roy Porter (eds), *Medicine and the Five Senses* (Cambridge: Cambridge University Press, 1992), 179–97.

Roy Porter and G. S. Rousseau (eds), *Sexual Underworlds of the Enlightenment* (Manchester: Manchester University Press, 1987).

Roy Porter and Mikuláš Teich (eds), *The Enlightenment in National Context* (Cambridge: Cambridge University Press, 1981).

Roy Porter and Mikuláš Teich (eds), *Sexual Knowledge, Sexual Science: The History of Attitudes to Sexuality* (Cambridge: Cambridge University Press, 1994).

The Works of Beilby Porteus, Late Bishop of London: With His Life by Robert Hodgson, new edn, 6 vols (London: T. Cadell and W. Davies, 1811).

F. Pottle (ed.), *Boswell's London Journal 1762–1763* (New Haven and London: Yale University Press, 1950).

F. Pottle (ed.), *Boswell in Holland 1763–1764* (London: Heinemann, 1950; New York: McGraw-Hill, 1950).

Marie-Christine Pouchelle, *The Body and Surgery in the Middle Ages* (Cambridge: Polity Press, 1989).

D'Arcy Power, *The Foundations of Medical History* (Baltimore, Md.: Johns Hopkins University Press, 1931), Lecture vi, '*Aristotle's Master-Piece*'.

John Power, *Essays on the Female Oeconomy* (London, 1821).

I. E. E. Prebble, 'Changing Pattern of Venereal Diseases: A Comparison between 1935 and 1960', *British Journal of Venereal Diseases*, xxviii (1962), 86–8.

M. Price, *To the Palace of Wisdom* (New York: Doubleday, 1964).

I. N. Orpwood Price and J. A. Burgess, 'Is a New Deal in the Control of Venereal Disease Necessary?', *British Journal of Venereal Diseases*, xx (1944), 19–30.

Frank K. Prochaska, *Women and Philanthropy in Nineteenth Century England* (Oxford: Oxford University Press, 1980).

Martin Pugh, *Women and the Women's Movement in Britain 1914–1959* (London: Macmillan, 1992).

G. R. Quaife, *Wanton Wenches and Wayward Wives: Peasants and Illicit Sex in Early Seventeenth Century England* (London: Croom Helm, 1979).

Claude Quétel, *The History of Syphilis*, trans. Judith Braddock and Brian Pike (Oxford: Basil Blackwell, 1990).

Maurice Quinlan, *Victorian Prelude: A History of English Manners, 1700–1830* (London: Cassell; New York: Columbia University Press, 1941).

D. D. Raphael, *British Moralists 1650–1800*, 2 vols (Oxford: Oxford University Press, 1969).

Dean Rapp, 'The Early Discovery of Freud by the British General Public', *Social History of Medicine*, iii (1990), 217–43.

J. Redwood, *Reason, Ridicule and Religion* (London: Thames and Hudson, 1976).

The Viscountess Rhondda, *This Was My World* (London: Macmillan, 1933).

P. G. Ritterbush, *Overtures to Biology* (New Haven: Yale University Press, 1964).

Isabel Rivers (ed.), *Books and their Readers in Eighteenth Century England* (Leicester: Leicester University Press, 1982).

K. B. Roberts, *The Fabric of the Body: European Traditions of Anatomical Illustration* (Oxford and New York: Clarendon Press, 1992).

Paul Robinson, *The Modernization of Sex: Havelock Ellis, Alfred Kinsey, William Masters and Virginia Johnson* (London: Elek, 1976; New York: Harper and Row, 1976).

Shirley A. Roe, *Matter, Life and Generation: Eighteenth-Century Embryology and the Haller–Wolff Debate* (Cambridge: Cambridge University Press, 1981).

J. Roger, *Les Sciences de la vie dans la pensée Française du XVIIIe siècle* (Paris: Colin, 1963).

K. M. Rogers, *The Troublesome Helpmate: A History of Misogyny in Literature* (Seattle: University of Washington Press, 1966).

Pat Rogers, *Grub Street: Studies in a Subculture* (London: Methuen, 1972).

C. H. Rolph (ed.), *Women of the Streets: A Sociological Study of the Common Prostitute* (London: Secker and Warburg, for and on behalf of the British Social Biology Council, 1955).

C. H. Rolph (ed.), *The Trial of Lady Chatterley: Regina v. Penguin Books Limited* (Harmondsworth: Penguin, 1961).

June Rose, *Marie Stopes and the Sexual Revolution* (London: Faber and Faber, 1992).

Theodore Rosebury, *Microbes and Morals* (New York: Viking Press, 1971).

G. S. Rousseau, 'Science and the Discovery of the Imagination in Enlightened England', *Eighteenth Century Studies*, iii (1969), 109–35.

G. S. Rousseau, 'Nerves, Spirits and Fibres: Towards Defining the Origins of Sensibility; with a Postscript, 1976', *The Blue Guitar*, ii (Rome, 1976), 125–53.

G. S. Rousseau, 'Psychology', in G. S. Rousseau and Roy Porter (eds), *The Ferment of Knowledge* (Cambridge: Cambridge University Press, 1980), 143–210.

G. S. Rousseau, 'Nymphomania, Bienville and the Rise of Erotic Sensibility', in P.-G. Boucé (ed.), *Sexuality in Eighteenth Century Britain* (Manchester: Manchester University Press, 1982), 95–119.

G. S. Rousseau, 'The Pursuit of Homosexuality in the Eighteenth Century: "Utterly Confused Category" and/or Rich Repository?', *Eighteenth-Century Life*, ix (1985), 132–68.

G. S. Rousseau, 'The Sorrows of Priapus: Anticlericalism, Homosocial Desire and Richard Payne Knight', in G. S. Rousseau and Roy Porter (eds), *Sexual Underworlds of the Enlightenment* (Manchester: Manchester University Press, 1987), 101–55.

G. S. Rousseau and Roy Porter (eds), *The Ferment of Knowledge* (Cambridge: Cambridge University Press, 1980).

Aline Rousselle, *Porneia: On Desire and the Body in Antiquity*, trans. Felicia Pheasant (New York: Basil Blackwell, 1988).

C. H. F. Routh, 'On the Moral and Physical Evils likely to follow if Practices Intended to Act as Checks to Population be not Strongly Discouraged and Condemned', *Medical Press and Circular* (1878, repr. London, 1879).

Constance Rover, *Love, Morals, and the Feminists* (London: Routledge and Kegan Paul, 1970).

Sheila Rowbotham and Jeffrey Weeks, *Socialism and the New Life: the Personal and Sexual Politics of Edward Carpenter and Havelock Ellis* (London: Pluto Press, 1977).

Beryl Rowlands, *Medieval Woman's Guide to Health: The First English Gynecological Handbook* (Kent, Ohio: Kent State University Press, 1981).

A. L. Rowse, *Homosexuals in History* (London: Weidenfeld and Nicolson, 1977).

G. Rudé, *Wilkes and Liberty* (Oxford: Clarendon Press, 1962).

Alan Rusbridger, *A Concise History of the Sex Manual, 1886–1986* (London and Boston: Faber and Faber, 1986).

Cynthia Eagle Russett, *Sexual Science: The Victorian Construction of Womanhood* (London and Cambridge, Mass.: Harvard University Press, 1989).

Michael Ryan, *The Philosophy of Marriage in its Social, Moral and Physical Relations* (London: Ballière, 1843).

C. Ryskamp and F. A. Pottle (eds), *Boswell: the Ominous Years 1774–1776* (London: Heinemann, 1963; New York: McGraw-Hill, 1963).

William Salmon, *Synopsis Medicinae* (London: C. Jones, 1671).

William Salmon, *Seplasium. The Compleat English Physician* (London: Gilliflower and Sawbridge, 1693).

William Salmon, *The Family-Dictionary* (London: H. Rhodes, 1696).

William Salmon, *The Country Physician, or A Choice Collection of Physick Fitted for Vulgar Use* (London: John Taylor, 1703).

William Salmon, *Collectanea Medica, the Country Physician* (London: J. Taylor, 1703).

William Salmon, *Botanologia. The English Herbal* (London: N. Rhodes and J. Taylor, 1710).

Jonathan Sawday, *The Mirror and the Knife: The Renaissance Culture of Dissection* (London: Routledge, forthcoming).

Mary Scharlieb and F. A. Sibly, *Youth and Sex: Dangers and Safeguards for Girls and Boys* (London: T. C. and E. C. Jack, 1913).

Londa Schiebinger, 'Skeletons in the Closet: The First Illustrations of the Female Skeleton in Eighteenth-Century Anatomy', in Catherine Gallagher and Thomas Laqueur (eds), *The Making of the Modern Body: Sexuality and Society in the Nineteenth Century* (Berkeley: University of California Press, 1987), 42–82.

Londa Schiebinger, *Nature's Body: Gender in the Making of Modern Science* (Boston, Mass.: Beacon Press, 1993).

Londa Schiebinger, 'Mammals, Primatology and Sexology', in Roy Porter and Mikuláš Teich (eds), *Sexual Knowledge, Sexual Science: The History of Attitudes to Sexuality* (Cambridge: Cambridge University Press, 1994), 184–209.

Dr A. R. Schofield and Dr P. Vaughan-Jackson, *What a Boy Should Know* (London: Cassell, 1913).

George Ryley Scott, *Scott's Encyclopaedia of Sex: A Practical Encyclopaedia Arranged in Alphabetical Order, Explanatory of Everything Pertaining to Sexual Physiology, Psychology and Pathology* (London: T. Werner Laurie, 1939).

George Ryley Scott, *A History of Prostitution from Antiquity to the Present Day*, revised and illustrated limited edn (London: Torchstream Books, 1954).

Wally Seccombe, *Weathering the Storm: Working-Class Families from the Industrial Revolution to the Fertility Decline* (London and New York: Verso, 1993).

James A. Secord, 'Newton in the Nursery: Tom Telescope and the Philosophy of Tops and Balls, 1761–1838', *History of Science*, xxiii (1985), 127–51.

L. A. Selby-Bigge, *British Moralists*, 2 vols (Oxford: Oxford University Press, 1897).

J. Sergeant, *Solid Philosophy* (London: R. Clavil, 1697).

Emma U. H. Seymour, 'Bodying Forth the Mind: Mind, Body and Metaphor, 1590–1640' (PhD thesis, University of Cambridge, 1993).

Carole Shammas, *The Pre-Industrial Consumer in England and America* (Oxford: Clarendon Press, 1990).

Mary Lyndon Shanley, *Feminism, Marriage, and the Law in Victorian England, 1850–1895* (Princeton, NJ: Princeton University Press, 1989).

S. Shapin, 'The Social Uses of Science', in G. S. Rousseau and Roy Porter (eds), *The Ferment of Knowledge* (Cambridge: Cambridge University Press, 1980), 93–142.

S. Shapin, 'History of Science and its Sociological Reconstructions', *History of Science*, xx (1982), 157–211.

Barbara J. Shapiro, *Probability and Certainty in Seventeenth Century England*

(Princeton, NJ: Princeton University Press, 1983).

Jane Sharp, *The Midwives Book, or the Whole Art of Midwifry Discovered* (London: Simon Miller, 1671).

Marion Shaw, ' "To Tell the Truth of Sex": Confession and Abjection in Late Victorian Writing', in Linda M. Shires (ed.), *Rewriting the Victorians: Theory, History and the Politics of Gender* (London: Routledge, 1992), 86–100.

Edward Shorter, *The Making of the Modern Family* (New York: Basic Books, 1975; London, Collins, 1976).

Edward Shorter, *A History of Women's Bodies* (New York: Basic Books; London: Allen Lane, 1982; Harmondsworth: Penguin, 1983).

Elaine Showalter, *Sexual Anarchy: Gender and Culture at the 'Fin de Siècle'* (New York: Viking Penguin, 1990; London: Bloomsbury, 1991).

Penelope Shuttle and Peter Redgrove, *The Wise Wound: Menstruation and Everywoman* (London: Gollancz, 1978).

Ebenezer Sibly, *The Medical Mirror; or, Treatise on the Impregnation of the Human Female. Shewing the Origin of Diseases, and the Principles of Life and Death* (London, 1794).

G. L. Simons, *Sex and Superstition* (London: Abelard-Schuman, 1973).

Irving Singer, *The Nature of Love*, 3 vols (Chicago: University of Chicago Press, 1984–7).

Sinibaldus, *Geneanthropeiae, sive de Hominis Generatione Decateuchon* (Rome, 1642).

Eliot Slater and Moya Woodside, *Patterns of Marriage: A Study of Marriage Relationships in the Urban Working Classes* (London: Cassell, 1951).

F. B. Smith, 'Sexuality in Britain, 1800–1900: Some Suggested Revisions', in Martha Vicinus (ed.), *A Widening Sphere: Changing Roles of Victorian Women* (Bloomington and London: Indiana University Press, 1977), 182–98.

F. B. Smith, *The People's Health, 1830–1910* (London: Croom Helm, 1979).

F. B. Smith, 'The Contagious Diseases Acts Reconsidered', *Social History of Medicine*, iii (1990), 73–86.

Kenneth Smith, *The Malthusian Controversy* (London: Routledge and Kegan Paul, 1951).

N. Smith, 'Sexual Mores in the Eighteenth Century: Robert Wallace's "Of Venery"', *Journal of the History of Ideas*, xxxix (1978), 419–33.

Virginia S. Smith, 'Cleanliness: the Development of an Idea and Practice in Britain 1770–1850' (PhD thesis, University of London, 1985).

Carroll Smith-Rosenberg, 'The Hysterical Woman: Sex Roles and Conflict in Nineteenth-Century America', *Social Research*, xxxix (1972), 652–78.

Carroll Smith-Rosenberg, 'Puberty to Menopause: The Cycle of Femininity in Nineteenth-Century America', in M. Hartman and L. Banner (eds), *Clio's Consciousness Raised* (New York: Harper and Row, 1974), 23–37.

Carroll Smith-Rosenberg, *Disorderly Conduct: Visions of Gender in Victorian America* (New York: Knopf, 1985).

Carroll Smith-Rosenberg and Charles Rosenberg, 'The Female Animal: Medical and Biological Views of Woman and Her Role in Nineteenth-Century America', *Journal of American History*, lx (1973), 332–56.

Carroll Smith-Rosenberg and Charles Rosenberg, 'The Female Animal: Medical and Biological Views of Woman and her Role in Nineteenth Century America', in J. W. Leavitt (ed.), *Women and Health in America* (Madison:

University of Wisconsin Press, 1984).

Ann Snitow, Christine Stansell and Sharon Thompson (eds), *Desire: The Politics of Sexuality* (London: Virago, 1984).

Samuel Solomon, *A Guide to Health, or, Advice to Both Sexes in Nervous and Consumptive Complaints, Scurvy, Leprosy and Scrofula, and on A Certain Disease and Sexual Debility, in which is added An Address to Boys, Young Men, Parents, Tutors, and Guardians of Youth*, 2nd edn (Stockport: the author, *c.* 1800).

Samuel Solomon, *An Account of that Most Excellent Medicine, The Cordial Balm of Gilead* (Stockport: Clarke, *c.* 1801).

R. A. Soloway, *Birth Control and the Population Question in England, 1870–1930* (Chapel Hill and London: University of North Carolina Press, 1982).

R. A. Soloway, *Demography and Degeneration: Eugenics and the Declining Birthrate in Twentieth Century Britain* (Chapel Hill: University of North Carolina Press, 1990).

Keith Soothill and Sylvia Walby, *Sex Crime in the News* (London: Routledge, 1991).

Patricia Meyer Spacks, ' "Ev'ry Woman is at Heart a Rake" ', *Eighteenth Century Studies*, viii (1974–5), 27–46.

Patricia Meyer Spacks, *The Female Imagination: A Literary and Psychological Investigation of Women's Writing* (New York: Knopf, 1975; London: Allen and Unwin, 1976).

A. Spencer (ed.), *Memoirs of William Hickey*, 6th edn, 4 vols (London: Hurst and Blackett, 1923–5).

Dale Spender, *Man Made Language* (London: Routledge and Kegan Paul, 1980).

Lyman Beecher Sperry, *Confidential Talks with Husband and Wife: A Book of Information and Advice for the Married and the Marriageable* (London and Edinburgh: Oliphant Anderson and Ferrier, 1900).

John Spinke, *Quackery Unmasked* (London: D. Brown, 1709).

John Spinke, *Venus's Botcher* (London: D. Brown, 1711).

Margaret Spufford, *Small Books and Pleasant Histories. Popular Fiction and its Readership in Seventeenth-Century England* (London: Methuen; Athens, Ga: University of Georgia Press, 1981).

P. Stallybrass and A. White, *The Politics and Poetics of Transgression* (Ithaca, NY: Cornell University Press, 1986).

Dorothy A. Stansfield, *Thomas Beddoes, M.D. 1760–1808, Chemist, Physician, Democrat* (Dordrecht: Reidel, 1984).

The State and Sexual Morality (London: Allen and Unwin, 1920).

Carol Z. Stearns and Peter N. Stearns, 'Victorian Sexuality: Can Historians Do It Better?', *Journal of Social History*, xviii (iv) (1985), 625–34.

Carolyn Steedman, *Childhood, Culture and Class in Britain: Margaret McMillan, 1860–1931* (London: Virago, 1990).

F. Steegmuller (ed.), *The Letters of Gustave Flaubert*, Vol. I (Cambridge, Mass.: Belknap Press of Harvard University Press, 1980; London: Faber and Faber, 1981).

Wilhelm Stekel, *Impotence in the Male: The Psychic Disorders of Sexual Function in the Male*, authorised English version by Oswald H. Boltz, 2 vols (New York: Liveright, 1927).

J. Stengers and A. Van Neck, *Histoire d'une grande peur: la masturbation* (Brussels: University of Brussels Press, 1984).

Laurence Sterne, *The Life and Opinions of Tristram Shandy*, ed. C. Ricks (Harmondsworth: Penguin, 1967).

Alan Graham Stewart, 'The Bounds of Sodomy: Textual Relations in Early Modern England' (PhD thesis, University of London, 1993).

Lawrence Stone, *The Family, Sex and Marriage in England 1500–1800* (London: Weidenfeld and Nicolson, 1977).

Lawrence Stone, *The Road to Divorce: England, 1530–1987* (Oxford: Oxford University Press, 1990).

Lawrence Stone, *Uncertain Unions: Marriage in England 1660–1753* (Oxford: Oxford University Press, 1992).

Lawrence Stone, *Broken Lives: Separation and Divorce in England 1660–1857* (Oxford: Oxford University Press, 1993).

Marie Stopes, *Married Love. A New Contribution to the Solution of Sex Difficulties. With a Preface by Dr Jessie Murray and Letters from Professor E. H. Starling FRS, and Father Stanislaus St John, SJ* (London: A. C. Fifield, 1918; later edns by G. P. Putnam's Sons).

Marie Stopes, *A New Gospel: A Revelation of God Uniting Physiology and the Religion of Man* (London: G. P. Putnam's Sons, 1920).

Marie Stopes, *Wise Parenthood. The Treatise on Birth Control For Married People. A Practical Sequel to 'Married Love' with an Introduction by Arnold Bennett* (London: G. P. Putnam's Sons, 1918; 11th edn 1923).

Marie Stopes, *Contraception (Birth-Control): Its Theory, History and Practice: a Manual for the Medical and Legal Professions* (London: John Bale, Sons and Danielsson, 1924).

Marie Stopes, *The First 5000* (London: John Bale, Sons and Danielsson, 1925).

Marie Stopes, *A Banned Play and a Preface on the Censorship* (London: John Bale, Sons and Danielsson, 1926).

Marie Stopes, *Sex and the Young* (London: Gill, 1926).

Marie Stopes, *Enduring Passion. Further New Contributions to the Solution of Sex Difficulties, Being the Continuation of 'Married Love'* (London: G. P. Putnam's Sons, 1928; 2nd edn 1929).

Marie Stopes, *Mother England: A Contemporary History self-written by those who have no historian* (London: John Bale, Sons and Danielsson, 1929).

Marie Stopes, *Change of Life in Men and Women* (London: G. P. Putnam's Sons, 1936).

C. Strachey (ed.), *The Letters of the Earl of Chesterfield to his Son*, 2 vols, 3rd edn (London: Methuen, 1932).

R. Straus, *The Unspeakable Dr Curll* (New York: Kelley, 1970).

John Styles, *An Essay on the Character, Immoral and Antichristian Tendency of the Stage* (London, printed for the author, 1806).

Susan Rubin Suleiman (ed.), *The Female Body in Western Culture: Contemporary Perspectives* (Cambridge, Mass.: Harvard University Press, 1986).

Maureen Sutton, *'We Didn't Know Aught': A Study of Sexuality, Superstition and Death in Women's Lives in Lincolnshire during the 1930s, '40s and '50s* (Stamford: Paul Watkins, 1992).

Frances Swiney, *The Cosmic Procession, or the Feminine Principle in Evolution: Essays of Illumination*, Higher Thought Series (London: Ernest Bell, 1906).

Frances Swiney, *The Bar of Isis, or The Law of the Mother* (London: C. W. Daniel, 1907; 3rd edn 1912).

Frances Swiney, *Woman and Natural Law*, 2nd edn (London: C. W. Daniel, 1912).

Reay Tannahill, *Sex in History* (New York: Stein and Day, 1980).

T. Tanner, *Adultery in the Novel* (Baltimore, Md.: Johns Hopkins University Press, 1979).

C. Taylor, *Sources of the Self. The Making of Modern Identity* (Cambridge: Cambridge University Press, 1989).

Gordon Rattray Taylor, *Sex in History* (London: Thames and Hudson, 1953; new edn, 1959).

Gordon Rattray Taylor, *The Angel-Makers: A Study in the Psychological Origins of Historical Change* (London: Heinemann, 1958; New York: E. P. Dutton, 1974).

Laurie Taylor, 'The Unfinished Sexual Revolution', *Journal of Biosocial Science*, iii (1971), 473–92.

O. Temkin, *Galenism* (Ithaca, NY: Cornell University Press, 1973).

L. Terman, *Psychological Factors in Marital Happiness* (New York: McGraw-Hill, 1939).

M. Thale (ed.), *The Autobiography of Francis Place* (Cambridge: Cambridge University Press, 1972).

B. This, *La Requête des enfants à naître* (Paris: Editions du Seuil, 1982).

Donald Thomas, *A Long Time Burning: The History of Literary Censorship in England* (London: Routledge and Kegan Paul, 1969).

Keith Thomas, 'The Double Standard', *Journal of the History of Ideas*, xx (1959), 195–216.

Keith Thomas, *Religion and the Decline of Magic* (London: Weidenfeld and Nicolson, 1971).

Keith Thomas, *Man and the Natural World* (London: Allen Lane, 1983).

C. J. S. Thompson, *The Mystery and Lore of Monsters* (London: Williams and Norgate, 1930).

Roger Thompson, *Unfit for Modest Ears: A Study of Pornographic, Obscene and Bawdy Works Written or Published in England in the Second Half of the Seventeenth Century* (London: Macmillan, 1979).

Stella Tillyard, *Aristocrats* (London: Chatto and Windus, 1994).

S. A. A. D. Tissot, *Onanism or, a Treatise upon the Disorders Produced by Masturbation: or, the Dangerous Effects of Secret and Excessive Venery*, trans. A. Hume (London: for Varenne, 1761).

Janet Todd, *Sensibility: An Introduction* (London: Methuen, 1986).

C. Tomalin, *The Life and Death of Mary Wollstonecraft* (London: Weidenfeld and Nicolson, 1974).

Sylvana Tomaselli, 'The Enlightenment Debate on Women', *History Workshop Journal*, xx (1985), 101–24.

Bridget A. Towers, 'Health Education Policy, 1916–1926: Venereal Disease and the Prophylaxis Dilemma', *Medical History*, xxiv (1980), 70–87.

R. T. Trall, *Sexual Physiology and Hygiene: An Exposition Practical, Scientific, Moral, and Popular of Some of the Fundamental Problems in Sociology* (1st edn USA *c.* 1888; Glasgow: T. D. Morison; London: Simpkin, Marshall, Hamilton and Kent, 1908).

Eric Trudgill, *Madonnas and Magdalens: the Origins and Development of Victorian Sexual Attitudes* (New York: Holmes and Meier, 1976).

Randolph Trumbach, 'London's Sodomites: Homosexual Behavior and

Western Culture in the Eighteenth Century', *Journal of Social History*, xi (1977), 1–33.

Randolph Trumbach, 'Sodomitical Subcultures, Sodomitical Roles, and the Gender Revolution of the Eighteenth Century: The Recent Historiography', in R. P. Maccubbin (ed.), *Unauthorized Sexual Behavior during the Enlightenment* (Williamsburg, Va.: College of William and Mary, 1985), *Eighteenth-Century Life*, ix (1978), 109–21.

Randolph Trumbach, *The Rise of the Egalitarian Family: Aristocratic Kinship and Domestic Relations in Eighteenth Century England* (New York: Academic Press, 1978).

Randolph Trumbach, 'Modern Prostitution and Gender in *Fanny Hill*: Libertine and Domesticated Fantasy', in G. S. Rousseau and Roy Porter (eds), *Sexual Underworlds of the Enlightenment* (Manchester: Manchester University Press, 1987), 69–85.

Randolph Trumbach, 'Review Essay: Is There a Modern Sexual Culture in the West; or, Did England Never Change between 1500 and 1900?', *Journal of the History of Sexuality*, i (ii) (1990), 296–309.

Randolph Trumbach, 'Sex, Gender and Identity in Modern Cultures: Male Sodomy and Female Prostitution in 18th Century London', in Ad van der Woude (ed.), *The Role of the State and Public Opinion in Sexual Attitudes and Demographic Behaviour* (Paris: International Commission of Historical Demography, 1990), 271–374.

Bryan S. Turner, *The Body and Society: Explorations in Social Theory* (Oxford: Basil Blackwell, 1984).

Bryan S. Turner, 'The Practices of Rationality: Michel Foucault, Medical History and Sociological Theory', in R. Fardon (ed.), *Power and Knowledge: Anthropological and Sociological Approaches* (Edinburgh: Scottish Academic Press, 1985), 193–213.

Bryan S. Turner, *Medical Power and Social Knowledge* (Beverly Hills, Calif.: Sage Publications, 1987).

E. B. Turner, 'The History of the Fight against Venereal Disease', *Science Progress*, xi (1916–17), 83–8.

Cornelie Usborne, *The Politics of the Body in Weimar Germany: Women's Reproductive Rights and Duties* (Ann Arbor: University of Michigan Press; London: Macmillan, 1992).

Carole S. Vance (ed.), *Pleasure and Danger: Exploring Female Sexuality* (Boston and London: Routledge and Kegan Paul, 1984).

Th. H. Van de Velde, *Ideal Marriage: Its Physiology and Technique*, trans. F. W. Stella Browne (Holland, 1926; London: Heinemann Medical Books, 1928).

A. Vartanian, *La Mettrie's L'Homme Machine* (Princeton, NJ: Princeton University Press, 1960).

N. Venette, *Le Tableau de l'amour conjugal* (New York: Garland, 1984); English trans., *The Mysteries of Conjugal Love Reveal'd* (London: S. N., 1712).

N. Venette, *Conjugal Love Reveal'd, In the Nightly Pleasure of the Marriage Bed and the Advantages of that Happy State, in an Essay Concerning Humane Generation, done from the French of Monsieur Venette, by a Physician*. Seventh Edition, Amor Omnibus Idem. (London: printed for the author, and sold by Tho. Hinton, at the White Horse, in Water Lane, Blackfryars, *c.* 1720).

N. Venette, *The Pleasures of Conjugal Love Explained in an Essay Concerning Human*

Generation, done from the French by a Physician. Amor Omnibus Idem. (London: printed for P. Meighan at Gray's Inn Gate, in Holborn, T. Griffiths at Charing Cross, T. Lapworth at the Anodyne Necklace without Temple Bar, n. d.).

N. Venette, *Conjugal Love; Or the Pleasures of the Marriage Bed Considered. In Several Lectures On Human Generation. From the French of Venette*, 20th edn (London: printed for the booksellers, 1750).

N. Venette, *La Génération de l'homme*, new edn, 2 vols (Paris: no publisher, 1764).

Martha Vicinus (ed.), *Suffer and Be Still: Women in the Victorian Age* (Bloomington: Indiana University Press, 1972).

Martha Vicinus (ed.), *A Widening Sphere: Changing Roles of Victorian Women* (Bloomington: Indiana University Press, 1977).

Martha Vicinus, 'Sexuality and Power: A Review of Current Work in the History of Sexuality', *Feminist Studies*, viii (1982), 133–56.

David Vincent, 'Love and Death and the Nineteenth Century Working Class', *Social History*, v (1980), 223–47.

Mary F. Wack, *Lovesickness in the Middle Ages: The 'Viaticum' and Its Commentaries* (Philadelphia: University of Pennsylvania Press, 1990).

Peter Wagner, 'The Pornographer in the Courtroom: Trial Reports about Cases of Sexual Crimes and Delinquencies as a Genre of Eighteenth Century Erotica', in P.-G. Boucé (ed.), *Sexuality in Eighteenth Century Britain* (Manchester: Manchester University Press, 1982), 120–40.

Peter Wagner, 'Researching the Taboo: Sexuality and Eighteenth-Century Erotica', *Eighteenth-Century Life*, iii (1983), 108–15.

Peter Wagner, 'The Veil of Science and Mortality: Some Pornographic Aspects of the ONANIA', *British Journal for Eighteenth Century Studies*, iv (1983), 179–84.

Peter Wagner, 'The Discourse on Sex – or Sex as Discourse: Eighteenth Century Medical and Paramedical Erotica', in G. S. Rousseau and Roy Porter (eds), *Sexual Underworlds of the Enlightenment* (Manchester: Manchester University Press, 1987), 46–68.

Peter Wagner, *Eros Revived: Erotica of the Enlightenment in England and America* (London: Secker and Warburg, 1988).

Margaret A. Wailes, 'The Social Aspect of the Venereal Diseases: Contact Tracing and the Prostitute', *British Journal of Venereal Diseases*, xxi (1945), 17–21.

Kenneth M. Walker, *Marriage: A Book for the Married and About to be Married* (London: Secker and Warburg for the British Social Hygiene Council, 1951).

Judith R. Walkowitz, *Prostitution and Victorian Society: Women, Class and the State* (Cambridge and New York: Cambridge University Press, 1980).

Judith R. Walkowitz, *City of Dreadful Delight: Narratives of Sexual Danger in Late-Victorian London* (London: Virago, 1992).

A. Wallas, *Before the Bluestockings* (London: Allen and Unwin, 1929).

Prof. W. H. Walling, *Sexology* (Philadelphia: Puritan Publishing Co., 1902).

Major G. O. Watts and Major R. A. Wilson, 'A Study of Personality Factors among Venereal Disease Patients', *Canadian Medical Association Journal*, liii (1945), 119–22.

M. A. Waugh, 'Attitudes of Hospitals in London to Venereal Disease in the 18th and 19th Centuries', *British Journal of Venereal Diseases*, xlvii (1971), 146–50.

Andrew Wear, 'The Popularization of Medicine in Early Modern England', in

Roy Porter (ed.), *The Popularization of Medicine, 1650–1850* (London: Routledge, 1992), 17–41.

Leslie D. Weatherhead (assisted by Dr Marion Greaves), *The Mastery of Sex through Psychology and Religion* (London: Student Christian Movement Press, 1931).

Lorna Weatherill, *Consumer Behaviour and Material Culture, 1660–1760* (London: Routledge, 1988).

P. Webb, *The Erotic Arts* (London: Secker and Warburg, 1975)

Sidney Webb, *The Decline in the Birth Rate* (London: Fabian Society, 1907).

Jeffrey Weeks, *Coming Out: Homosexual Politics in Britain from the Nineteenth Century to the Present* (Totowa, NJ: Barnes and Noble, 1977; London: Quartet, 1977).

Jeffrey Weeks, 'Havelock Ellis and the Politics of Sex Reform', in Sheila Rowbotham and Jeffrey Weeks (eds), *Socialism and the New Life: The Personal and Sexual Politics of Edward Carpenter and Havelock Ellis* (London: Pluto Press, 1977), 139–85.

Jeffrey Weeks, *Sex, Politics and Society: The Regulation of Sexuality since 1800* (London: Longman, 1981).

Jeffrey Weeks, *Against Nature: Essays in History, Sexuality and Identity* (London: Rivers Oram Press, 1991).

Otto Weininger, *Sex and Character*, authorized trans. from the 6th German edn (London: Heinemann, 1906).

C. McC. Weis and F. A. Pottle (eds), *Boswell in Extremes* (New York: McGraw-Hill, 1970).

René J. A. Weiss, *Criminal Justice: The True Story of Edith Thompson* (London: Hamish Hamilton, 1988).

Kaye Wellings *et al.*, *Sexual Behaviour in Britain. The National Survey of Sexual Attitudes and Lifestyles* (Harmondsworth: Penguin, 1994).

Rebecca West, 'The Tosh Horse', in *The Strange Necessity: Essays and Reviews* (London: Jonathan Cape, 1928), 319–25.

Rebecca West, *The Young Rebecca: Writings of Rebecca West 1911–1917*, selected and introduced by Jane Marcus (London: Macmillan, 1982).

Cynthia L. White, *Women's Magazines 1693–1968* (London: Michael Joseph, 1970).

The White Cross League, *The Blanco Book* (London: White Cross League, 1913).

William L. Whitwell, 'James Graham, Master Quack', *Eighteenth-Century Life*, iv (1977), 43–9.

J. Whorton, *Crusaders for Fitness* (Princeton, NJ: Princeton University Press, 1982).

H. F. Wijnman, '*Venus Minsieke Gasthuis*', in Herbert Lewandowski and P. J. Van Dronen, *Beschavingsen zedergeschiedenis van Nederland* (Amsterdam: N. V. Uitagevers-Maatschappy, 1983), 280–4.

John Wilkes, *Essay on Woman* (London: privately printed, 1763).

B. Willey, *The Seventeenth Century Background* (London: Chatto and Windus, 1934).

B. Willey, *The Eighteenth Century Background* (London: Chatto and Windus, 1940).

N. Williams, *Powder and Paint* (London: Longmans, 1957).

A. F. M. Willich, *Lectures on Diet and Regimen* (London, 1799).

M. Williford, 'Bentham on the Rights of Women', *Journal of the History of Ideas*, xxxvi (1975), 167–76.

W. David Wills, *Homer Lane: A Biography* (London: Allen and Unwin, 1964).

A. Wilson, 'William Hunter and the Varieties of Man-Midwifery', in W. F. Bynum and Roy Porter (eds), *William Hunter and the Eighteenth Century Medical World* (Cambridge: Cambridge University Press, 1985), 343–69.

Adrian Wilson, *The Making of Man-Midwifery: Women and Men in English Childbirth, 1700–1770* (London: University College Press, forthcoming 1995).

Dudley Wilson, *Signs and Portents: Monstrous Births from the Middle Ages to the Enlightenment* (London: Routledge, 1993).

Marris Wilson, *On Diseases of the Vesiculae Seminales and their Associated Organs, with Special Reference to the Morbid Secretions of the Prostatic and Urethral Mucous Membrane* (London: published for the author by Tallant and Allen, 1856).

Philip Wilson: ' "Out of Sight, out of Mind?": the Daniel Turner–James Blondel Dispute over the Power of the Maternal Imagination', *Annals of Science*, xlix (1992), 63–85.

W. K. Wimsatt and F. A. Pottle (eds), *Boswell for the Defence, 1769–1774* (New York: McGraw Hill, 1959).

E. Wind, *Pagan Mysteries in the Renaissance* (Harmondsworth: Penguin, 1967).

John J. Winkler, *Constraints of Desire: The Anthropology of Sex and Gender in Ancient Greece* (New York: Routledge, Chapman and Hall, 1990).

E. D. Wittkower, 'The Psychological Aspects of Venereal Disease', *British Journal of Venereal Diseases*, xxiv (1948), 59–67.

Josiah Woodward, *Rebuke of the Sin of Uncleanness* (London: printed and sold by Joseph Downing, 1704).

Virginia Woolf, *The Diary of Virginia Woolf*, Vol. I, *1915–1919*, ed. Anne Olivier Bell (London: Hogarth Press, 1977; Harmondsworth: Penguin, 1979).

Virginia Woolf, *The Diary of Virginia Woolf*, Vol. IV, *1931–1935*, ed. Anne Olivier Bell (London: Hogarth Press, 1982; Harmondsworth: Penguin, 1983).

Michael Worton and Judith Still (eds), *Textuality and Sexuality: Reading Theories and Practices* (Manchester: Manchester University Press, 1993).

Helena Wright, *The Sex Factor in Marriage. A Book for Those Who Are or Are About to be Married* (London: Williams and Norgate, 1930).

Helena Wright, *More About the Sex Factor in Marriage: A Sequel to 'The Sex Factor in Marriage'* (London: Williams and Norgate, 1947).

Keith Wrightson and David Levine, *Poverty and Piety in an English Village: Terling 1525–1700* (New York and London: Academic Press, 1979).

E. A. Wrigley and R. S. Schofield, *The Population History of England 1541–1871* (London: Edward Arnold, 1981).

T. J. Wyke, 'Hospital Facilities for, and Diagnosis and Treatment of, Venereal Disease in England, 1800–1870', *British Journal of Venereal Diseases*, xlix (1973), 78–85.

T. J. Wyke, 'The Manchester and Salford Lock Hospital, 1818–1917', *Medical History*, xix (1979), 73–86.

F. Yates, *The Art of Memory* (London: Routledge and Kegan Paul, 1966).

R. M. Young, 'Science *is* Social Relations', *Radical Science Journal*, v (1977), 65–129.

Wayland Young, *Eros Denied: Studies in Exclusion* (London: Weidenfeld and Nicolson, 1965).

T. Zeldin, *France, 1848–1945. Ambition, Love, Politics* (Oxford: Clarendon Press, 1973).

Jan Ziolkowski, *Alan of Lille's Grammar of Sex: the Meaning of Grammar to a Twelfth-Century Intellectual* (Cambridge, Mass.: Medieval Academy of America, 1985).

Index